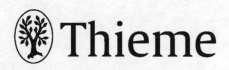

Essentials of Anesthesiology

Puneet Khanna, MD
Associate Professor
Department of Anesthesiology, Pain Medicine and Critical Care
All India Institute of Medical Sciences (AIIMS)
New Delhi, India

Shashikant Sharma, MD
Senior Resident
Department of Anesthesiology, Pain Medicine and Critical Care
All India Institute of Medical Sciences (AIIMS)
New Delhi, India

Thieme
Delhi • Stuttgart • New York • Rio de Janeiro

Publishing Director: Ritu Sharma
Development Editor: Dr Gurvinder Kaur
Director-Editorial Services: Rachna Sinha
Project Manager: Shipra Sehgal
Vice President Sales and Marketing: Arun Kumar Majji
Managing Director & CEO: Ajit Kohli

Thieme Medical and Scientific Publishers Private
Limited.
A - 12, Second Floor, Sector - 2, Noida - 201 301,
Uttar Pradesh, India, +911204556600
Email: customerservice@thieme.in
www.thieme.in

Cover design: © Thieme
Cover image source: © Thieme

Typesetting by RECTO Graphics, India

Printed in India by Sai Printo Pack Pvt Ltd, New Delhi.

5 4 3 2 1

ISBN: 978-93-90553-90-7
eISBN: 978-93-90553-95-2

Important note: Medicine is an ever-changing science undergoing continual development. Research and clinical experience are continually expanding our knowledge, in particular, our knowledge of proper treatment and drug therapy. Insofar as this book mentions any dosage or application, readers may rest assured that the authors, editors, and publishers have made every effort to ensure that such references are in accordance with the state of knowledge at the time of production of the book.

Nevertheless, this does not involve, imply, or express any guarantee or responsibility on the part of the publishers in respect to any dosage instructions and forms of applications stated in the book. Every user is requested to examine carefully the manufacturers' leaflets accompanying each drug and to check, if necessary, in consultation with a physician or specialist, whether the dosage schedules mentioned therein or the contraindications stated by the manufacturers differ from the statements made in the present book. Such examination is particularly important with drugs that are either rarely used or have been newly released in the market. Every dosage schedule or every form of application used is entirely at the user's own risk and responsibility. The authors and publishers request every user to report to the publishers any discrepancies or inaccuracies noticed. If errors in this work are found after publication, errata will be posted at www.thieme.com on the product description page.

Some of the product names, patents, and registered designs referred to in this book are in fact registered trademarks or proprietary names even though specific reference to this fact is not always made in the text. Therefore, the appearance of a name without designation as proprietary is not to be construed as a representation by the publisher that it is in the public domain.

Thieme addresses people of all gender identities equally. We encourage our authors to use gender-neutral or gender-equal expressions wherever the context allows.

The views and opinions expressed in this book are solely those of the contributing authors and editors and are not advocated by any institution.

Dedicated to the teachers and residents of Department of Anesthesiology for
their endeavor to disseminate and acquire knowledge; my parents for their blessings;
my daughter, Ziva, for being patient and tolerant during the loss of many precious moments;
and finally, to my wife Ishita for being understanding and encouraging.

Puneet Khanna, MD

Dedicated to my parents, my wife, my teachers, and my students.

Shashikant Sharma, MD

Contents

Contents

Preface

The practice of anesthesia, which began somewhere in 1850, has revolutionized patient care and is growing and evolving rapidly. In the modern era, anesthesia care providers are no more confined to the operation theater but are spread across every corner of the patient care facility.

As a subject, anesthesia is a combination of anatomy, physiology, pharmacology, and disease pathophysiology, and this peculiarity of the subject has the effect of beautifying it as a specialty. Saving a life during cardiac arrest and taking care of chronic pain for the patient's lifetime make anesthesia providers unique among health care professionals.

This book, which comes in a comprehensive yet compact format, orients undergraduates, students preparing for postgraduate entrance examination, and anesthesia technicians to anesthesia basics, including anatomy, physiology, pharmacology, drugs, types of equipment, and management of specific ailments of all the organ systems.

The chapters in this book are simplified by way of tables, flowcharts, and appropriate figures, thereby making the reading and understanding of the subject easy. This book includes chapters on artificial intelligence and updates of the Cardiopulmonary Resuscitation Guidelines 2020 by the American Heart Association (AHA).

This book is thoroughly updated, comprehensive, and will meet the requirements of medical students preparing for theory as well as practical examinations, especially those preparing for various postgraduate entrance tests. It covers most of the frequently asked topics in MCQs of various postgraduate entrance examinations. Candidates preparing for PG entrance examinations will find it to be an authentic reference source. This book will also be very helpful for OT technicians and critical care and anesthesia nursing staff.

The authors have put in their best efforts while writing this book; however, the scope of errors remains. It would be particularly useful if readers were to point out any grammatical errors or controversies whatsoever, in order to make the changes at the earliest. We will be more than happy to rectify the errors and make the book a better one. So, kindly communicate such errors by writing to k.punit@yahoo.com.

We would like to thank Thieme Medical and Scientific Publishers Private Limited for their valuable efforts in bringing this book to fruition.

Puneet Khanna, MD
Shashikant Sharma, MD

Acknowledgments

We would like to thank Dr Akhil Kant Singh and Dr Damarla Haritha who helped in proofreading the book.

We are extremely indebted to the faculty, senior residents, and junior residents for helping us shape this book in its present form. Our special thanks to our friends for their support and faith. We would also like to acknowledge our colleagues and juniors for their continuous support.

We are also indebted to Thieme India team for their continuous help in completion of the book.

Nothing can be complete without extending our gratitude to the one who has powered us from within to complete this work, *God Almighty*.

Puneet Khanna, MD
Shashikant Sharma, MD

Contributors

Abhishek Singh, MD
Assistant Professor
Department of Anesthesiology, Pain Medicine
and Critical Care
All India Institute of Medical Sciences (AIIMS)
New Delhi, India

Ajay Singh, MD
Assistant Professor
Department of Anesthesiology
Postgraduate Institute of Medical Education and
Research
Chandigarh, India

Ajisha Aravindan, MD
Assistant Professor
Department of Anesthesiology, Pain Medicine
and Critical Care
All India Institute of Medical Sciences (AIIMS)
New Delhi, India

Ajit Kumar, MD
Associate Professor
Department of Anesthesiology, Pain Medicine
and Critical Care
All India Institute of Medical Sciences (AIIMS)
Rishikesh, Uttarakhand, India

Akhil Kant Singh, MD
Assistant Professor
Department of Anesthesiology, Pain Medicine
and Critical Care
All India Institute of Medical Sciences (AIIMS)
New Delhi, India

Anju Gupta, MD
Assistant Professor
Department of Anesthesiology, Pain Medicine
and Critical Care
All India Institute of Medical Sciences (AIIMS)
New Delhi, India

Ankur Sharma, MD
Assistant Professor
Department of Anesthesiology, Pain Medicine
and Critical Care
All India Institute of Medical Sciences (AIIMS)
Jodhpur, Rajasthan, India

Aravind B. Guledagudd, MD
Senior Resident
Department of Anesthesiology
Government Medical College & Hospital
Chandigarh, India

Arush Singla, MD
Senior Resident
Department of Anesthesiology
Government Medical College & Hospital
Chandigarh, India

Arushi Goyal, MD
Senior Resident
Department of Anesthesiology
Government Medical College & Hospital
Chandigarh, India

Avishek Roy, MD
Senior Resident
Department of Anesthesiology, Pain Medicine
and Critical Care
All India Institute of Medical Sciences (AIIMS)
New Delhi, India

Bhavya Krishna, MD
Senior Resident
Department of Anesthesiology, Pain Medicine
and Critical Care
All India Institute of Medical Sciences (AIIMS)
New Delhi, India

Damarla Haritha, MD
Senior Resident
Department of Anesthesiology, Pain Medicine
and Critical Care
All India Institute of Medical Sciences (AIIMS)
New Delhi, India

Ganasekran Srinivasan, MD
Assistant Professor
Department of Anesthesiology
Jawaharlal Institute of Postgraduate Medical
Education & Research
Puducherry, India

Gourav Mittal, MD
Senior Resident
All India Institute of Medical Sciences (AIIMS)
New Delhi, India

Heena Garg, MD
Senior Resident
Department of Anesthesiology, Pain Medicine
and Critical Care
All India Institute of Medical Sciences (AIIMS)
New Delhi, India

Kritika Saini, MD
Senior Resident
Department of Anesthesiology, Pain Medicine
and Critical Care
All India Institute of Medical Sciences (AIIMS)
Rishikesh, Uttarakhand, India

Michelle Sirin Lazzar, MD
Senior Resident
Department of Anesthesiology
Postgraduate Institute of Medical Education and
Research
Chandigarh, India

Mritunjay Kumar, MD
Assistant Professor
Department of Anesthesiology, Pain Medicine
and Critical Care
All India Institute of Medical Sciences (AIIMS)
New Delhi, India

Neel Prakash, MD
Senior Resident
Department of Anesthesiology
Sanjay Gandhi Postgraduate Institute of Medical
Sciences
Lucknow, Uttar Pradesh, India

Neha Garg, MD
Assistant Professor
Department of Anesthesiology
Institute of Liver and Biliary Sciences
New Delhi, India

Nikita Goel, MD
Assistant Professor
Department of Anesthesiology
Postgraduate Institute of Medical Education and
Research
Chandigarh, India

Nishant Patel, MD
Assistant Professor
Department of Anesthesiology, Pain Medicine
and Critical Care
All India Institute of Medical Sciences (AIIMS)
New Delhi, India

Niyati Arora, MD
Senior Resident
Department of Anesthesiology, Pain Medicine
and Critical Care
All India Institute of Medical Sciences (AIIMS)
Rishikesh, Uttarakhand, India

Praveen Talawar, MD
Associate Professor
Department of Anesthesiology, Pain Medicine
and Critical Care
All India Institute of Medical Sciences (AIIMS)
Rishikesh, Uttarakhand, India

Puneet Khanna, MD
Associate Professor
Department of Anesthesiology, Pain Medicine
and Critical Care
All India Institute of Medical Sciences (AIIMS)
New Delhi, India

Ranjitha Nethaji, MD
Senior Resident
Department of Anesthesiology
Mahatma Gandhi Medical College and Research
Institute
Pondicherry, India

Ravishankar Kumar, MD
Senior Resident
Department of Anesthesiology, Pain Medicine
and Critical Care
All India Institute of Medical Sciences (AIIMS)
Rishikesh, Uttarakhand, India

Richa Saroa, MD
Associate Professor
Department of Anesthesiology
Government Medical College & Hospital
Chandigarh, India

Ridhima Sharma, MD
Assistant Professor
Department of Anesthesiology
Superspeciality Paediatric Hospital and
Postgraduate Teaching Institute
Noida, Uttar Pradesh, India

Ripon Choudhary, MD
Assistant Professor
Department of Anesthesiology
GB Pant Hospital
New Delhi, India

Rohan Magoon, MD
Assistant Professor
Department of Cardiac Anesthesia
Atal Bihari Vajpayee Institute of Medical Sciences
New Delhi, India

Roshan, MD
Senior Resident
Department of Anesthesiology, Pain Medicine
and Critical Care
All India Institute of Medical Sciences (AIIMS)
Rishikesh, Uttarakhand, India

Ruchi Kapoor, MD
Associate Professor (CHS)
Department of Anesthesiology
University College of Medical Sciences and GTB
Hospital
New Delhi, India

Sandeep Sahu, MD
Professor
Department of Anesthesiology
Sanjay Gandhi Postgraduate Institute of Medical
Sciences
Lucknow, Uttar Pradesh, India

Sanjeev Palta, MD
Professor
Department of Anesthesiology
Government Medical College & Hospital
Chandigarh, India

Shashikant Sharma, MD
Senior Resident
Department of Anesthesiology, Pain Medicine
and Critical Care
All India Institute of Medical Sciences (AIIMS)
New Delhi, India

Souvik Dey, MD
Senior Resident
Department of Cardiac Anesthesia
Atal Bihari Vajpayee Institute of Medical Sciences
New Delhi, India

Tanvir Samra, MD
Associate Professor
Department of Anesthesiology
Postgraduate Institute of Medical Education and
Research
Chandigarh, India

Tazeen Khan, MD
Senior Resident
All India Institute of Medical Sciences (AIIMS)
New Delhi, India

Ushkiran Kaur, MD
Senior Resident
Department of Anesthesiology
Sanjay Gandhi Postgraduate Institute of Medical
Sciences
Lucknow, Uttar Pradesh, India

Vijaybabu Adabala, MD
Senior Resident
Department of Anesthesiology, Pain Medicine
and Critical Care
All India Institute of Medical Sciences (AIIMS)
Rishikesh, Uttarakhand, India

Competency Mapping Chart

Competency code	COMPETENCY The student should be able to	Page no
AS4.6	Observe and describe the principles and the steps/techniques involved in daycare anesthesia	319
AS4.7	Observe and describe the principles and the steps/techniques involved in anesthesia outside the operating room	309, 312
Regional Anesthesia		
AS5.1	Enumerate the indications for and describe the principles of regional anesthesia (including spinal, epidural, and combined)	112, 114, 119, 121, 122
AS5.2	Describe the correlative anatomy of the brachial plexus, subarachnoid, and epidural spaces	112, 119, 127
AS5.3	Observe and describe the principles and steps/techniques involved in peripheral nerve blocks	125, 126
AS5.4	Observe and describe the pharmacology and correct use of commonly used drugs and adjuvant agents in regional anesthesia	120
AS5.5	Observe and describe the principles and steps/techniques involved in caudal epidural in adults and children	122
AS5.6	Observe and describe the principles and steps/techniques involved in common blocks used in surgery (including brachial plexus blocks)	127, 130, 133
Postanesthesia Recovery		
AS6.1	Describe the principles of monitoring and resuscitation in the recovery room	390, 392
AS6.2	Observe and enumerate the contents of the crash cart and describe the equipment used in the recovery room	390
AS6.3	Describe the common complications encountered by patients in the recovery room, their recognition, and principles of management	393
Intensive Care Management		
AS7.1	Visit, enumerate, and describe the functions of an intensive care unit	400
AS7.2	Enumerate and describe the criteria for admission and discharge of a patient to an intensive care unit	400, 420
AS7.3	Observe and describe the management of an unconscious patient	402
AS7.4	Observe and describe the basic setup process of a ventilator	398
AS7.5	Observe and describe the principles of monitoring in an intensive care unit	401
Pain and Its Management		
AS8.1	Describe the anatomical correlates and physiologic principles of pain	325
AS8.2	Elicit and determine the level, quality, and quantity of pain and its tolerance in patient or surrogate	325
AS8.3	Describe the pharmacology and use of drugs in the management of pain	326
AS8.4	Describe the principles of pain management in palliative care	331
AS8.5	Describe the principles of pain management in the terminally ill	331
Fluids		
AS9.1	Establish intravenous access in a simulated environment	Practicals/ Viva voce

Competency code	COMPETENCY The student should be able to	Page no
AS9.2	Establish central venous access in a simulated environment	Practicals/ Viva voce
AS9.3	Describe the principles of fluid therapy in the preoperative period	31
AS9.4	Enumerate blood products and describe the use of blood products in the preoperative period	40
Patient Safety		
AS10.1	Enumerate the hazards of incorrect patient positioning	Practicals/ Viva voce
AS10.2	Enumerate the hazards encountered in the perioperative period and steps/techniques taken to prevent them	Practicals/ Viva voce
AS10.3	Describe the role of communication in patient safety	Practicals/ Viva voce
AS10.4	Define and describe common medical and medication errors in anesthesia	388

Section I
Preliminaries in Anesthesia

CHAPTER 1

Anatomy, Physiology, and Applied Physics

Mritunjay Kumar

Introduction

The training of an anesthesiologist would be incomplete without acquiring the concept of anatomy and physiology of the respiratory system. Evaluation of the respiratory system and optimization of any associated medical illness is integral to anesthetic care. This chapter is an overview of important anatomical features of the respiratory system and the relevant physiological aspects.

Anatomy and Physiology of Respiratory System (AS4.2)

The respiratory system comprises the following:

- Upper airway—nose, mouth, nasal cavity, paranasal sinuses, pharynx, and larynx.
- Lower airway—trachea, bronchi, bronchioles, alveolar ducts, and alveoli.

1. Nose and nasal cavity

The airway begins at the nostril. The nose can be divided into two regions—the external nose and internal nasal cavity. Alae nasi are the lateral margins of the nostrils. Flaring of alae nasi indicates airway obstruction or respiratory distress. Distance from alae nasi to tragus or external auditory meatus is used for oropharyngeal airway size selection and temperature probe insertion.

The nasal cavity humidifies, warms, filters, and acts as a conduit for inspired air. About 10,000 L of air passes through the nose every 24 hours. Great vascularity of the nose helps in maintaining the constant temperature of the gases. The source of humidification is from the transudation of fluid through the mucosal epithelium, secretory glands, and goblet cells. The daily volume of nasal

secretions is about 1 L, three-fourth of which is used in saturating the inspired air. Tracheal intubation and high fresh gas flow bypass this humidification system, making usage of HME (heat and moisture exchanger) filters necessary. Prolonged exposure of lower respiratory tract to this nonhumidified air leads to dehydration of mucus, altered ciliary function, inspissation of secretion, atelectasis, and ventilation-perfusion mismatch.

For nasotracheal intubation, tube passage inferior to inferior turbinate is preferred. The tube should be directed backward along the floor of the nose. The mucosa of the nose and the posterior pharyngeal wall is very vascular and may easily be torn; so force should not be used during insertion. Tearing through mucosa may lead to the passage of the tube into retropharyngeal space and injury to posterior ethmoidal vessels (Woodruff's plexus), leading to serious hemorrhage.

2. Pharynx

Pharynx starts at the base of the skull and extends up to the inferior border of the cricoid cartilage (C6 vertebrae). It is 12- to 14-cm long and 3.5-cm wide at its base. Its width is 1.5 cm at the pharyngoesophageal junction, which is the narrowest part of the digestive system.

The posterior pharyngeal wall is made up of buccopharyngeal fascia, which separates pharyngeal structures from retropharyngeal space. Improper and forced placement of gastric or tracheal tubes can result in laceration of this fascia.

3. Nasopharynx

It extends from the posterior nasal aperture to the posterior pharyngeal wall above the soft palate. The area where it ends at soft palate is called velopharynx and is a common site for airway obstruction in both awake and anesthetized patients. The roof of the nasopharynx is at an acute angle with the posterior pharyngeal wall, which can be straightened by extension of the head to facilitate the passage of any nasal tube. Adenoids are located in its roof, frequently hypertrophied during childhood, and may cause obstruction or hemorrhage while passing any tube through the nose. Retropharyngeal and peritonsillar abscess pose as a serious anesthetic challenge.

4. Oropharynx

It extends from soft palate to epiglottis and also includes tonsil, uvula, and epiglottis.

Mallampatti classification is based on visualization of the soft palate, fauces, uvula, and tonsillar pillars in the oral cavity in relation to the tongue.

Airway obstruction during sleep, decreased consciousness, and general anesthesia is caused by collapsible soft tissue around the pharynx. Jaw thrust and neck extension helps to create space between the epiglottis and posterior pharyngeal wall. The laryngoscope blade tip lies in vallecula (a space between epiglottis and base of tongue) during the classical Macintosh laryngoscopy.

Three narrowest portions of the pharynx are retropalatine space, retroglossal space, and retro-epiglottic space (**Fig. 1.1**). Excessive fat deposition around these spaces and muscles would result in inefficient contraction of pharyngeal dilator muscles, leading to pharyngeal airway obstruction during sedation and anesthesia.

On each side of the laryngeal inlet is a deep depression called the piriform fossa, which is a common point for foreign body lodging.

5. Larynx

Larynx lies opposite C3 to C6 vertebra in adult and C1 to C4 vertebra in children. The average measurements of the larynx in adults are shown in **Table 1.1**.

The laryngeal view during laryngoscopy is shown in **Fig. 1.2**.

Table 1.1 Dimensions of the larynx in adults

Parameters	Male	Female
Vertical length	44 mm	36 mm
Transverse diameter	43 mm	41 mm
Anteroposterior diameter	36 mm	26 mm

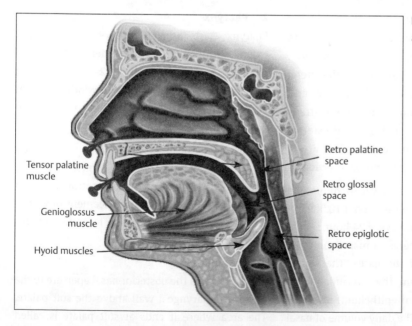

Tensor palatine muscle

Genioglossus muscle

Hyoid muscles

Retro palatine space

Retro glossal space

Retro epiglotic space

Fig. 1.1 Anatomy of upper airway.

Larynx consists of cartilages and muscles. There are three unpaired cartilages, namely, thyroid, cricoid, and epiglottis. The three paired cartilages are arytenoid, corniculate, and cuneiform. The musculature of larynx comprises intrinsic and extrinsic muscles (**Table 1.2**).

The innervation of the larynx is summarized in **Table 1.3**.

The injuries to nerves supplying the larynx can cause mild hoarseness to respiratory stridor, requiring tracheostomy. The injuries to nerves of the larynx and corresponding manifestations are summarized in **Table 1.4**.

Cords are also in cadaveric position during anesthesia with muscle relaxants.

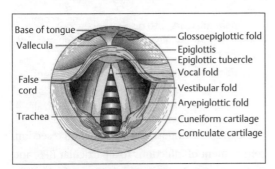

Fig. 1.2 Laryngeal view during laryngoscopy.

Backward upward rightward pressure (BURP) and optimum external laryngeal maneuvers (OELM) are used to improve the view of the glottis during laryngoscopy and tracheal intubation. Sellick's maneuver is downward pressure applied over cricoid cartilage to prevent passive regurgitation.

6. Trachea

It extends from C6 (cricoid cartilage) to the carina (T4–T5). Its length is 11 to 13 cm in adults. The mean anteroposterior and transverse diameters of the trachea in adults are 20 and 17 mm, respectively. The other important features are as follows:

- The trachea has 16 to 22 horseshoe bands (c-shaped) of cartilages.

- Posterior tracheal wall lacks cartilage and is supported by the trachealis muscle.

- The division of the trachea into right and left main stem bronchi corresponds to the level of T5 posteriorly and Louis angle of the sternum anteriorly. Right bronchus takes off at an angle of 25°, while left at an angle of 45° from the carina.

Table 1.2 Muscles of larynx

Intrinsic muscles	
1. *Those acting on the vocal cords*	
• Abductor	• Posterior cricoarytenoid
• Adductor	• Lateral cricoarytenoid, transverse and oblique arytenoid
• Tensor (elongation)	• Cricothyroid, vocalis (partly)
• Relaxor (shortening)	• Thyroarytenoid, vocalis (partly)
2. *Those acting on laryngeal inlet*	
• Openers	• Thyroepiglotticus, thyroarytenoid
• Closer	• Aryepiglotticus, oblique arytenoid
Extrinsic muscles	
Elevators of larynx	*Depressor of larynx*
• Stylohyoid	• Sternohyoid
• Mylohyoid	• Sternothyroid
• Geniohyoid	• Omohyoid

Table 1.3 Nerve supply of larynx

Sensory supply	
Up to vocal cords	The internal branch of superior laryngeal nerve
Below vocal cords	Recurrent laryngeal nerve
Motor supply	
All muscles (except cricothyroid)	Recurrent laryngeal nerve
Cricothyroid	External branch of superior laryngeal nerve

Table 1.4 Injuries to nerves of the larynx

Nerve injured	Manifestations
Unilateral paralysis of recurrent laryngeal nerve	Hoarseness of voice
Bilateral partial paralysis of recurrent laryngeal nerve	Abductors go first leading to adduction of vocal cords and consequent stridor
Complete paralysis of bilateral recurrent laryngeal nerve	Cords are adducted due to tensing action of cricothyroid (which is supplied by the superior laryngeal nerve) The patient presents with respiratory distress, aphonia, and stridor, and management requires tracheostomy
Complete paralysis of both recurrent and superior laryngeal nerve	Cords are held in midposition (cadaveric position)

- The right main bronchus is shorter (2.2 cm in length compared to 5 cm of left main bronchus), broader (15 mm compared to 13 mm of left), straighter, and more in line with trachea in adults. That is why aspiration is more common on the right.

7. Bronchopulmonary segments

Each bronchopulmonary segment (BPS) has its own segmental bronchus and arteries. The venous and lymphatic vessels pass through intersegmental planes. BPSs are 10 in the right lung and 8 to 9 in the left lung.

Mnemonic to memorize the following:

Right—"**A PALM S**eed **M**akes **A**nother **L**ittle **P**alm" (superior to inferior—apical, posterior, anterior, lateral, medial, superior, medial basal, anterior basal, lateral basal, posterior basal).

Left—"**ASIA ALPS**" (apicoposterior, superior lingular, inferior lingular, anterior, anteromedial basal, lateral basal, posterior basal, superior basal).

These BPSs are important for segmental resection, confinement of infections to a particular BPS, and for postural drainage and bronchoscopy.

Dichotomous division starts with trachea and continues till alveolar sacs, making it to 23 divisions or generations in total. On average, each alveolar sac contains 17 alveoli. So, finally, there are 300 million alveoli in an average adult, which provides a membrane area of 50 to 100 m^2 for gas exchange. The thin side of the alveolocapillary membrane is less than 0.4-mm wide and is the site of the gas exchange. The thick team with a width of 1 to 2 mm provides structural support for the alveolus.

Functions of the respiratory system include the following:

- Air distribution and blood flow for gas exchange.
- Oxygenation of body tissue.

- Extraction of carbon dioxide.
- Maintain constant homeostasis for metabolic needs.

Muscles of Respiration

The principal muscle for respiration is the diaphragm. During normal inspiration, the contraction of diaphragm and external intercostal muscles increases intrathoracic volume. During forceful inspiration, accessory muscles like sternocleidomastoid, scalenes, and pectoralis major muscles also act.

Normal expiration is a passive process due to elastic recoil of lung, while during forceful expiration, abdominal (rectus abdominis, external and internal oblique, and transversus abdominis) and internal intercostal muscles aid in the downward movement of the ribs.

Regulation of Respiration

Respiration is regulated by pneumotaxic center and apneustic center located in the pons and PreBotzinger complex, and dorsal and ventral respiratory groups situated in the medulla. Central chemoreceptors located in the medulla and peripheral chemoreceptors in carotid and aortic bodies also play significant roles in the regulation of respiration.

Lung Volumes

Lung volumes or respiratory volumes are the volume of gas in the lungs at a particular time of the respiratory cycle. Lung capacities are calculated from a summation of different lung volumes. The different lung volumes are summarized in **Table 1.5**.

While tidal volume, inspiratory reserve volume (IRV), and expiratory reserve volume (ERV) are measured by spirometry, residual volume, function residual capacity (FRC), and total lung capacity (TLC) are calculated by body plethysmography, nitrogen washout, and helium dilution technique.

Dead Space

It is also known as physiological dead space and comprises anatomical and alveolar dead space.

- **Anatomic dead space**: It is the fraction of tidal volume that remains in the conducting airways. It is around 30% of tidal volume (150 mL or 2 mL/kg).
- **Alveolar dead space**: The alveoli that are ventilated but not perfused constitute alveolar dead space.

The anesthetic implication of dead space can be understood through following:

- Anesthesia circuits, masks, and humidifiers increase the anatomical dead space.
- Endotracheal tubes and tracheostomy tubes bypass the upper airways and decrease the anatomical dead space.
- Lateral position during anesthesia results in more ventilation to nondependent lung but increased blood flow to dependent lung, leading to V/Q mismatch and consequent increase in alveolar dead space.
- Intermittent positive pressure ventilation and use of positive end-expiratory pressure (PEEP) increase both anatomical and alveolar dead space.

Both cessation of blood flow to the alveoli (as in pulmonary embolism) or excessive alveolar ventilation (as in chronic obstructive pulmonary disease [COPD]) will lead to an increase in dead space. Physiological dead space may be measured with *Bohr's method*, and anatomical dead space may be measured by *Fowler's method*.

Table 1.5 Lung volumes

Lung volume	Definition	Normal value
TV	The volume that can be inhaled or exhaled during a normal breath	6 to 10 mL/kg. Usually, it is 10% of VC breath but may go up to 50% of VC breath during exercise
IRV	The maximal additional volume that can be inspired above the TV	The normal adult value is 1,800–3,200 mL
ERV	The maximal additional volume that can be expired below the TV	The normal adult value is 800–1,200 mL. ERV may be reduced due to *obesity, pregnancy, ascites or after upper abdominal surgeries*
RV	The volume of air remaining in the lungs after a *maximal* exhalation	Its normal value in adults is about 1,200 mL (20–30 mL/kg). *RV may be increased in obstructive lung disease due to incomplete emptying and air trapping. High RV leads to high inflation pressures and decreases venous return during mechanical ventilation, increasing the risk of barotrauma*
FRC	The amount of air remaining in the lungs after a *normal* exhalation FRC = RV + ERV	The normal value is about 1,800–2,400 mL. *FRC is effort independent.* FRC is increased in obstructive lung disease and decreased in restrictive disorders
IC	The maximum volume of air that can be inhaled following a resting state IC = IRV + TV	2,300–3,700 mL in adults
VC	The total amount of air exhaled after a maximal inhalation VC = TV + IRV + ERV	The normal value of VC is 60–70 mL/kg (4–5 L in adults)
FEV	The volume of air a person can exhale during a forced breath	Volume, thus, exhaled during 1st, 2nd, and 3rd seconds are called $FEV1$, $FEV2$, $FEV3$, and so on. FVC is the total amount of air exhaled during the FEV test performance
TLC	The maximum volume of air the lungs can accommodate after maximum inspiration. It is the summation of all the four primary lung volumes TCL = TV + IRV + ERV + RV	Its normal value is 4–6 L in adults (normally 5,800 in males and 4,300 in females). TLC may be increased in obstructive lung disease and decreased in restrictive disorders

Abbreviations: ERV, expiratory reserve volume; FEV, forced expiratory volume; FRC, function residual capacity; IC, inspiratory capacity; IRV, inspiratory reserve volume; RV, residual volume; TLC, total lung capacity; TV, tidal volume; VC, vital capacity.

Respiratory Mechanics, Compliance, Airway Resistance, and Pressure-Volume (PV) Curve

a. Respiratory mechanics

Movement of lungs is determined by elastic resistance of tissue and gas–liquid interface and nonelastic resistance to gas flow. Lung and chest walls tend to recoil in opposite directions, balancing each other. The lung tissue has a high content of elastic fiber and surface tension forces acting at the air–fluid interface in alveoli.

Surface tension forces reduce the area of interface and favor alveolar collapse. According to *Laplace law*, pressure = $2T/R$ (T = surface tension, R = radius of the alveoli here). So, chances of alveolar collapse are directly proportional to its surface tension, but inversely proportional to alveolar size. Thus, the smaller the size, the more collapse. Surfactants are secreted by type 2 pneumocytes and lower surface tension in alveoli. It facilitates gas flow from the larger to the smaller alveolus. In smaller airways, surfactants are more, which decreases surface tension and thus prevents collapse. In larger airways, surfactants are less concentrated, which leads to increased surface tension and thus prevents overdistension.

b. Compliance

Lung compliance is the change in volume in the lungs for a given change in transpulmonary or transmural pressure ($\Delta V/\Delta P$). Compliance is inversely proportional to elastance or elastic resistance.

Normal lung compliance is 200 to 300 mL/cm of H_2O (2–3 L/kPa). The total respiratory compliance, which is a summation of lung and chest wall compliance, is normally 70 to 80 mL/cm H_2O.

Static compliance is the compliance at the end of inspiration, when there is no gas flow, like during an inspiratory pause. *Dynamic compliance* is measured during a normal tidal breath, during actual gas flow.

The static compliance curve can be used to select the ideal level of PEEP for a patient on mechanical ventilation (above the lower inflection point—point at which most of the collapsed alveoli open and below upper inflection point to prevent overdistention).

Lung compliance decreases in pulmonary edema, atelectasis, fibrosis, and decreased surfactants. It increases due to emphysema and increased lung volumes.

Compliance of chest wall reduces due to obesity, conditions causing generalized edema, pleural effusion, and joint disorders like ankylosing spondylitis.

c. Resistance

Resistance to gas flow occurs due to the friction caused by air movement in the respiratory system.

Resistance = driving pressure/resultant gas flow

Normal total airway resistance is about 0.5 to 2 cm H_2O/L/s in a spontaneously breathing persons, with the largest contribution (80%) coming from medium-sized bronchi (before the seventh generation) (airway resistance) along with some sliding of lung and chest wall tissue elements during inspiration or expiration (tissue resistance).

The presence of an endotracheal tube adds to the airway resistance. Resistance to the gas flows further increases at high flow rates, increase in the length of the tube, incorporation of angle (s) on the way to gas flow, sudden changes in the diameter of the tube, and at branches.

Resistance to the fluid flow in a cylinder can be calculated by Poiseuille's law:

$$R = 8 \times \text{length} \times \text{fluid viscosity}/\pi \times (\text{radius})^4$$

d. PV curve

PV curve describes the mechanical behavior of the lungs and chest wall during inspiration and expiration. It informs us about changes in the patient's lung compliance, air leaks, patient-ventilator dyssynchrony, and increased work of breathing (**Fig. 1.3**).

Right shift in PV curve—fibrotic lung disease and interstitial and alveolar edema.

Left shift—emphysema, chronic bronchitis, asthma.

Oxygen and Carbon Dioxide Physiology

Oxygen Transport

Oxygen is the substrate used by cells in maximum quantity and is a key factor for aerobic metabolism and cell integrity. The decreased supply of O_2 to tissues leads to anaerobic metabolism, which generates lactic acid and only 2 ATPs compared to 38 ATPs in aerobic metabolism. The delivery of oxygen from the atmosphere to cells requires a pressure gradient dependent movement of oxygen through the following steps:

a. Atmosphere to alveoli

Room air has 21% oxygen and 79% nitrogen. As we breathe air into our lungs, the nose and conducting airways warm and humidify the air, such that it is fully humidified and warmed to 37°C by the time it reaches alveoli. Water vapor at 37°C exerts a partial pressure of 47 mm Hg. Thus, the partial pressure of oxygen in warmed and humidified air at sea level will be 150 mm Hg $(760 - 47) \times 21/100 = 150$ mm Hg.

b. Alveoli to pulmonary capillaries

Once CO_2 is added to the alveolar gas, the partial pressure of oxygen drops even further:

From simplified alveolar gas equation:

Partial pressure of O_2 in alveoli (PAO_2)

$= PIO_2 - (PaCO_2 / $ respiratory quotient$)$

$= 150 - (40 / 0.8) = 150 - 50 = 100$ mm Hg

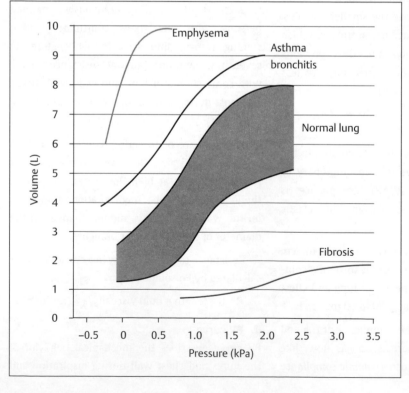

Fig. 1.3 Pressure volume curve.

PAO_2 is the driving pressure that causes oxygen to enter from alveoli into the blood in pulmonary capillaries and determines arterial O_2 concentration (PaO_2) too.

c. Alveolar – arterial gradient (A – a gradient)

PAO_2 – PaO_2 (A – a) gradient reflects the overall efficiency of O_2 uptake from alveoli to arterial blood and helps to assess the integrity of the alveolar-capillary unit.

A – a gradient is useful in determining the source of *hypoxemia* (intrapulmonary or extra-pulmonary). A normal A – a gradient for a young adult nonsmoker breathing air is between 5 and 10 mm Hg. A – a gradient increases with age at a rate of 1 mm Hg/decade. An abnormally increased A – a gradient suggests a defect in *diffusion*, V/Q (*ventilation/perfusion ratio*) mismatch, or *right-to-left shunt.*

d. Transport of oxygen

Oxygen in the blood is transported in two forms:

- Chemically combined
  - ▶ 1 g of Hb when fully saturated contains 1.34 mL of oxygen.
- Physically dissolved

At PO_2 of 100 mm Hg, only about 0.003 mL O_2 is dissolved in each mL of blood.

The physically dissolved oxygen is not sufficient to meet the metabolic demand for oxygen, even at rest. However, dissolved O_2 in plasma acts as a pathway for the supply of O_2. O_2 in the blood is first transferred to the cells, while its place is rapidly being taken up by more O_2 is liberated from the Hb. Functions of hemoglobin are as follows:

- It facilitates O_2 transport.
- It facilitates CO_2 transport.
- Has an important role as a tissue O_2 buffer.
- It transports NO.

A total of 97 to 98% of O_2 in the blood is carried in combination with Hb (only 2–3% dissolved in plasma).

O_2 content of blood (CaO_2) can be calculated by formula $1.34 \times Hb \times \% Sat + 0.0031 \times PO_2$.

1 g Hb binds 1.34 mL of oxygen—Hüffner's constant, 1.39 for in vitro (pure Hb) form.

When Hb is 100% saturated, 100 mL of arterial blood carries roughly 20.4 mL of oxygen (20.1 mL as Oxy Hb + 0.3 mL in plasma). Some important points for consideration here are:

- Oxygen delivery (DO_2)—The volume of oxygen (in milliliters) that reaches the systemic capillaries each minute.
- Total or "global" oxygen delivery (DO_2) = cardiac output (Qt) × O_2 content of the blood (CaO_2).

The normal DO_2 in adults at rest is 900 to 1,100 mL/min.

e. Unloading O_2 in tissues

Arterial blood that reaches systemic capillaries has a partial pressure of 95 mm Hg. The partial pressure of O_2 in the interstitial tissue fluid surrounding tissue cell is 40 mm Hg. A pressure gradient of 55 mm Hg (95 – 40) causes oxygen to move from systemic capillaries into the interstitium.

An average 70-kg adult consumes about 250 mL of oxygen per minute.

- Oxygen extraction ratio (VO_2 / DO_2): It is the fraction of delivered O_2 and which is consumed. The value in normal adult is 0.2 to 0.3. The oxygen which is not extracted by the tissues returns to the lungs in the mixed venous blood. Mixed venous saturation (SvO_2), which is measured in the pulmonary artery, represents the pooled venous saturation from all organs. SvO_2 is influenced by changes in both DO_2 and VO_2. Normal SvO_2 value is > 65%.

Critical DO_2: The degree of oxygen delivery, below which supply is inadequate to meet oxygen demand = 4 to 8 mL/kg/min.

f. Diffusion of oxygen from tissue fluid into cells

Tissues are continuously utilizing oxygen; as a result, the PO_2 in peripheral tissue cells is much lower than PO_2 in systemic capillaries. Normal intracellular PO_2 varies between 5 and 40 mm Hg (average about 23 mm Hg). An intracellular PO_2 of 1 to 3 mm Hg is sufficient to fully support intracellular aerobic metabolic activities. Below this level, oxygen consumption falls, and various members of the electron transport chain tend to revert to the reduced state. The critical PO_2 varies between different organs and different species, but, as an approximation, a mitochondrial PO_2 of about 1 mm Hg (0.13 kPa) may be taken as the level below which there is a serious impairment of oxidative phosphorylation and a switch to anaerobic metabolism—*Pasteur point*.

Oxygen flux is the amount of O_2 leaving the left ventricle per minute in the arterial blood. It represents O_2 delivered to the tissues. It depends on cardiac output, arterial O_2 saturation, and Hb concentration. *The lowest tolerable value of O_2 flux is 400 mL/min.* Oxygen flux is decreased in anemia, congestive heart failure, and acidosis and increased during exercise, pain, shivering, and thyrotoxicosis.

g. Oxyhemoglobin dissociation curve (ODC)

It is a graphical illustration (**Fig. 1.4**) of the percentage of Hb that is chemically bound to O_2 at each O_2 pressure. It plots PO_2 of the plasma with the percent of hemoglobin saturation.

This curve is S-shaped since the reactions of the four subunits of hemoglobin with oxygen occur sequentially and not simultaneously. The fall in PO_2 below 60 mm Hg produces a rapid decrease in the amount of O_2 bound to hemoglobin, leading to a significant reduction in O_2 delivery to the tissue.

P50 is the partial pressure at which the hemoglobin is 50% saturated with oxygen. Its value is 26.6 mm Hg in adults. It is a conventional

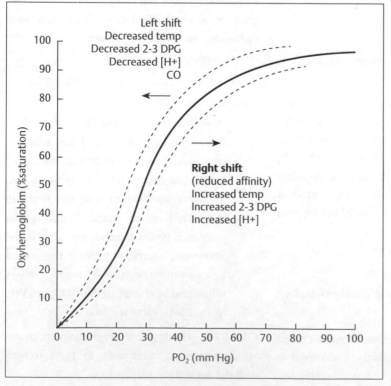

Fig. 1.4 Oxygen dissociation curve.

measure of hemoglobin affinity for oxygen. An increased P50 indicates a rightward shift or decreased affinity. A lower P50 indicates a leftward shift or decreased affinity. A variety of factors can affect the oxygen dissociation curve (**Table 1.6**).

Bohr Effect

Bohr effect was described by a Danish physiologist Christian Bohr. Hemoglobin–oxygen binding affinity is inversely related both to acidity and to the concentration of carbon dioxide.

In *systemic capillaries*, higher PCO_2 (because of local CO_2 production) causes a decrease in pH compared to arterial blood which, in turn, causes a rightward shift of the ODC and decreased affinity of Hb for O_2, resulting in offloading of O_2 to the tissues. Conversely, in the lungs, in *pulmonary capillaries*, lower PCO_2 causes a rise in pH; therefore, the O_2 affinity of Hb is increased to encourage uptake.

Double Bohr Effect

In the placenta, gaseous exchange takes place directly between two different bloodstreams: maternal and fetal. This provides a situation wherein the Bohr effect has double benefits. The CO_2 liberated by fetal blood shifts the ODC of maternal blood to the right. The lowering of PCO_2 of fetal blood shifts its own ODC to the left.

Carbon Dioxide Transport

The amount of CO_2 present in the body is a function of both CO_2 elimination and CO_2 production.

While the removal of CO_2 depends on pulmonary blood flow and alveolar ventilation, the production of CO_2 (VcO_2) parallels O_2 consumption (VO_2), according to the respiratory quotient (RQ). Under normal resting conditions, the collective RQ of the human body is 0.8. Transport of CO_2 happens in our body with the help of the following mechanisms:

a. As bicarbonate

This constitutes 70 to 90 % of total CO_2 transport. This occurs mainly in red blood cells (RBCs). CO_2 combines with water to form carbonic acid (H_2CO_3), which then dissociates to form H^+ and bicarbonate spontaneously. Carbonic anhydrase enzyme present in RBCs and blood vessels makes this reaction 25,000 times faster, so that conversion of HCO_3^- and H^+ back into CO_2 and H_2O can occur in the pulmonary capillaries during the very brief pulmonary capillary transit time to facilitate effective CO_2 elimination. Chloride shift is the process of exchange of intracellular HCO_3^- with chloride.

b. As carbamate

It accounts for roughly 13% of CO_2 transported in the blood.

c. As dissolved gas in the plasma

It contributes to 10% of total CO_2 being transported in the blood. CO_2 is 10 to 20 times more soluble in water compared to O_2. In plasma, CO_2 exists both as dissolved and as H_2CO_3 ($H_2O + CO_2$). The CO_2 in solution is related to PCO_2 by the use of Henry's law. Total dissolved CO_2 in solution = PCO_2 X a, where a is the solubility coefficient of

Table 1.6 Factors affecting oxygen dissociation curve

Leftward shift	Rightward shift
• Decreased $PaCO_2$	• Increased $PaCO_2$
• Alkalosis	• Acidosis
• Hypothermia	• Increased temperature
• Decreased 2, 3-DPG	• Increased 2, 3-DPG
• Fetal Hb	• Pregnancy
• CO poisoning	• Inhalational anesthetics
• Methemoglobin, etc.	

CO_2 in plasma (0.03 mmol/L/mm Hg at 37°C) = 1.2 mmol/L.

d. As carbonic acid—minimal amount

Breathing O_2 sometimes induces hypercapnia in patients with severe chronic lung disease because of the following reasons:

- Impairment of hypoxic pulmonary vasoconstriction (HPV) by elevated O_2 allows diminished efficiency of CO_2 exhalation.

- Haldane effect—For a given PCO_2, the CO_2 content of the blood increases as PO_2 falls and vice versa. It is the shift in the CO_2 dissociation curve which is caused by the degree of oxygenation of Hb. Low PO_2 shifts the CO_2 dissociation curve to the left, so that blood is able to pick up more CO_2 (as occurs in capillaries of rapidly metabolizing tissues). Oxygenation of Hb (as occurs in the lungs) reduces the affinity of Hb for CO_2, and the CO_2 dissociation curve is shifted to the right, thereby increasing CO_2 removal.

Hypoxic Pulmonary Vasoconstriction

HPV is a reflex constriction of intrapulmonary arteries in response to the low regional partial pressure of oxygen (PO_2) or alveolar hypoxia. This vasoconstriction is contrary to the systemic circulation, which typically vasodilates in response to hypoxia. HPV reduces blood flow in areas of the lung where PO_2 is low, so that circulation is redistributed to reach to the well-oxygenated area. HPV is biphasic with a second more powerful response occurring after approximately 45 minutes and is active in utero too. Although the role of HPV in normal lungs is controversial, it has a beneficial role to play in stable asthma, COPD, acute lung injury, and one-lung ventilation during various thoracic surgeries. It is reported that people who are susceptible to develop high altitude pulmonary edema had more intense HPV response. In different hypoxic conditions, augmentation of HPV is desirable.

HPV is more intense in the fetal and neonatal circulations and in the presence of metabolic and respiratory acidosis. Almitrine and a_1 agonists such as norepinephrine or phenylephrine can augment HPV. Factors which attenuate HPV include the following:

- Alkalosis.

- Hypothermia.

- Acetazolamide.

- Drugs causing pulmonary vasodilation like:
  - Inhaled nitric oxide, phosphodiesterase inhibitors (sildenafil, etc.).
  - Nitric oxide donors (sodium nitroprusside, nitroglycerine).
  - Hydralazine, prostacyclin, calcium channel blockers (verapamil, nifedipine).
  - Endothelin antagonists (ET_A and ET_B receptor blocker—sitaxsentan; ET_A receptor blocker—bosentan).
  - Inhalational agents (halothane > isoflurane, sevoflurane, desflurane).

Applied Physics in Anesthesia

The principles of physics are often employed in anesthesia equipment and procedures. The important laws and principles are described below:

- Gas laws
  - **Boyle's law**: It states that at a constant temperature, the volume of a given gas is inversely related to its pressure, that is, $P \alpha\, 1/V$.
  - **Charles' law:** It says that at constant pressure, the volume of gas is directly proportional to the temperature, that is, $V \alpha\, T$.
  - **Graham's law:** It states that the rate of diffusion of a gas is inversely proportional to the square root of their molecular weight.

- ▶ **Gay–Lussac's law**: It says that at a constant volume, the pressure is proportional to the temperature.
- Avogadro number: It is the number of molecules contained in 1 g molecular weight of a substance, and it is equal to 6.23×10^{23} molecules.
- Critical temperature: It is the temperature above which a gas cannot be liquefied irrespective of the pressure applied.
- The flow of gases: The flow of a gas can be laminar or turbulent, depending upon the Reynolds number. The laminar flow occurs in a straight tube and at Reynolds number less than 2000. It is more affected by the viscosity of gas and follows Haegen–Poiseulli's law. At the same time, the turbulent flow occurs at very high flow rates and when gas passes through constrictions/bends. Turbulent flow occurs at Reynolds's number more than 4000. It is more affected by the density of the gas.
- Venturi principle: It is based on Bernoulli's law and says that when a gas or fluid passes through a tube of varying diameter, the lateral pressure exerted by fluid is minimum where the velocity (kinetic energy) is maximum. The devices based on venturi principles are as follows:
  - ▶ Venturi masks.
  - ▶ Venturi nozzles.
  - ▶ Sander's jet injectors.
  - ▶ Atomizers.
  - ▶ Modern vaporizers.
  - ▶ Nebulization chambers.
- Coanda effect: The constriction at bifurcation causes sticking of blood/gas to one side of bifurcation due to a rise in velocity and reduction in pressure. This is known as the Coanda effect. Situations where Coanda effects are seen:
  - ▶ Maldistribution of gases due to mucus plug at the bifurcation in the airway tree.
  - ▶ Unequal flow due to atherosclerotic plaque in the vascular tree.
- Poynting effect: The mixing of liquid nitrous oxide at low pressure with oxygen at high pressure leads to the formation of gas of nitrous oxide (inside Entonox cylinder). Therefore, both nitrous oxide and oxygen are in the gaseous state in the cylinder.

Conclusion

The anatomy and physiology of the respiratory system is not consistent across different age groups. It also changes during pregnancy. The knowledge of the same and its anesthetic implication is important for safe and smooth management of patients during the perioperative period.

CHAPTER 2

Historical Milestones in Anesthesia

Ridhima Sharma and Ripon Choudhary

Introduction

On October 16, 1846 (considered as the era of the beginning of anesthesia), *William TG Morton* gave the first successful public demonstration of anesthesia using ether at the Massachusetts General Hospital, and that is why October 16 is celebrated as world anesthesia day. This chapter covers the historical evolution of various anesthetic agents, be it inhalational, intravenous (IV), and muscle relaxants.

Inhaled Anesthetic Agents

The muddle experienced by the surgeon during surgery played a pivotal role in the development of "inhalational agents." Active physical resistance, crying, and screaming by the patients were distracting during the surgery and, overall, increased the mortality and morbidity.

In the 15th century, Paracelsus was aware of the soporific action of ether, a compound synthesized from sulfuric acid and alcohol by the chemist Valerius Cordus (called as volatile liquid "sweet vitriol"). Paracelsus observed the effect of ether on chickens and stated that "it quiets all suffering without harm and relieves all pain." Various inhalational anesthetic agents are briefly explained below.

Chloroform

The propensity to explode in ether prompted the search of alternative inhaled agents, including chloroform ($CHCl_3$). David Waldie suggested $CHCl_3$ (prepared in 1931) to James Young Simpson. Simpson and his friends at a dinner party on November 4, 1847 inhaled it and promptly felt unconscious and within 2 weeks submitted his discovery to *The Lancet*.

The entity of $CHCl_3$ had gained popularity when *John Snow* used it for the pain-free delivery of Queen Victoria.

Nitrous Oxide

The annals of nitrous oxide (N_2O) backdated with its isolation in 1772 by Joseph Priestly. Over the decade, *Humphry Davy accidentally noted its analgesic property*. The idea of using N_2O with oxygen was credited to Edmund Andrews (1824–1904) and provided analgesia without cyanosis. He also advocated the use of liquid N_2O in iron flasks. Paul Bert (1833–1886) demonstrated the effect of surgical anesthesia without hypoxia when delivered at a pressure greater than 1 atmosphere.

Frederick Hewitt (1857–1916) devised an anesthesia machine to deliver N_2O and oxygen at variable proportions.

Diethyl Ether

William TG Morton gave a successful public demonstration of ether at the Massachusetts General Hospital. It is an excellent muscle relaxant.

Inhaled Fluorinated Anesthetics

A survey on 166 gases concluded that fluorine substitution for halogens increased stability and reduced the boiling point and toxicity. The first fluorinated anesthetic (1954), namely, fluroxene or trifluoromethyl vinyl ether, was discovered and later on withdrawn (1974) due to toxic metabolite found in animals.

In 1954, Charles Suckling synthesized halothane. James Raventos (1905–1983) studied the pharmacological properties of halothane, which later on was widely accepted clinically across the world in 1956 by Michael Johnstone. Some of the flourinated inhalational anesthetic agents are as follows:

- **Methoxyflurane:** In 1960, methoxyflurane followed halothane and remained popular for a decade. However, due to its high fluoride content, nephrotoxicity (high-output renal failure), and risk of oxalate stone, the search for the ideal volatile agent started.

- **Enflurane and isoflurane:** Ohio Medical products developed enflurane and isoflurane about 40 years ago. Enflurane utilization was limited due to its cardiodepressant, fluorine nephrotoxicity, and its epileptiform activities, while isoflurane has been widely used since that time.

- **Desflurane and sevoflurane:** *Desflurane* was one of the last volatile anesthetics to be manufactured and had high vapor pressure (fast induction, recovery, and pungent smell). Furthermore, the Travenol laboratories synthesized *sevoflurane* more than 40 years ago with rapid recovery and form an unstable component in soda lime.

Although William Ramsay in the 1940s (noble gas) isolated xenon and considered very close to ideal gas, it is still not used widely due to scarcity in availability and is also very expensive.

Intravenous Anesthetics

The discovery of IV anesthetic agents began with barbiturates, and later on, phencyclindine derivatives, benzodiazepines and etomidate joined the series. These are commonly used agents for induction as well as maintenance of anesthesia with unique physicochemical properties and pharmacodynamics. The historical track of these agents is discussed in this chapter.

Thiopentone

IV anesthesia dates back from the introduction of thiopentone in 1934, preceded by hexobarbital in 1932.

Sodium thiopental (sodium pentothal) was discovered by Ernest H. Volwiler and Donalee L. Tabern, working in collaboration with Abbott Laboratories. On March 8, 1934, Dr Ralph M. Water used it for the first time in human beings. Although Water was the first to clinically use thiopentone, Dr John S. Lundy (June 18, 1934) was the first to press and responsible for the large popularity of the drug.

Methohexitone

The discovery of methohexitone was credited to the Lilly Research Laboratories (1956); Chernish and colleagues described it to be more potent than thiopentone with rapid recovery.

Phencyclidine Derivatives

Phencyclidine is also known as angel dust and is known to have mind-altering effects. It can also cause altered perception of sounds, violent behavior, and hallucinations. Ketamine is one of the derivatives of it with unique anesthetic effect.

Ketamine

Ketamine history dates back to the 1950s at Parke-Davis and Company's laboratories in Detroit, Michigan, USA. On March 26, 1956, Maddox (chemist) discovered the process of synthesis of phencyclidine. Later on, Chen and Dr Domino studied the effects of the drug on animals and found them in a cataleptic state with their eyes open and poor muscle relaxation. Domino's wife Toni, later on, suggested the term *"dissociative anesthesia."*

Propofol

Propofol's first clinical trials in 1977 by Kay and Rolly were initially formulated using Cremophor

EL (solubilizing agent) but later changed to intralipid due to anaphylactic reactions and pain on injection. Later on, a commercial preparation of propofol (Diprivan, AstraZeneca, Wilmington, DE, USA) was formulated as a fat emulsion containing 10% soyabean oil with long-chain triglycerides.

Etomidate

The first literature on etomidate was published in 1965 by Janssen Pharmaceuticals (a division of Ortho-McNeil-Jannsen Pharmaceuticals, Titusville, New Jersey, USA) as an arylalkyl imidazole-5-carboxylate esters. Initially, it was developed as an antifungal agent. In 1983, various academic publications revealed adrenal toxicity.

Benzodiazepines

Benzodiazepines' discovery dates back to 1957, when Leo Sternbach (chemist), serendipitously discovered the first benzodiazepines (diazepam) while working in the Hoffmann-La Roche laboratories, New Jersey. Chlordiazepoxide (benzheptoxdiazine derivative) was discovered in 1957 from an earlier project. The drug has sedative, anticonvulsant, and muscle relaxation properties.

Midazolam is a rapid-onset, short-acting benzodiazepine patented by Hoffmann-La Roche in 1976.

History of Opioid Discovery

The word opium is derived from the Greek word "juice." In 1805, Friedrich Wilhelm Adam Ferdinand Serturner was the first to isolate morphine (Morpheus, the Greek God to sleep) from poppy. In that era, the invention of a hypodermic needle (hollow) and syringes by Charles Gabriel and Alexander Wood allowed subcutaneous application.

The use and misuse of morphine during the American Civil War (1861–1865) and the French-German War (1870–1871), known as soldiers' disease, spurred the researcher to find an alternative with low risk of abuse:

Methadone was discovered during World War II (Germany) and used as a substitute for drug addiction.

Fentanyl: Paul AJ Janssen, in 1953, discovered fentanyl (40 times more active than morphine). Subsequently, drugs with strong potency and similar compounds were discovered like carfentanil, sufentanil, and alfentanil.

Muscle Relaxants

Homer and Virgil mentioned poison arrows. The word toxin is derived from the Greek root toxon (bow). Curare was used for hunting game from centuries by South American Indians.

Bovet divided the curares into pachycurares (nondepolarizing mechanism of action) and leptocurares (depolarizing action). Suxamethonium is the only leptocurares. Furthermore, Benjamin Brodie found that the use of artificial ventilation of the lung could keep the rabbits alive who were paralyzed with curare. Some of the common muscle relaxants are briefly explained below.

Gallamine

Gallamine is the first synthetic muscle relaxant discovered by Daniel Bovet (Pasteur Institute in Paris).

Suxamethonium

In 1949, Daniel Bovet was the first to describe the paralysis induced by suxamethonium and was awarded the Nobel Prize for Medicine in 1957 for his contribution to the field.

Pancuronium

In the 1960s, malouetine (disquaternary steroidal alkaloid) was isolated from the bark of a plant Malouetia bequaertiana and found to have curare-like effects. In 1964, Hewett and Savage synthesized pancuronium from two quaternary ammonium groups.

Vecuronium

Savarese and Kitz discovered vecuronium in 1975 with properties of rapid onset and recovery.

Atracurium

In 1981, Stenlake and colleagues, in a collaboration between the University of Strathclyde and Wellcome Laboratories, synthesized atracurium (benzylisoquinoline).

Mivacurium

Savarese and colleagues in the USA had synthesized mivacurium, an ester-linked benzylisoquinoline metabolized by plasma cholinesterase.

Rocuronium

Rocuronium is a deacetoxy analog of vecuronium and was discovered by Bowman in 1988.

Rapacuronium

It is an analog of vecuronium with rapid onset, close to that of suxamethonium. It was withdrawn from the market because of multiple reports of severe bronchospasm.

The Historical Journey of Local Anesthetics

The discovery of local anesthetics paved the era of regional anesthesia, and their use in modern anesthesia practice is growing exponentially with better pain management and improved patient's outcome. Given below is a detailed description of discovery of local anesthetics.

Cocaine

The indigenous people of Peru had the knowledge of a wonderful plant (Khoka) whose leaves were considered as a stimulant when chewed. Between 1859 and 1860, Niemann coined the term cocaine.

Karl Damian Ritter von Schroff (pharmacologist) described cocaine as a narcotic and found to make skin insensible after its topical application.

Sigmund Freud was the first to postulate the idea of using cocaine clinically for its local anesthetic properties and mentioned this to his colleagues. In 1884, Carl Koller clinically demonstrated the analgesic properties of cocaine in the eye.

A. Eihorn (1898) synthesized *"nirvaquine,"* the first local anesthetic (amino amide). It was eventually withdrawn due to local tissue irritation.

Eihorn synthesized *benzocaine* and *procaine* in 1900 and 1905, respectively. Procaine was used for spinal anesthesia and local infiltration. The low potency with slow onset and recovery has made it unpopular for the peripheral and central neuraxial blocks.

Chloroprocaine results from chlorine substitution on the aromatic ring of procaine. It has a rapid onset and a short duration of action. It was used in short procedures in epidural anesthesia. Prolonged block due to unintentional subarachnoid administration declined its use after the 1980s.

Tetracaine, an ester-type local anesthetic, was discovered in 1930. It can be used as an isobaric, hypobaric, or hyperbaric solution for spinal anesthesia with 1.5- to 2.5-hour duration of action. Tetracaine can be used as an effective topical airway anesthetic.

In 1931, *Cinchocaine* was introduced as a local anesthetic and was withdrawn immediately due to a considerable level of toxicity.

Lofgren in 1948 prepared *lidocaine* which was the first amide local anesthetic to be used clinically; the high potency and rapid onset made it an attractive choice for peripheral as well as central neuraxial blocks. The use of *lidocaine has been associated with transient neurologic symptoms and cauda equina syndrome.*

Mepivacaine was introduced for clinical use in 1957.

Prilocaine was introduced in 1960. It is primarily used for infiltration, peripheral nerve block, and peridural anesthesia. It produces less vasodilatation than lidocaine and has a lesser potential for systemic toxicity at similar doses. *The most alarming adverse effect is methemoglobinemia.*

The isolation of *bupivacaine* in 1963 created a revolution in the history of regional anesthesia. It is a long-acting local anesthetic used for infiltration, peripheral nerve block, and epidural and spinal anesthesia. The use of bupivacaine is associated with significant cardiotoxicity.

In 1972, *etidocaine* (long-acting local anesthetic) was introduced. The profound motor blockade has led to the diminished use of etodicaine in the modern day of practice.

Ropivacaine was evaluated in clinical trials, starting in 1990 and introduced clinically in 1996, and has a better sensorimotor dissociation at lower doses. It is short-acting and less cardiotoxic than bupivacaine.

Conclusion

To summarize, the practice of anesthesia keeps on growing with discovery of newer agents and will continue to evolve in the future too. The discovery of newer agents with better safety profile will improve the patient's care in coming years.

CHAPTER 3

Preoperative Checkup

Neha Garg

Introduction (AS3.1)

Anesthetizing a patient without a preoperative check is like traveling in an airplane without a pilot. Preoperative assessment is the cornerstone of perioperative care by anesthesiologists. Relevant history, including comorbidities, the medications, and past surgical history with associated anesthetic complications, can be obtained during preoperative evaluation. This information can be supplemented with the findings of physical examination and necessary investigations to formulate an optimal anesthetic plan. Also, preoperative checkup helps anesthetists to build rapport and gain the confidence of the patients. The preoperative checkup includes the following steps:

- Preoperative assessment.
- Premedication and instruction.
- Assessment of airway and plan for anticipated difficult airway.

Preoperative Assessment

It is done for the following:

- Know about the patient's comorbidities and their functional status, which can significantly impact anesthetic care.
- To optimize the patients for their comorbid illness before an elective surgery.
- To formulate an anesthesia plan by deciding the drugs to be used and the type of anesthesia.
- Stratify the patient.
- Take consent.

It involves a thorough history taking and examination of the patient.

History (AS3.2)

History-taking during the preoperative period is required to obtain information about the patient's medical, surgical, and medication details, which guide the anesthetic management during the perioperative period. The history-taking should focus on:

- Demographic details including the age, weight, and body mass index (BMI).
- Comorbid illnesses such as diabetes mellitus, hypertension, thyroid disorders, seizure disorder, and coronary artery disease.
- Medication history (types and duration of each drug the patient is taking).
- Personal history (smoking, alcoholism).
- History of allergy (including allergy to any food items or any medication).
- History of previous surgery (regional anesthesia [RA] or general anesthesia [GA], complications, etc.) is taken.
- Family history: The unexpected death of a first-degree relative under GA makes the probability of malignant hyperthermia high.

Examination (AS3.3)

Head-to-toe examination of the patient is done, with an emphasis on the cardiorespiratory system. Abnormal findings in any organ system should be properly evaluated and optimized before taking the patient for elective surgery. The important head-to-toe findings that require further evaluation are as follows:

- Central nervous system:
  - ▶ Altered sensorium and behavior.

- ▸ Sensory and or motor deficit.
- ▸ Abnormal gait and cranial nerve palsy.
- Cardiovascular system:
  - ▸ Irregular heart rate (except for sinus arrhythmia).
  - ▸ The difference in blood pressure of two limbs.
  - ▸ Presence of carotid bruit and murmurs on auscultation.
- Abdomen:
  - ▸ Any lump or swelling.
  - ▸ Presence of tenderness.
- Musculoskeletal system:
  - ▸ Limitation of movement at any joint may complicate patient positioning during transfer and under anesthesia.
  - ▸ Limitation of movement at the cervical spine makes laryngoscopy and intubation difficult.
- Respiratory system:
  - ▸ Altered thoracic spine curvature suggests scoliosis.
  - ▸ Presence of wheeze/crepitation (may be due to lower respiratory tract infection).

Breath-holding time is commonly done to assess the cardiorespiratory reserve of the patients. The patients are instructed to hold breath after deep inspiration and the time is noted (till the patients are able to hold the breath) in the following manner:

- ≥25 seconds: Good reserve.
- 25 to 15 seconds: Borderline.
- <15 seconds: Poor reserve.

The detailed examination of upper respiratory tract along with its clinical implication has been described later on in this chapter.

After history-taking and physical examination, risk stratification is done, based on the American Society of Anesthesiologists (ASA) classification system. Patients are classified under increased risk of morbidity and mortality by this classification (**Table 3.1**).

Premedication and Preoperative Instruction (AS3.5, AS3.6)

The premedication and preoperative instructions include the following:

- Consent.
- Nil per oral (NPO): 8 hours for solid, 6 hours for liquid, 2 hours for clear fluid like water, and nonpulpy juices like Appy. In infants, 6 hours for formula feed and 4 hours for breast milk.
- Antianxiety medication: Tablet alprazolam at bedtime and in the morning in only highly anxious patients, hypertensive patients with a history of arrhythmia, etc.
- Most of the time, reassurance and counseling the patient reduces anxiety, and drugs are not needed.
- In children, syrup midazolam, clonidine, dexmedetomidine may be used.
- Antiaspiration prophylaxis: H2 receptor blockers or proton pump inhibitors (PPI) at bedtime and in the morning in high-risk cases like obesity and intra-abdominal tumors. Other drugs like metoclopramide and antacids like sodium citrate can also be used.
- Others: Antisecretory medications like glycopyrrolate in difficult airway cases where fiberoptic intubation is planned, nebulization with salbutamol for asthmatic patients.

Patients with comorbid illnesses are on a variety of medications which undergo myriad interactions with anesthetic agents and can adversely affect patient's outcome. It is imperative to acquaint with pharmacology as well as their interaction with anesthetic agents. **Table 3.2** highlights important medications and their timings with surgery.

Table 3.1 ASA physical status classification

ASA class[a]	Definition	Examples
I	A normal healthy patient	Healthy, nonsmoking, no or minimal alcohol use

II	A patient with mild systemic disease	• The mild disease only without substantive functional limitations
		• Examples include (but not limited to):
		  ○ Current smoker
		  ○ Social alcohol drinker
		  ○ Pregnancy
		  ○ Obesity (30 < BMI < 40)
		  ○ Well-controlled DM/HTN
		  ○ Mild lung disease

III	A patient with severe systemic disease	• Substantive functional limitations
		• Examples include:
		  ○ Poorly controlled DM/HTN/COPD
		  ○ Morbid obesity (BMI > 40)
		  ○ Active hepatitis
		  ○ Alcohol abuse or dependence
		  ○ Implanted pacemaker
		  ○ Premature infant (PCA < 60 weeks)
		  ○ ESRD on regular dialysis
		  ○ History of: CAD/MI/CVA > 3 months

IV	A patient with severe systemic disease that is a constant threat to life	Examples include: • History of: CAD/MI/CVA < 3 months • ESRD not on regular dialysis • Ongoing cardiac ischemia or severe valvular dysfunction • Sepsis, DIC
V	A moribund patient who is not expected to survive without the operation	Examples: • Ruptured abdominal/thoracic aneurysm • Massive trauma • Intracranial bleed with mass effect
VI	A declared brain-dead patient whose organs are being removed for the purpose of the donation	

Abbreviations: ASA, American Society of Anesthesiologists; BMI, body mass index; CAD, coronary artery disease; COPD, chronic obstructive pulmonary disease; CVA, cerebrovascular accident; DIC, disseminated intravascular coagulation; DM, diabetes mellitus; ESRD, end-stage renal disease; HTN, hypertension; MI, myocardial infarction; PCA, postconceptional age.
Note: [a]The addition of "E" denotes emergency surgery: An emergency is defined as existing when a delay in treatment of the patient would lead to a significant increase in the threat to life or body part.

Investigations (AS3.4)

Investigation before surgery is not mandatory in all patients. It needs to be tailored based on patient's needs as well as surgical factors. The investigations may include blood (complete blood count [CBC]), serum electrolytes, kidney function test (KFT), liver function test (LFT), coagulation studies, ECG, and chest X-ray; more advanced testing may be warranted in a specific group of patients.

The investigations are done on an individual basis. Hemoglobin level estimation is important in anemic patients. Similarly, CBC, serum electrolytes, renal function test, and coagulation profile are valuable for patients afflicted with

Table 3.2 Preoperative medications

Medication	Instructions
Antihypertensive	Continue on the day of surgery except for ACEIs and ARBSs
Beta-blockers, digoxin	Continue
Thyroid medications	Continue
Opioids	Continue
Oral contraceptive pills	Continue
Eye drops	Continue
Anticonvulsants	Continue
Asthma medications	Continue
Corticosteroids (oral/inhaled)	Continue
Statins	Continue
Aspirin	Continue in patients with prior PCI, high-grade ischemic heart disease, and significant CVD. Otherwise, discontinue 3 days before surgery
P2Y12 inhibitors (clopidogrel, ticlopidine, ticagrelor, prasugrel)	*No need to stop in patients undergoing cataract surgery (topical or GA)* For other cases: • Clopidogrel/ticagrelor: 5–7 days before surgery • Prasugrel: 7–10 days before surgery • Ticlopidine: 10 days before surgery
Insulin	For all patients, discontinue all short-acting insulin on the day of surgery (except insulin administered by continuous pump): • *Type 2 DM*: None to half of long-acting or combination insulin on the day of surgery • *Type 1 DM*: One-third of long-acting insulin on the day of surgery
Oral hypoglycemic agents	[a] Discontinue on the day of surgery (exception: SGLT2 inhibitors should be discontinued 24 h before surgery) [a] *The drugs which do not cause an increase in insulin level (e.g., metformin) can be continued even on the day of surgery*
Diuretics	Discontinue on the day of surgery *except for thiazides*
Sildenafil	Discontinue 24 h before surgery
COX-2 inhibitors	Continue on the day of surgery unless the surgeon is concerned about bone healing
NSAIDs	Discontinue 48 h before surgery
Warfarin	Discontinue 5 days before surgery
Antidepressants, anxiolytics	Continue
MAO inhibitors	[b] Continue (but avoid meperidine and ephedrine during the perioperative period)

Abbreviations: ACEIs, angiotensin converting enzyme inhibitors; ARBs, angiotensin II receptor blockers; CVD, cardiovascular disease; DM, diabetes mellitus; GA, general anesthesia; MAO, monoamine oxidase inhibitors; NSAIDs, nonsteroidal anti-inflammatory drugs; PCI, percutaneous intervention; SGLT2, sodium glucose transport protein 2.

Notes: [a] The drugs which do not cause an increase in insulin level (e.g., metformin) can be continued even on the day of surgery. [b] MAO inhibitors used to be stopped 3 weeks before surgery but discontinuing them for such long duration increases patient's morbidity.

chronic kidney disease. Fasting blood sugar is the most important diagnostic as well as monitoring parameter for diabetic patients. ECG is done when there is a history of chest pain and palpitations. Advanced investigations such as echocardiography and pulmonary function tests may also be done when needed.

Airway Assessment (AS3.4)

The evaluation of the airway is the most important and vital skill which every anesthetist must acquire. With repeated assessment of patients, anesthetists should be able to anticipate the level of difficulty in the airway and learn the skills to manage them. Improper evaluation and planning of the airway can endanger a patient's life.

The normal intubation position is sniffing the morning air position. In a sniffing position, *there is an extension at the atlantoaxial joint and flexion at the lower cervical joint.* This position brings the oral, pharyngeal, and laryngeal axis in line to ease intubation.

The evaluation of the airway by anesthetists should follow a proper sequence, so as not to miss any component of the airway, which can, later on, complicate airway management. This can be achieved in the following ways:

Assess the factors for difficult bag and mask ventilation:

- Look for the presence of facial hair, obesity, being edentulous, advanced age, and history of snoring.

- Dentition should be assessed, and dentures should be removed before intubation. However, dentures may be left in place for noninvasive airway management.

Assess mouth opening: Ask the patient to open their mouth completely. Normal mouth opening is 3 to 4 fingerbreadths (patient's own fingerbreadth).

Mallampati (MMP) grading: It is used to assess the size of the oropharyngeal cavity, with respect to tongue size, and predict the ease of endotracheal intubation (**Fig. 3.1**).

Neck movement (flexion and extension): This testing method is also known as Delikan test. Ask the patient to flex and extend the neck. It can be graded in the following manner:

- Chin above the occiput in extension: Normal.

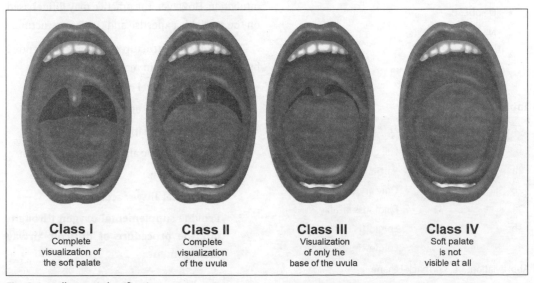

Class I	Class II	Class III	Class IV
Complete visualization of the soft palate	Complete visualization of the uvula	Visualization of only the base of the uvula	Soft palate is not visible at all

Fig. 3.1 Mallampati classification.

Notes: Intubation becomes difficult as grade increases and is not possible in grade 4 MMP. Another grading defined is 0 in which even the epiglottis is visible. However, intubation is difficult in this case.

- Chin at the level of occiput: Mildly restricted.
- Chin below the occiput: Severely restricted.

Assess thyromental distance: The distance between thyroid notch and mental prominence in neck extension.

- ≥6.5 cm: Easy laryngoscopy.
- 6.5 to 6 cm: Laryngoscopy may be difficult.
- ≤6 cm: Difficult laryngoscopy.

Assess neck circumference: The intubation becomes difficult if it is ≥ 42 cm for males and ≥ 39 cm for females.

- **Cormack–Lehane (CL) grading:** For laryngeal view by direct laryngoscopy (**Table 3.3**).

Causes of Difficult Airway

Unanticipated as well as anticipated difficult airways often make anesthetists sweat because of the fear of losing the airway in case of failure. Proper evaluation to assess the level of difficulty and corresponding preparation avoid such situations.

Difficult mask ventilation: It can be remembered by the mnemonic "BONES."

- *B*—beard.
- *O*—obese.
- *N*—no teeth.
- *E*—elderly.
- *S*—snorers.

Table 3.3 CL grades

CL grade	Findings
1	Full glottis visible
2a	Partial glottis visible
2b	Only arytenoids seen
3a	Epiglottis liftable
3b	Epiglottis not liftable
4	Epiglottis not seen

Abbreviation: CL, Cormack-Lehane.

Difficult supraglottic airway: It can occur due to restricted mouth opening, restricted upper airway, and stiff lungs with poor compliance.

Difficult intubation: It can happen in case of limited mouth opening, thyromental distance less than 6 cm, retrognathia, micrognathia, cleft palate, thyroid swelling, submandibular abscess or hematoma, obesity, protruded incisors, and cervical spine injury.

Difficult surgical airway: It can happen due to coagulation abnormality, agitated patient, flexion deformity of the neck, and vascular lesion at the site intended for tracheostomy.

Plan for Anticipated Difficult Airway

A good history taking and proper airway evaluation make the chances of missing a difficult airway negligible. Once a difficult airway is encountered during preoperative evaluation, a structured plan with the involvement of an experienced anesthetist is a must. Patients should be explained about the level of difficulty, and the airway management plan should be discussed to make the patient cooperative (especially for awake procedure). *The standard practice for an anticipated difficult airway is awake fiberoptic intubation.* However, the practice may differ based on the available expertise and the infrastructure.

The following structured plan recommended by ASA is acceptable in most situations:

1. **Assess the level of difficulty:**
   - Patient consent/cooperation.
   - Mask ventilation.
   - Supraglottic airway device insertion.
   - Intubation.
   - Surgical airway access.
2. **Provide supplemental oxygen throughout the procedure of difficult airway management.**

3. **Consider the merits and feasibility of available choices**:

   - Awake intubation versus intubation after induction of GA.

   - Noninvasive technique versus invasive technique as the first choice.

   - Preservation versus abolition of spontaneous respiration.

   - Video-assisted laryngoscopy as an initial approach to intubation.

4. **Formulate primary and alternative plans:**

   - Plan for awake intubation (**Flowchart 3.1**).

   - Intubation after induction of GA: The plan for intubation after induction of GA is shown in **Flowchart 3.2**.

Plan for Unanticipated Difficult Airway

Many a time, a normal-appearing airway is found to be difficult during laryngoscopy and intubation. The approach suggested by Difficult Airway Society (DAS) guidelines is quite simple and handy. The difficult airway trolley is the cornerstone of difficult airway management, and it contains airway equipment in the sequence the planned airway handling is done. An organized, difficult airway trolley is as follows:

- It should have a top surface and four to five drawers.

- Mobile and robust.

- Airway equipment stocked in a logical sequence.

- Clearly labeled.

- Easily cleanable.

- Attached documents (DAS/modified local guidelines, a checklist for restocking, and logbook for daily checking).

The arrangement of a difficult airway trolley is shown in **Table 3.4**.

The algorithm for adult airway management for difficult airway (unanticipated) is shown in **Flowchart 3.3**.

The discussion concerning the management of the unanticipated difficult airway in children and pregnancy is beyond the scope of this book. The readers are requested to refer to the latest guidelines for further knowledge.

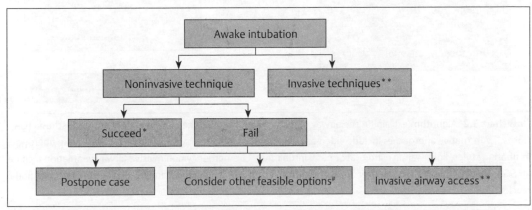

Flowchart 3.1 Algorithm explaining the awake intubation plan. Notes: *Confirm ventilation, intubation, and supraglottic airway (SGA) placement with exhaled CO_2; **Invasive airway device include surgical or percutaneous airway, jet ventilation, and retrograde intubation; # Other feasible options are surgery utilizing facemask or SGA, local anesthesia infiltration, or regional blocks.

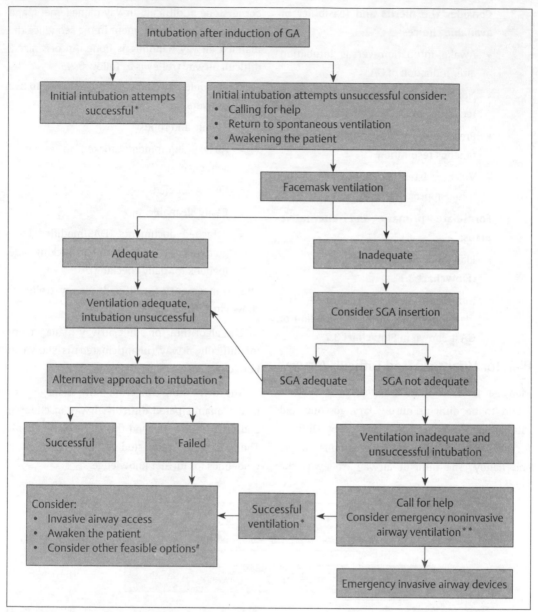

Flowchart 3.2 Algorithm explaining the airway management plan after the induction of general anesthesia (GA). Notes: * Alternative approaches include video-assisted laryngoscopy, supraglottic airway (SGA), awake fiberoptic, intubating stylet, light wand, blind oral or nasal intubation; ** emergency noninvasive airway ventilation include an SGA; # other feasible options are: Surgery utilizing facemask or SGA, local anesthesia infiltration, or regional blocks.

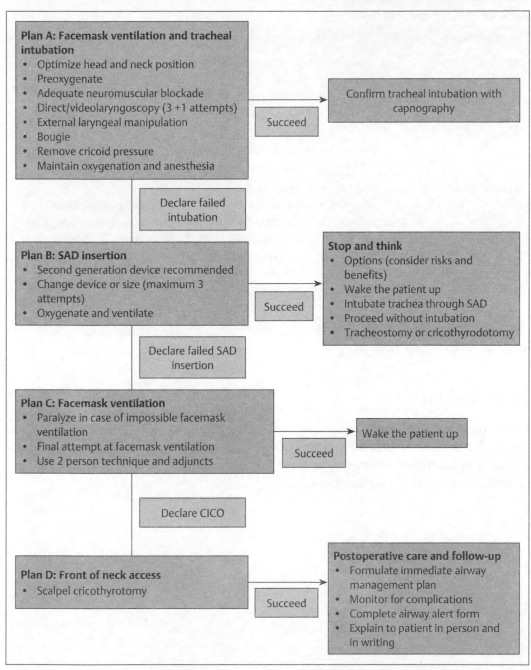

Flowchart 3.3 Unanticipated difficult airway in adults (Difficult Airway Society [DAS] guidelines). Abbreviations: CICO, cannot intubate cannot oxygenate; SAD, supraglottic airway device.

Table 3.4 Difficult airway trolley

Compartment of trolley	Contents
Top of trolley	Flexible intubating fiberscopes
Side of the trolley	• Bougie • Aintree intubating catheter • Airway exchange catheter
Drawer 1 (plan A)	• Bougie, short handle laryngoscope • Straight blade/McCoy blade • Video laryngoscope
Drawer 2 (plan B)	• LMA size: 3, 4, 5 • Intubating LMA (size: 3, 4, 5), Aintree intubating catheter • Fiberoptic adjuvants (Berman/Ovasappian airways, mucosal atomization devices, nasal sponge, 4 and 10% lignocaine)
Drawer 3 (plan C)	• Facemask: Various sizes • Oropharyngeal airways: Various sizes • Nasopharyngeal airways: Various sizes • LMA/ProSeal LMA: various sizes (3, 4, 5)
Drawer 4 (plan D)	Cricothyroidotomy set

Abbreviation: LMA, laryngeal mask airway.

Conclusion

Before surgery, preoperative evaluation of the patient provides an optimal window to formulate an appropriate anesthetic plan based on demography, comorbidities, medications, and airway assessment. It also provides a platform to help patients reduce their anxiety and anesthetists gaining the patient's confidence. It is the most important skill that every anesthetist should master with time.

CHAPTER 4

Fluids (AS9.3)

Damarla Haritha and Puneet Khanna

Introduction

Fluid therapy is an integral component of perioperative care by anesthesia providers. Administration of fluid helps to prevent dehydration, maintains effective circulatory volume, and ensures adequate tissue perfusion during the period when the patient is unable to achieve these goals through normal oral intake.

Therefore, a basic knowledge of different types of fluids, their physicochemical properties, and their pathophysiological effects is necessary to achieve optimal patient care.

Water constitutes 60% of total body weight in the average adult, varying with age, gender and body composition (**Box 4.1** and **Table 4.1**).

The human plasma maintains its osmolarity in a very narrow range (280–290 mosm/L). The administration of fluids with different osmolarity

> **Box 4.1 Distribution of total body water between fluid compartments**
>
> - Intracellular (55%).
> - Extracellular (45%).
>   - Functional (27.5%).
>   - Interstitial (20%).
>   - Intravascular (7.5%).
>   - Plasma (5.5%).
>   - Subglycocalyceal layer (SGL) (2%).
>   - Sequestered[a] (17.5%).
>   - Bone and connective tissue (15%).
>   - Transcellular (2.5%).

Note: [a] "sequestered" extracellular compartment refers to water present in bone and dense connective tissue or within transcellular compartment and therefore not readily available for equilibration with other fluid compartments.

can alter the plasma osmolarity, leading to water shift from or into cells. Change in plasma osmolarity can also stimulate or suppress the hypothalamic osmoreceptors, therefore altering the thirst response.

So, it would be noteworthy to overview the concept of osmolality, osmolarity, and tonicity (**Table 4.2**).

A given fluid can be isotonic, hypotonic, or hypertonic with respect to a reference solution.

Isotonic solution has identical osmolality as the reference solution. *No movement of water across the semipermeable membrane occurs.*

Hypotonic solution has lesser osmolality than that of the reference solution. *Water moves into cells when kept inside hypotonic solution and results in cellular edema.*

Hypertonic solution has higher osmolality than that of the reference solution. *Water moves out of cells when kept inside hypertonic solution and leads to cellular dehydration and shrinkage.*

The fluids commonly used during perioperative period belong either to crystalloid or the colloid category. **Table 4.3** illustrates crystalloids and colloids.

Crystalloids

Crystalloids are solutions of electrolytes or small particles and are the most commonly used fluids in the perioperative period during resuscitation and intensive care. The comparative composition of various crystalloids is depicted in **Table 4.4**. **Table 4.5** lists the properties, indications, and side effects of crystalloids.

Table 4.1 Age-related variation in total body water and extracellular fluid as percentage of body weight

Age	TBW (%)	ECF (%)	Blood volume (%)
Neonate	80	45	9
6 months	70	35	
1 year	60	28	
5 year	65	25	8
Young adult (male)	60	22	7
Young adult (female)	50	20	7
Elderly	50	20	

Abbreviations: ECF, extracellular fluid; TBW, total body water.

Table 4.2 Differentiating features between osmolality, tonicity, and osmolarity

Osmolality	Tonicity	Osmolarity
• It is defined as the number of moles per kg of solvent • *It is not affected by temperature* • Plasma osmolality is calculated as (moles/kg) = 2 × Na + (glucose/18) + (urea/2.8) Na is in mmol/L, glucose and urea in mg/dL	• It is the number of effective osmoles • The solute particles which can move freely across a membrane do not contribute to osmolality (e.g., urea and glucose) • It can be calculated by subtracting glucose and urea concentration from calculated osmolality	• It is defined as the number of moles per liter of solution • *It is affected by temperature* • It is calculated as: osmolarity in (mmoles/L) = (concentration in mg/dL × 10)/molecular weight

Table 4.3 Comparison of crystalloids and colloids

Crystalloids	Colloids
Crystalloid is a solution of electrolytes or smaller particles	Colloid consists of larger size particles in a solution of electrolytes
They expand intravascular volume for lesser duration because of short intravascular half-life[a]	They expand intravascular compartment for longer duration
Cheap	Expensive
Move easily between intravascular and interstitial compartment, therefore can precipitate edema	Stay mainly in intravascular compartment and decreases cerebral and pulmonary edema
Do not interfere with clotting, blood grouping	• Can interfere with clotting • *Dextrans can interfere with blood grouping by causing rouleaux formation*
Usually do not cause renal dysfunction, but infusion of large doses of 0.9% NaCl can cause renal dysfunction (due to hyperchloremic metabolic acidosis)	Colloid can cause renal dysfunction
No allergy potential (unless contaminated)	Allergic reactions are common
Examples: 0.9% NaCl, ringer lactate, and plasmalyte	Examples: Hydroxyethyl starch, albumin, gelatins, and dextrans

Note: [a] The studies on effects of fluids on red blood cells (RBC) dilution and change in hematocrit suggests that the crystalloids do not leave the intravascular compartment immediately but move in to subglycocalyceal layer (SGL), which is a subcompartment of intravascular chamber (volume 700–1,000 mL), while the colloids remain in the intravascular chamber and therefore cause more dilution of hematocrit than crystalloids.

Table 4.4 Comparative composition of various crystalloids

Fluid	Na	K	Cl	Ca	Mg	HCO₃	Lactate	Acetate	Gluconate	Glucose (g/L)	Osmolarity (mosm/L)
Plasma	140	5	100	4.4	2	24	1	-	-	1	285
0.9% NaCl	154	-	154	-	-	-	-	-	-	-	308
5% Dextrose	-	-	-	-	-	-	-	-	-	50	252
25% Dextrose	-	-	-	-	-	-	-	-	-	250	1,260
50% Dextrose	-	-	-	-	-	-	-	-	-	500	2,520
0.45% NaCl	77	-	77	-	-	-	-	-	-	-	154
5% Dextrose/0.45% NaCl	77	-	77	-	-	-	-	-	-	-	406
Ringer lactate	130	4	109	3	-	-	28	-	-	-	273
Plasmalyte A	140	5	98	-	3	-	-	27	23	-	293

Note: Units of electrolytes: meq/L.

Table 4.5 Properties, indications, and side effects of crystalloids

Crystalloid	Properties	Indication	Side effects/concerns
0.9% NaCl	• Osmolarity: 308 (slightly hypertonic) • SID: "0" • pH: 6.0 • **Normal saline:** Because in in vitro experiments, it was found to maintain RBC integrity like plasma • *Compatible with blood*	• Maintain effective blood volume and blood pressure in emergencies • Hypovolemic shock • Hypochloremic metabolic alkalosis, hyponatremia • Fluid in DKA • Renal failure • Hypercalcemia • Fluid challenge in prerenal ARF • Irrigation fluid • Vehicle for drugs	• Increased chloride content can cause hyperchloremic metabolic acidosis • Hypernatremia
Ringer's lactate	• pH 6.5 • Osmolarity: 273 (slightly hypoosmolar)	• Fluid of choice in postoperative patients, burns, fracture • Fluid of choice in diarrhea-induced dehydration in pediatrics • Maintenance of fluid during surgery	• *Clot formation with blood (ringer lactate volume should be at least 50% of blood volume to cause clot formation)* • Accumulation of lactate in patients with hepatic insufficiency • Hypoosmolar: Cannot be used in patients with increased ICP • Can cause hyperkalemia
5% Dextrose	• Osmolarity: 252	• Cheapest fluid to provide calories • In hepatic failure patients to prevent hypoglycemia • For correction of hypernatremia to provide free water • Administration of drugs • Prevention of ketosis in starvation, vomiting, diarrhea	• Can aggravate cerebral edema in neurosurgery patients • Increased blood sugar can aggravate ischemic brain injury and promote anerobic metabolism, leading to lactate production • Worsens hyponatremia and water intoxication • As it is hypotonic, it can cause RBC lysis and clumping • Cannot be used in diabetic patients
DNS (5% dextrose/0.9% NaCl)	• Osmolarity: 560 • Hypertonic	• Conditions with both salt depletion and hypovolemia • Correction of vomiting-induced alkalosis and hypochloremia with calories • *Compatible with blood transfusion*	• Can cause anasarca: CI in cardiac, hepatic, renal cause • Cannot be used in severe hypovolemic shock

Table 4.5 *(Continued)*

Crystalloid	Properties	Indication	Side effects/concerns
1/2 DNS (5% dextrose/ 0.45% NaCl)	• Osmolarity: 406 • Hypertonic	• Fluid therapy in pediatrics • Maintenance of fluid in postoperative period	• Hyponatremia
10% dextrose, 25% dextrose	• Osmolarity (10% D): 504 • Osmolarity (25% D): 1260	• Hypertonic crystalloids: Useful in faster replacement of glucose, as in hypoglycemic coma • Given in liver disease • Nutrition in patients on maintenance fluid • Treatment of hyperkalemia with insulin	• Dehydration • Diabetes mellitus • Glycosuria
Hypertonic saline 1.8%, 3%, 7%, 5%	• 3% NaCl, osmolarity: 1046	• Plasma volume expansion • Correction of hypoosmolar hypernatremia • Treatment of raised ICP in neurosurgery • 11.5% used as sclerosant	• High osmolarity can cause endothelial damage; it requires central venous catheter for infusion
Plasmalyte	• pH 7.4 • Caloric content: 21 kcal/L • Gluconate and acetate act as buffers • Acetate-lesser respiratory quotient, so decreased CO_2 production	• Balanced salt solution without Ca^{2+}, so compatible with blood • Hepatectomy and liver transplant	• Hyperkalemia • Severe renal failure • Mg^{2+} counteracts vasoconstrictive response of hypovolemia
Sterofundin	• Na: 145, K: 4.0, Mg: 2.0 • Cl: 127.0, Ca^{2+}: 5.0 • Acetate: 24 • Malate: 5.0 • Osmolarity: 309 • pH 5.0–5.9	• No lactate: Can be used in liver disease • Can be used in Cl loss: Gastric outlet obstruction	

Abbreviations: ARF, acute renal failure; Cl, chloride; CI, contraindicated; DKA, diabetic ketoacidosis; DNS, dextrose normal saline; ICP, intracranial pressure; RBC, red blood corpuscles; SID, strong ion difference.

Colloids

Colloids are suspensions of high-molecular weight solute molecules (>30,000 Da) in normal saline and remain largely in the intravascular space by creating colloid oncotic pressure.

Colloids can be either natural or artificial. Examples of natural colloids include fresh frozen plasma (FFP), 5%, 20%, 25% albumin, and 4%, 5% plasma proteins, whereas examples of artificial colloids include dextrans, gelatins and hydroxyethyl starch (HES).

The behavior of a colloid after intravenous infusion depends upon the following characteristics:

- Molecular weight.
- Size of the molecule.
- Osmolarity.
- Colloid oncotic pressure.
- Intravascular half-life (it depends on molecular weight and renal elimination).
- Electrolyte content.
- Acid base composition.
  - ▶ Albumin, gelatin: Physiological pH.
  - ▶ Rest: Acidic.

Individual Colloids

Properties, indications, advantages and disadvantages of human albumin, dextrans, and gelatins are shown in **Table 4.6**.

Table 4.6 Comparison of properties of different colloids

Colloid Criteria	Human albumin	Dextrans	Gelatins
Characteristic features	• A natural colloid • Constitute 50–60% of plasma proteins • Consists of single peptide chain (585 amino acids) • Molecular weight: 69,000 Da • Synthesized in liver • After administration: Volume expansion lasts for 16–24 h • Preparations: 5%, 20%, 25%	• Dextrans are highly branched polysaccharide molecules • It is produced by conversion of sucrose to dextran by the enzyme dextran sucrase (*comes from bacterium leuconostoc mesenteroides*) • Preparations: 　○ Dextran 40 (10%)– MW– 40 KD 　○ Dextran 70 (6%)– MW– 70 KD	• Gelatins are prepared by boiling the animal connective tissues • Succinylated/modified gelatins (gelofusin, plasmagel): *Compatible with blood transfusion because of low calcium content* • Urea cross-linked (polygeline): Hemacel • Oxypolygelatins (gelifundol) • Volume expansion: 70–80% • Duration of action shorter than starch and albumin
Indications	• Treatment of shock due to plasma loss • Fluid resuscitation in intensive care unit • Acute management of burns • Spontaneous bacterial peritonitis • Hypoalbuminemia (*paracentesis/liver cirrhosis/after liver transplant*)	• To improve microcirculation (microsurgical reimplantation) • Extracorporeal circulation during cardiopulmonary bypass	• Hypovolemia (due to blood loss) • Acute normovolemic hemodilution • Extracorporeal circulation– cardiopulmonary bypass • Volume preloading prior to regional anesthesia

(Continued)

Table 4.6 *(Continued)*

Colloid Criteria	Human albumin	Dextrans	Gelatins

Advantages	• Natural colloid: So less side effects
	• Acts as an antioxidant
	• Volume expansion greater than gelatins and dextrans
		• Volume expansion: 100–150%
		• Improves microcirculation by:
		  ○ Decreasing viscosity of blood
		  ○ Decreasing RBC aggregation
			• Cheaper (than albumin/starch)
			• No upper limit of transfusion
			• No renal impairment

Disadvantages	• Expensive • Can cause interstitial edema in case of shock (*due to increased capillary permeability*)	• *Anaphylactic reactions (more than HES and gelatins)* • *Coagulation abnormalities (decreases platelet adhesion, decreases factor VII level and increased fibrinolysis)* • *Interferes with blood grouping (coats RBC surface and interfere with cross-matching)* • *Acute renal failure (causes tubular plugging, leading to acute renal failure)*	• Anaphylactoid reactions • Interference with coagulation (controversial)

Abbreviations: HES, hydroxyethyl starch; RBC, red blood corpuscles.

Hydroxyethyl Starch

HES is a derivative of amylopectin (source being maize and potato). *Hydroxyl (OH) groups of glucose units of amylopectin are substituted (mainly at C2 and C6 positions) with ethyl to prevent rapid in vivo hydrolysis by amylase.* The salient properties of HES are listed in **Table 4.7**.

The indications, advantages and disadvantages of HES are tabulated in **Table 4.8**.

▌Fluid Management

Fluid management during intraoperative period includes replacement of fasting fluids, maintenance of fluid, and replacement of losses.

Hourly maintenance fluid is calculated, based on the Holliday–Segar formula. It is also known as the 4-2-1 rule:

Up to 10 kg = 4 mL/kg/h

10–20 kg = 2 mL/kg/h

>20 kg = 1 mL/kg/h

Fasting fluid is calculated as (number of hours of fasting × hourly maintenance fluid requirement). As much as 50% of that is given during the 1st hour, 25% in 2nd hour, and the remaining 25% in the 3rd hour.

Anesthesia and surgical stress cause release of growth hormone (GH), cortisol and catecholamines leading to hyperglycemia. Therefore, dextrose-free

Table 4.7 Salient properties of HES

Degree of substitution	Molar substation ratio	C2/C6 ratio	MW
It is the ratio of number of substitute glucose molecules to the total number of glucose molecules	It is the ratio of number of OH-ethyl radical groups present to total number of glucose molecules	Total number OH ethyl radicals at C2 to total number OH ethyl radicals at C6 Based on the ratio, HES can be: • Tetrastarch (0.4) • Pentastarch (0.5) • Hexastarch (0.6) *Increased ratio: Slower metabolism: More long-lasting effect*	High MW: 450–480 KDa Medium MW: 200 KDa Low MW: 70 KDa Smaller MW HES: Rapidly excreted Large MW HES: • More prolonged effect • More renal dysfunction due to accumulation • Coagulopathy

Abbreviations: HES, hydroxyethyl starch; MW, molecular weight.

Table 4.8 Indications, advantages, and disadvantages of HES

Indications	Advantages	Disadvantages
• Rapid stabilization of hemodynamics • Anti-inflammatory properties	• Less expensive than albumin • Maximum allowable volume is 30–50 mL/kg/day	• **Coagulation**: It causes molecular weight-dependent decrease in Von Willebrand factor and factor VIII, resulting in decreased clot strength • **Accumulation in tissues**: Can persist in skin, muscle, liver, and reticuloendothelial system for years after infusion and causes pruritus • **Renal dysfunction**: Causes AKI in patients with existing renal injury • **Can increase amylase concentration:** No clinically significant impact

Abbreviation: AKI, acute kidney injury.

solutions should be used. Considering the composition (nearly physiological) and cost of ringer lactate, it is considered as fluid of choice for maintenance.

For replacement of losses during surgery, crystalloids are preferred over colloids because of the following reasons:

• Crystalloids replace intravascular as well extravascular volume, whereas colloids remain mainly in the intravascular compartment.

• Crystalloids do not interfere with clotting.

• Crystalloids do not cause renal dysfunction.

• Crystalloids are cheap.

Recent studies have identified SGL layer as an integral part of intravascular compartment and provided a new edge to distribution of crystalloids after infusion. Previously, 70% of infused crystalloid was thought to leave the intravascular compartment. But now, it is said that only 40 to 50% crystalloid leave the intravascular compartment after infusion. Therefore, the crystalloids should be replaced in 1.5:1 ratio (previously 3:1). It means, for each milliliter of blood, loss should be replaced by 1.5 mL of crystalloid.

The fluid administration according to conventional 4-2-1 rule and 3:1 replacement often leads to fluid overload. Goal-directed fluid

Table 4.9 Fluid therapy in various clinical scenarios

Clinical scenario	Fluid therapy
Cardiac failure	Fluid administration should be guided by GDT
Liver failure	• GDT should be used • Metabolism of lactate and acetate is reduced. So, caution with using balanced salt solutions
Renal failure	• GDT is preferred • Crystalloid without potassium should be used • Hyperchloremic acidosis by infusion of normal saline can cause hyperkalemia • Colloids (especially HES) can cause renal dysfunction
Cerebral and pulmonary edema	• Avoid dextrose containing solutions in patients with cerebral edema (*hyperglycemia causes neuronal injury*) • Colloids can safely be used in patients with ARDS and cerebral edema if required
Shock	Crystalloids preferred over colloids
Sepsis	Caution with colloids (chances of renal dysfunctions are very high in sepsis)
Burns	• Fluid replacement is guided by Parkland's formula • For first 24 h, ringer lactate at 4 mL/kg/% body surface burn area should be given. 50% of total fluid is given over 8 h and remaining 50% over next 16 h

Abbreviations: ARDS, acute respiratory distress syndrome; GDT, goal-directed fluid therapy; HES, hydroxyethyl starch.

therapy (GDT) has now dramatically changed the practice of fluid administration with improved patient outcomes. GDT is based on measurement of dynamic cardiac parameters, for example:

- Stroke volume variation (SVV) (using transthoracic or transesophageal echocardiography).
- Pulse pressure variation (PPV) (using arterial waveform).

  Variation in SVV and PPV of >10 to 15% suggests fluid responsiveness (i.e., hypovolemia).

- Flow time through aorta (using esophageal Doppler).

Pulmonary artery occlusion pressure (PAOP) can also be used to guide fluid therapy (<8– hypovolemia, >18– hypervolemia).

It is important to note that the measurement of central venous pressure (CVP) has poor correlation with fluid status.

Table 4.9 provides important information regarding consideration of fluid therapy in various clinical scenarios.

Conclusion

Fluids are drugs, and their composition and dose have a significant impact on a patient's physiology and outcome.

All anesthesia providers must be clear about the composition of various crystalloids and colloids and use them in appropriate doses, based on the patient's profile and clinical scenario.

CHAPTER 5

Blood Transfusion (AS9.4)

Shashikant Sharma and Puneet Khanna

Historical Background

Blood transfusion, often a life-saving strategy, historically dates back to the Egyptian and Roman era. Egyptians took a blood bath as a recuperative measure, while the Romans drank the blood of fallen gladiators to cure epilepsy. Deviating from such ancient rituals, Jean-Baptiste Denis performed the first animal-to-human transfusion in 1667, where he administered the blood of a lamb to a 15-year-old boy. Unfortunately, the practice of animal-to-human transfusion led to increased mortality, which put a halt on the transfusion practice for the next 150 years. The first well-documented transfusion with human blood happened on September 26, 1818, followed by multiple reports on transfusion in obstetric hemorrhages. Lack of knowledge of blood groups and screening tests resulted in transfusion-related infectious as well as noninfectious complications in the 19th century.

The discovery of blood groups by Karl Landsteiner in 1900 and advanced techniques equipped with highly sensitive and rapid tests to screen the blood products has made the blood transfusion practice safe in the modern era.

The practice of blood transfusion has been evolving for the last many decades, dominated by the administration of whole blood and fresh frozen plasma (FFP) to the administration of component therapy through the 1970s and 1980s. Since 2010 onward, the practice has shifted from simply correcting anemia and coagulopathy to patient-centered, multipronged approach in relation to evidence-based transfusion medicine, which is termed as patient blood management (PBM).

Although a life-saving strategy, blood transfusion is not without complications. Therefore, a thorough knowledge of blood components and transfusion-related complications is imperative to ensure patient safety and improved outcomes.

Blood Components

The constituents of blood include red blood cells, white blood cells, platelets, and a variety of proteins including coagulation factors. The whole blood after collection from the donor can be fragmented into its components (PRBC, platelets, cryoprecipitate, and fresh frozen plasma).

The individual components after separation are stored in the blood bank at an appropriate temperature in storage devices like freezers, refrigerators, and platelet incubators. These products are released as and when they are requested as per the need of patients and discarded after expiry if not used. The description of individual components is as follows:

1. **Packed red blood cells (PRBCs):** Contain the same amount of hemoglobin as the whole blood, but due to plasma removal, the hematocrit of PRBC is approximately 60%. It is stored at 1 to 6°C in the blood bank to decrease the metabolic activity of red blood cells. Crystalloids and colloids facilitate the transfusion of PRBC. The calcium content (e.g., calcium in Ringer lactate may precipitate clotting) and the tonicity (hypotonic and hypertonic fluids can cause swelling and shrinkage of red blood cells, respectively) are important in choosing the appropriate fluid. The recommended solutions compatible with

PRBC are 5% dextrose with 0.45/0.9% saline, 0.9 saline, and Normosol-R with pH 7.4.

PRBC is stored in specific anticoagulant/ preservative solutions to increase shelf life. The commonly used preservative solutions are as follows:

- Citrate-phosphate-dextrose (CPD): 21 days.
- Citrate-phosphate-dextrose-adenine (CPDA): 35 days.
- Additives (AS1, AS3, AS5): 42 days.
- AS7: 56 days (approved by FDA in 2015; commercially not available).

The additive solutions do prolong the storage duration of PRBC, but as the duration of storage increases, they add to biochemical changes, which are collectively known as *red cell storage lesions*. During storage, red blood cells metabolize glucose to lactate, hydrogen ions accumulate, and pH decreases. Failure of Na^+K^+ ATPase pump at 1 to 6°C leads to the gain of intracellular sodium and transfer of potassium from cells to plasma. With time, there is a progressive decrease in ATP, nitric oxide, and 2,3-diphosphoglycerate (2,3-DPG) levels in addition to increased RBC fragility.

Although hemoglobin level has traditionally been used as a trigger to transfuse PRBC, many other factors, such as cardiovascular status, age, anticipated additional blood loss, arterial oxygenation, mixed venous oxygenation, intravascular blood volume, and cardiac output, should be considered to decide upon the need for further transfusion.

ABO compatibility is a must, and one unit of PRBC transfusion raises Hb by 1 g/dL (hematocrit by 3%). The current recommendations regarding PRBC transfusion are as follows:

- In healthy adults and most children, the threshold for red cell transfusion is 7 g/dL.
- A restrictive transfusion strategy (hemoglobin level of 7–9 g/dL) is not acceptable for preterm infants or children with cyanotic heart disease, severe hypoxemia, active blood loss, or hemodynamic instability.
- Red blood cells contain multiple antigens on their surface, which can interact with antibodies present in the serum of recipients, leading to serious hemolytic reactions. Therefore, it is mandatory to do compatibility testing before attempting transfusion, except for the situations where there is no time to compatibility tests (emergent need for blood products in case of trauma, obstetric hemorrhage). The most important and common antigen groups are ABO-Rh. **Table 5.1** shows

Table 5.1 Compatible blood groups

Blood group	Red blood cells	Plasma antibodies	Can donate blood to	Can receive blood from
A	Antigen A	Anti B	Group A, AB	Group A, O
B	Antigen B	Anti A	Group B, AB	Group B, O
AB (universal recipient)	Antigen A and B	Nil	AB	A, B, O, AB
O (universal donor)	Nil	Anti A and Anti B	A, B, O, AB	O

Note: In case of emergency transfusion where compatibility testing is not possible, O-ve PRBC can be transfused.

major blood groups and the compatible donors and recipients.

2. **Platelets:** Platelet concentrates are obtained either as pooled from four to six donors (known as random donor platelet) or by apheresis from a single donor (known as single donor platelet). Platelets are stored at 20 to 24°C to improve post-transfusion in vivo recovery (as cold exposure inactivates platelets). Platelets are highly sensitive to changes in pH. Constant and gentle agitation promotes gas exchange between platelets and containers, which helps in maintaining the pH. At room temperature, platelet concentrates can be used up to 7 days. Storage at room temperature makes platelet concentrates susceptible to bacterial contamination; hence, they are implicated in septic complications after transfusion. Whenever possible, ABO-compatible platelets should be transfused, but it is not necessary. One unit of apheresis platelets should increase the platelet count in adults by 30,000 to 40,000, while that of random donor platelet increases platelet count by 5,000 to 10,000. The various indications of platelet transfusions are tabulated in **Table 5.2**.

3. **Fresh frozen plasma (FFP):** It is the most frequently used plasma product. It is generally frozen within 8 or 24 hours of donation. It contains all plasma proteins, mainly factors V and VIII. Shelf life is for 12 months when stored at < −18°C. Thawed plasma is stored at 1 to 6°C up to 5 days. The indications for FFP transfusions are:

- International normalized ratio (INR) > 1.6.
- Reversal of effect of warfarin in an emergency situation.
- Disseminated intravascular coagulopathy (DIC).
- Thrombotic microangiopathies.
- Plasma protein deficiency.

Each unit of FFP increases the level of each clotting factor by 2 to 3%. The initial volume of transfusion is 10 to 15 mL/kg. ABO compatibility for FFP transfusion is not mandatory but highly desirable.

4. **Cryoprecipitate:** It is derived from thawed plasma at 1 to 6°C. It contains factor VIII, Von Willebrand factor, factor XIII, fibrinogen, and fibronectin. It can be stored for up to 12 months at < −18°C. When the product is requested for use, it should be thawed at 30 to 36°C. As per current recommendations by the American Academy of Blood Bank (AABB), one bag of cryoprecipitate must contain at least 150 mg of fibrinogen and 80 U of factor VIII. One bag of cryoprecipitate raises fibrinogen levels by 5 to 10 mg/dL. The indications for cryoprecipitate infusion are:

- Massive blood loss during cardiac surgery.

Table 5.2 Indication of platelet transfusion in adults

Indications (prophylactic transfusion)	Platelet count ($\times 10^3$ per μL)
Major surgery and invasive procedure, no active bleeding	≤50
Surgery on the brain or posterior eye with no bleeding diathesis	≤100
Ongoing bleeding and planned for surgery	<50 (usually) >100 (rarely)
Stable patients with no bleeding	<10

- Massive transfusion (trauma and obstetric hemorrhage).
- Deficiency of factors VIII (to be used when recombinant factors are not available) and XIII.
- Von Willebrand disease.
- Congenital dysfibrinogenemia.

Transfusion-Related Complications

As emphasized at the beginning of this chapter, transfusion of blood products is not without complications. The transfusion-related complications can either be infectious or noninfectious. With due availability of rapid and sensitive screening tests, the incidence of infectious complications has decreased dramatically, with no impact on noninfectious complications. The transfusion-related complications (noninfectious) are tabulated in **Table 5.3**.

The discussion of transfusion-related complications would be incomplete without elaborating on some of the important complications.

Acute Transfusion Reactions

1. *Acute hemolytic reactions*:
   - Hemolytic transfusion reactions are immune-mediated, recipient's antibodies' targeted destruction of transfused RBCs.

- The most common reason being ABO incompatibility due to clerical error.
- The destruction of red cells starts immediately, and most of the transfused red cells are destroyed within 24 hours of transfusion. The blood as low as 10 mL is enough to produce hemolytic reactions.
- Pain and burning sensation at the site of transfusion is the earliest clue to the possible hemolytic reaction. Other manifestations include fever, chills, rigors, nausea, vomiting, dyspnea, and hypotension.
- Patients under anesthesia cannot report any of the above symptoms; however, tachycardia, fall in blood pressure, and persistent oozing from surgical sites are valuable indicators of acute hemolytic reaction.
- Treatment includes:
  - Immediately stop transfusion.
  - Confirm patient's and the blood product bag details.
  - Send the blood sample of the patient along with remaining blood to the blood bank.
  - Send blood sample to assay hemoglobin, platelet count, fibrinogen level, and activated partial thromboplastin time (APTT) to diagnose disseminated

Table 5.3 Noninfectious hazards of transfusion

Acute (within 24 h of transfusion)	Delayed (>24 h of transfusion)
• Acute hemolytic reaction • Allergic reaction • Anaphylactic reaction • Coagulation problems in massive transfusion • Febrile nonhemolytic reaction • Metabolic derangements • Mistransfusion (transfusion of the incorrect product to the incorrect recipient) • Septic or bacterial contamination • Transfusion-associated circulatory overload • Transfusion-related acute lung injury	• Delayed hemolytic reaction • Iron overload • Posttransfusion purpura • Transfusion-associated graft-versus-host disease • Transfusion-related immunomodulation

intravascular coagulopathy (DIC) and arrange the required blood products.

- ▶ Target urine output of 1 to 2 mL/kg/h with the administration of fluids and mannitol.
- ▶ Hemodialysis, if required.

2. *Allergic reactions*:
- Allergic reactions range from mild (urticarial) to life-threatening (anaphylactic) reactions and most commonly happen due to plasma proteins.
- Treatment of mild form includes antihistamines and steroids, while for anaphylactic variety, it requires immediately stopping transfusion, adrenaline, and steroids.

3. *Transfusion-related acute lung injury (TRALI)*:
- Patients presenting with hypoxemia and noncardiogenic pulmonary edema within 6 hours of transfusion with no other risk factor for lung injury suggests TRALI.
- Plasma-rich blood products collected from multiparous women are often associated with TRALI.
- The TRALI working group of the AABB recommends using male-predominant plasma for transfusions.

The treatment includes:
- Supplementation oxygenation to treat hypoxemia.
- Avoidance of fluid overload.
- Use of diuretics if the fluid overload is present.
- Lung-protective ventilation if the patient develops acute respiratory distress syndrome (ARDS).

4. *Febrile nonhemolytic transfusion reactions (FNHTR)*:
- Patients presenting with fever, chills, and rigor during the course of transfusion may indicate a febrile transfusion reaction.

- FNHTRs are caused by white cell microaggregates.
- Febrile reactions are usually mild and do not require treatment.

5. *Transfusion-associated circulatory overload (TACO)*:
- It is nonimmune-mediated and results when transfused blood volume is in excess of that the recipient's circulatory system can handle.
- *Susceptible patients group include* underlying cardiopulmonary compromise, renal failure, or chronic anemia, and infants or older patients.
- Signs and symptoms include tachycardia, cough, dyspnea, and hypertension.
- The treatment is diuresis to decrease volume overload.

Delayed Transfusion Reactions

Transfusion-associated graft-versus-host disease:
- Transfusion-associated graft-versus-host disease is donor's lymphocytes' mediated; an immune attack against the recipient's tissues and organs with the fatality of >90%.
- It is common in patients with Hodgkin disease, those receiving chemotherapy, and stem cell transplant.
- Symptoms include rash, fever, diarrhea, liver dysfunction, and pancytopenia occurring 1 to 6 weeks after transfusion.
- The use of gamma-irradiated blood products can prevent transfusion-associated graft-versus-host disease.

Infectious Complications of Blood Transfusion

Infections related to the transfusion of blood products do occur, and the chances are increased when blood products are collected from multiple donors (e.g., random donor platelets, cryoprecipitate). A few common infections related to blood transfusion are discussed in this chapter.

- Hepatitis: 90% of cases are due to hepatitis C, with an incidence of 1 in 2,00,000 to 1 in 9,00,000.

- Other viral diseases: HIV/AIDS, cytomegalovirus, human T cell lymphotropic virus, Epstein–Barr virus, and West Nile virus.

- Bacterial infections: Bacterial infections are not uncommon and can be due to staphylococcus, salmonella, yersinia, and rickettsial diseases.

- Parasitic infection: It can occur due to malaria, toxoplasma, and filaria.

Autologous blood transfusion provides an opportunity and a safer option to decrease transfusion-related complications. Also, it helps to conserve blood bank supply and an acceptable option in patients with rare blood group phenotype/alloantibodies. Autologous blood transfusion can be achieved in three ways:

- Preoperative autologous donation.
- Acute normovolemic hemodilution.
- Intraoperative cell salvage.

The comparative features of all these techniques are tabulated in **Table 5.4**.

Artificial Blood

Artificial blood products are substitutes for red blood cells, which are produced by chemical isolation or recombinant biochemical technology. These products carry oxygen to tissues and remove carbon dioxide but are unable to replicate other functions of natural blood. Artificial blood is reserved for situations like:

- Jehovah's witness (a community which does not consent for allogenic transfusion).
- Unavailability of compatible PRBCs.
- Bridge to stabilizing therapy.

Artificial blood products can be broadly categorized as perfluorocarbons (PFCs) or hemoglobin-based products.

Table 5.4 Techniques of autologous blood transfusion

Autologous donation	Acute normovolemic hemodilution	Intraoperative cell salvage
<ul><li>Blood is donated by patients preoperatively, which is stored in the blood bank and transfused when required during the perioperative period</li><li>Inclusion criteria:<ul><li>Donor's Hb should not be < 11 g/dL</li><li>There should be a gap of 72 h between the last donation and planned surgery to ensure adequate restoration of intravascular volume</li></ul></li></ul>	<ul><li>Whole blood is removed just prior to significant blood loss, and intravascular volume is simultaneously restored with either crystalloid (3 mL/kg) or colloid (1 mL/kg)</li><li>Blood is stored at room temperature for 8 h or at 4° for 24 h</li><li>Inclusion criteria:<ul><li>Likelihood of transfusion should be > 10%</li><li>Preoperative Hb should be at least 12 g/dL</li><li>Absence of significant organ dysfunction (liver/lung/kidney/heart)</li><li>Absence of infection and risk of bacteremia</li></ul></li></ul>	<ul><li>It involves collecting, processing, and transfusing blood lost by a patient during surgery</li><li>Inclusion criteria:<ul><li>Anticipated blood loss > 20%</li><li>Cross-match blood is unobtainable</li><li>Patient unwilling to accept allogenic blood</li><li>The procedure is likely to require more than one unit of PRBCs</li></ul></li></ul>

Abbreviation: PRBCs, packed red blood cells.

Table 5.5 Comparison of artificial blood with allogenic blood

Parameter	Artificial	Allogenic
Oxygen delivery	Rapid and consistent	Depends on 2,3-DPG
Risk of disease transmission	None	Significant (e.g., HIV, hepatitis, malaria, etc.)
Storage	Room temperature	Refrigeration
Shelf life	1–3 years	42 days
Preparation	Ready to use	Crossmatch
Compatibility	Universal	Type-specific
Duration of action	1–3 days	60–90 days

PFC is a biologically inert material, relatively inexpensive, with the capacity to dissolve about 50 times more oxygen than blood plasma. From a technological standpoint, they pose significant hurdles before they can be utilized as artificial blood:

- First, they are insoluble in water, which necessitates combining them with emulsifiers to make them functional.

- Second, their oxygen-carrying capacity is much less than hemoglobin-based products. This means that significantly more PFC must be used.

In contrast to PFC products where dissolving is the key mechanism, oxygen covalently bonds to hemoglobin-based products. The problem of blood typing is absent because of the lack of membrane in hemoglobin-based products. However, the use of raw hemoglobin is associated with the following issues:

- Raw hemoglobin is not stable in a solution.

- Hemoglobin gets broken down to smaller molecules which are toxic to organs.

Therefore, techniques like cross-linking molecules or using recombinant DNA technology are employed to make hemoglobin molecules more stable and less toxic. Examples include polyethylene glycol-modified liposome-encapsulated hemoglobin, nanoparticle and polymersome encapsulated hemoglobin, stabilized hemoglobin solutions, polymerized hemoglobin solutions, and conjugated hemoglobin solutions. Conjugation of hemoglobin helps in:

- Decreasing the antigenicity of hemoglobin.

- The slow rate of removal from the circulation.

- Lesser chance of recognition by the reticuloendothelial system.

The unique features of conjugated hemoglobin are their high oncotic pressure, which makes them very potent plasma-volume expanders, and their viscosity.

Although artificial blood is similar to natural blood in terms of delivering oxygen to tissues, it is noteworthy to overview the contrasting features of artificial blood (**Table 5.5**).

Conclusion

Blood is needed when the patient's oxygen delivery capacity becomes insufficient to meet the metabolic demand. The blood transfusion and related blood products stabilize hemodynamics, optimize oxygen-carrying capacity, and stop bleeding in patients with coagulopathy or thrombocytopenia. However, their use without appropriate indications and in excess doses could lead to serious adverse effects. Proper labeling of samples and transfusing the right product to the right patient at the right time is crucial to avoid untoward events.

CHAPTER 6

Monitoring in Anesthesia

Shashikant Sharma and Puneet Khanna

Introduction

Monitoring in anesthesia had been in place long before the introduction of clinical anesthesia. The importance of respiratory pattern was known since antiquity. Work by William Harvey, Stephen Holes, and Claude Bernard led to the discovery of cardiovascular monitoring. Despite advancing technology and the availability of sophisticated monitoring tools, anesthesia practitioners continue to witness anesthesia-related morbidity and mortality in patients receiving anesthesia. This fact highlights the central role of monitoring the patients during the perioperative period to improve the patient's safety and outcomes.

The expert recommendations to improve patient safety and outcomes during the perioperative period have been evolving continuously, and the latest one is by the American Society of Anesthesiologists (ASA), 2015.

Standards of ASA Monitoring (AS4.4, AS4.5)

It was first introduced in 1986 by ASA and last amended in October 2015. It includes two sets of recommendations:

1. Standard I
Qualified anesthesia personnel shall be present in the room throughout the conduct of all general anesthetics, regional anesthetics, and monitored anesthesia care.

Objective: Because of the rapid changes in patient status during anesthesia, qualified anesthesia personnel shall be continuously present to monitor the patient and provide anesthesia care.

2. Standard II
During all anesthetics, the patient's oxygenation, ventilation, circulation, and temperature shall be continually evaluated.

The objectives and techniques to monitor oxygenation, ventilation, circulation, and temperature are summarized in **Table 6.1**.

Cardiovascular Monitoring

Monitoring of the cardiovascular system (CVS) helps to identify disturbances in rhythm, myocardial injury, and fluctuation in blood pressure. Detailed information about pulmonary vasculature and cardiac function can be obtained with the help of advanced monitoring devices. It can be done in the following three ways:

- Noninvasive: Electrocardiogram (ECG), noninvasive blood pressure (NIBP).
- Semi-invasive: Transesophageal echocardiography (TEE).
- Invasive: Invasive blood pressure, central venous pressure (CVP), pulmonary capillary wedge pressure (PCWP).

Electrocardiogram

- Electrocardiogram monitoring helps in detecting rhythm abnormalities, myocardial injury, and cardiac arrest during the perioperative period.
- Lead II is the preferred lead for arrhythmia detection.
- Lead V5 alone will detect 75% of the ischemic episode; adding lead V4 increases this to 90%, and the combination of lead II, V4, and V5 add up to 96% detection rate.

Table 6.1 Standard II ASA recommendations

Parameter	Objective	Techniques
Oxygenation	To ensure adequate oxygen concentration in the inspired gas and the blood during all anesthetics	• Inspired oxygen concentration (using oxygen analyzer) • Blood oxygenation (using pulse oximeter)
Ventilation	To ensure adequate ventilation of the patient during all anesthetics	• Clinical signs such as chest excursion, observation of the reservoir breathing bag, and auscultation of breath sounds • Quantitative monitoring of the volume of expired gas • Capnography or capnometry with end-tidal CO_2 alarms
Circulation	To ensure the adequacy of the patient's circulatory function during all anesthetics	• Electrocardiogram • Arterial blood pressure and heart rate (at least every 5 mins) • Palpation of a pulse, auscultation of heart sounds, monitoring of a tracing of intra-arterial pressure, ultrasound peripheral pulse monitoring, or pulse plethysmography or oximetry
Temperature	To aid in the maintenance of appropriate body temperature during all anesthetics	• Every patient receiving anesthesia shall have temperature monitored when clinically significant changes in body temperature are intended, anticipated, or suspected

Abbreviation: ASA, American Society of Anesthesiologists.

• The use of monitors with features of automatic ST analysis is highly recommended.

Noninvasive Blood Pressure

• Works on the *principle of oscillometry* and record blood pressure at a set interval (interval should not be more than 5 mins).

• Oscillometry principle calculates mean arterial pressure first and derives systolic and diastolic pressure utilizing set algorithm.

• The length and width of the cuff should be 80 and 40% of the arm circumference, respectively.

• Too large cuff underestimates blood pressure while too small cuff overestimates it.

• Identifies fluctuations in blood pressure.

Invasive Blood Pressure

It is more accurate compared to NIBP and *is the gold standard for blood pressure monitoring*. It works on the principle of "*Wheatstone bridge*" and requires cannulation of one the accessible arteries like radial (most common site), ulnar, brachial, femoral, posterior tibial, and dorsalis pedis. *The cannulation of any of such arteries can lead to complications like bleeding, local hematoma, thrombosis, arterial spasm, digital ischemia, sepsis, and aneurysm formation.* Being an invasive procedure with a myriad complications, invasive monitoring should be employed in cases where indicated, for example, the following:

• Pheochromocytoma.

• Patients requiring vasopressors/inotropes.

• Frequent blood analysis is needed.

- Cardiopulmonary bypass.
- Unavailability of appropriate size BP cuff.
- Measurement of advanced dynamic parameters such as pulse pressure variation (PPV), stroke volume variation (SVV), and cardiac output using Flotrac device.

Although Allen's test has been in use for many years to assess the adequacy of contribution to circulation of hand by the ulnar artery, *it is not foolproof against the prevention of complications.* It is performed by occluding the radial and ulnar artery after complete exsanguination of the patient's hand. The time taken for the color of the hand to become normal after the release of pressure from the ulnar artery while maintaining pressure over the radial artery is interpreted as follows:

- Normal: < 7 seconds.
- Borderline: 7 to 14 seconds.
- Do not attempt radial artery cannulation →15 seconds.

Transesophageal/Transthoracic Echocardiography

Echocardiography is a real-time and highly sensitive tool in detecting cardiac functions and regional wall motion abnormality during the perioperative period. The use of echocardiography can aid in:

- Detection of any regional wall motion abnormality.
- Assessment of valvular dysfunction.
- Diagnosing heart failure (systolic, diastolic).
- Detection of air embolism (TEE is the most sensitive tool).

Transthoracic echocardiography (TTE) is non-invasive but limited by the window through the chest wall; on the other hand, TEE offers an excellent window, but being invasive requires the patient to be intubated.

Central Venous Pressure

CVP tracing is obtained by placing a venous catheter in central veins. The preferred vein is internal jugular, because it is valveless and in direct communication with the right atrium. The other sites are subclavian, basilic, and femoral veins. The CVP trace consists of "a," "c," "x," "v," and "y" waves, as shown in **Fig. 6.1**.

The waves of CVP are described as below:

a = due to atrial contraction.

c = due to the backward movement of tricuspid valves during its closure.

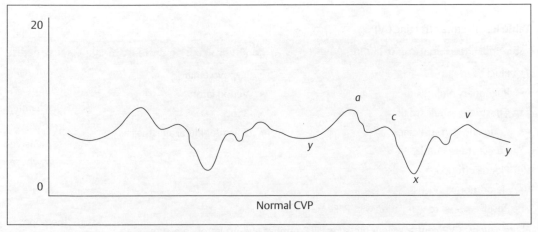

Fig. 6.1 Normal CVP trace. Abbreviation: CVP, central venous pressure.

x = due to ventricular systole.

v = due to ventricular filling.

y = due to tricuspid opening.

Indications of CVP are:

- Fluid management in shock.
- Major surgeries where large fluctuations in hemodynamics are expected.
- Open heart surgeries.
- Parenteral nutrition.
- Cardiac pacing.
- Aspiration of air embolus.

Normal CVP in adult is 3 to 10 cm H_2O (2–8 mm Hg).

The various conditions which affect CVP values are tabulated in **Table 6.2**.

The tip of the catheter should be at the junction of the internal jugular vein and the superior vena cava (*i.e., at 1–2 cm above the pericardial reflection*) to avoid rupture of the pericardium and consequent cardiac tamponade.

The cannulation of central veins is not without complications. The noteworthy complications are:

- Arterial puncture.
- Arrhythmias.
- Trauma to brachial plexus and phrenic nerve.

- Pneumothorax/hemothorax/chylothorax– more common with subclavian cannulation.
- Cardiac perforation/cardiac tamponade— life-threatening.
- Insertion site infection and sepsis.
- Arterial and venous thromboses.

Pulmonary Capillary Wedge Pressure

PCWP monitoring is achieved by placing a pulmonary artery catheter (Swan Ganz Catheter) and wedging it into the distal smallest branch of the pulmonary artery. *When properly placed, the tip of the catheter should be in the west's lung zone III.* Insertion of a pulmonary artery catheter can cause arrhythmias, rupture of the pulmonary artery, and death in the worst scenario.

The normal value is 4 to 12 mm Hg. PCWP of >18 mm Hg indicates cardiogenic pulmonary edema.

In today's practice, the only indications of pulmonary artery catheterization are:

- Refractory heart failure.
- Hemodynamic instability of unknown origin.

Other uses of pulmonary artery catheter are:

- Measurement of the pressure of cardiac chambers (except left ventricle).

Table 6.2 Factors affecting CVP

Conditions causing increase in CVP	Conditions causing decrease in CVP
• Fluid overload	• Hypovolemia
• Pulmonary embolism	• Venodilators
• Constrictive pericarditis	• Shock
• Coughing and straining	• Spinal/epidural anesthesia
• Cardiac tamponade	
• Pleural effusion	
• Hemothorax	
• Positive pressure ventilation with PEEP	

Abbreviations: CVP, central venous pressure; PEEP, positive end-expiratory pressure.

- Measurement of cardiac output (using the thermodilution technique).

- Sampling for mixed venous saturation.

- Titration of fluid therapy.

Respiratory Monitoring

Monitoring of respiratory system includes multiple tools like a pulse oximeter, capnography, blood gas analysis, lung volumes, oxygen analyzers, airway pressure monitoring, and apnea monitoring.

Pulse Oximetry

It works on the principle of **Beer's–Lambert law**, which states:

"the absorbance of light is directly proportional to the thickness of the media through which the light is being transmitted multiplied by the concentration of absorbing chromophore";

that is,

$$A = \varepsilon bc$$

where A is the absorbance, ε is the molar extinction coefficient, b is the thickness of the solution, and c is the concentration.

Pulse oximeter consists of a red and infrared light-emitting diode and a photodetector. There is a difference in wavelength of light absorbed by oxygenated blood (940 nm) and deoxygenated blood (660 nm). It measures the functional saturation of hemoglobin in arterial blood (S_aO_2), which ranges between 97 and 98% in normal healthy individuals. The accuracy of pulse oximeter lies between 70 and 100% saturation; below 70%, it becomes unreliable. The conditions where SpO_2 is relatively less compared to the actual value of S_aO_2 are:

- Hypotension.

- Anemia.

- Motion.

- Hemoglobin K.

- Dyes like methylene blue, indigo carmine, and indocyanine green.

- Nail polish—black, purple, and dark blue.

In methemoglobinemia, the SpO_2 is relatively fixed around 85%, while in carboxyhemoglobinemia, SpO_2 is falsely high.

The pulse oximeter is able to measure only oxygenated and deoxygenated hemoglobin but not other species like methemoglobin, sulfhemoglobin, and others. *Pulse co-oximeter can measure all types of hemoglobin species and hence able to characterize conditions such as methemoglobinemia and carboxyhemoglobinemia.*

Capnography

It is the continuous measurement of end-tidal (expired) carbon dioxide concentration ($EtCO_2$) in mm Hg and its waveform. The working principle is the absorbance of infrared light by carbon dioxide, and the normal value is 35 to 45 mm Hg. The monitoring methods include:

- Mainstream technique.

- Sidestream technique.

In sidestream technique, expiratory gases are delivered to the sample analyzer through the sampling line. *The disadvantages of these techniques are delayed response and blockade of sampling line with humidity.*

In the mainstream technique, the analyzer is placed in the expiratory limb. The benefit is of rapid response, but it adds to dead space.

It is a highly sensitive monitoring tool with use not only in the perioperative period but also in intensive care and during cardiac arrest, as shown in **Fig. 6.2**.

Blood Gas Analysis

A heparinized syringe: Preferably, a glass syringe is used to collect samples from easily accessible arteries like radial, femoral, or lower limb arteries. The sample should be immediately processed and

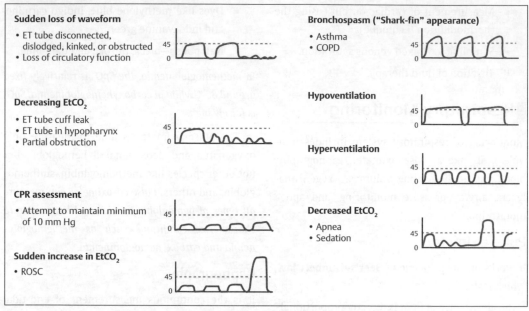

Fig. 6.2 Capnography waveforms. Abbreviations: COPD, chronic obstructive pulmonary disease; ET, endotracheal tube; EtCO$_2$, end-tidal carbon dioxide; ROSC, return of spontaneous circulation.

analyzed and be ice freezed if the delay of more than 10 to 15 minutes is anticipated in order to avoid false values. The PH, PaO$_2$, and PaCO$_2$ are directly measured, which gives us information about acid–base status, oxygenation, and ventilation. It is frequently used in:

- Cardiothoracic surgeries.
- Hypotensive anesthesia.

The modern gas analyzers are highly efficient in producing results in 1 to 2 minutes and require as low as 0.2 mL of blood.

Lung Volumes

Lung volumes are measured by a spirometer, and any discrepancy between inspired and expired tidal should alert the anesthesiologists about a possible leak.

Oxygen Analyzers

These devices are fitted in the inspiratory limb of the breathing circuit, which measures the actual fraction of oxygen being delivered to the patient. *They play a central role during low-flow anesthesia.*

Airway Pressure Monitoring

The pressure measured at the proximal end of the endotracheal tube (ETT) or supraglottic airway device should be less than 20 to 25 cm of H$_2$O in patients with normal lung compliance. A loss or decrease in airway pressure suggests disconnection or leak, respectively, while the rise in pressure is indicative of tube blockage, bronchospasm, or decrease in lung compliance.

Apnea Monitoring (Monitoring of Respiration)

Apnea is defined as the cessation of breathing for more than 10 seconds. Monitoring respiration can be done by capnography and airway pressure monitor in intubated patients, while in nonintubated patients, chest movements and airflow at nostrils (using acoustic probes) can be used.

Central Nervous System Monitoring

Central nervous system (CNS) monitoring equates to monitoring the depth of anesthesia. Signs and symptoms like tachycardia, hypertension, lacrimation, tachypnoea, coughing, laryngospasm, bronchospasm, and movement in response to noxious stimulus suggests a lighter plane of anesthesia. The monitoring tools include electroencephalogram (EEG), entropy, bispectral index (BIS), and patient-evoked responses.

Electroencephalogram

It is the recording of the electrical activity of the brain by applying electrodes on the surface of the scalp. The electrical activity of the brain keeps on changing physiologically like awake and sleep state, so it varies with the depth of anesthesia. *With increasing depth of anesthesia, high amplitude, low-frequency waves appear.*

*The effects of anesthetic agents and other factors on EEG are summarized in **Table 6.3**.*

Bispectral Index

It is the quantitative EEG used to monitor the depth of anesthesia and has been successful in reducing the risk of intraoperative awareness. Its value ranges between 0 and 100.

- BIS (40–60) = adequate depth of anesthesia.
- BIS (90–100) = completely awake.

- BIS (0) = complete suppression of cortical activity.

Entropy

It is the acquisition of EEG and facial electromyography (EMG) together to monitor the depth of anesthesia. It was introduced by GE healthcare, and it measures two entropy parameters—fast-acting response entropy (RE) and more steady and robust state entropy (SE). *Response entropy is sensitive to activation of facial muscles, and its value ranges between 0 and 100, while state entropy is either equal to or less than response entropy and suggests hypnotic effects of anesthetics on the brain.*

Evoked Response

It assesses the integrity of neuronal tissues during surgeries. The evoked responses can be:

- Somatosensory-evoked potentials (SSEP):

  It evaluates the sensory tract. Important monitoring tool in spine surgeries, repair of abdominal aortic aneurysm, and surgery on the somatosensory area of cortex.

- Auditory-evoked potential (AEP):

  It assesses the auditory pathway and is helpful in resection of acoustic neuroma and posterior fossa surgeries.

- Visual-evoked potential (VEP):

  It is for procedures involving visual tracts, for example, optic glioma, pituitary tumors.

Table 6.3 Factors affecting EEG

Anesthetic agents/other factors	Effect
• All anesthetics (inhaled or intravenous) with exceptions below	• Excitation in low dose and depression with the higher dose
Exceptions: • Opioids • Nitrous oxide/ketamine	• Depression only • Excitation only
Other factors: • Hypoxia/hypercarbia • Hypothermia and cerebral ischemia	• Excitation in the early phase and depression in the advanced stage • Progressive depression of EEG

- Motor-evoked response (MER):

  Useful for procedures where motor tracts are at risk of injuries, for example, surgery on spine/spinal cord.

Effects of anesthetic agents on the evoked response are:

- All anesthetics tend to decrease amplitude and increase latency with the following exceptions:

  ▶ Combination of opioids with propofol and dexmedetomidine is the preferred regimen in cases where evoked response monitoring is used (as propofol, opioid, and dexmedetomidine do not affect evoked responses).

  ▶ Ketamine and etomidate increase amplitude with no effect on latency.

  ▶ Midazolam and nitrous oxide increases the latency without affecting amplitude.

Temperature Monitoring

Homeothermic mammals maintain their core body temperature in a very narrow range, which is required for optimal cellular functions. Intraoperative hypothermia is not uncommon and occurs because of heat loss by various mechanisms such as the following:

- Vasodilation caused by anesthetics.
- Cold environment.
- Cold intravenous (IV) fluids.
- Heat loss from body through convection, evaporation, and radiation.

Common monitoring sites for core body temperature include the esophagus, nasopharynx, pulmonary artery, and tympanic membrane (most accurate for brain temperature).

The esophagus is the best site for the core temperature monitoring, but the most accurate measurement is obtained by a pulmonary artery catheter.

Hypothermia is defined as a decrease in core temperature of less than 35°C. The intraoperative hypothermia can have the following systemic manifestations:

- **CVS:** Bradycardia, hypotension, and cardiac arrhythmias at a temperature less than 28°.
- **CNS:** Decrease in cerebral metabolic rate with progressive slowing of EEG activity.
- **Respiratory:** Left shift of oxygen dissociation curve, decrease in minute ventilation, and respiratory arrest at less than 23°.
- **Blood:** Increased blood viscosity and decreased activity of clotting factors.
- **Kidney:** Decrease in glomerular filtration rate (GFR) and renal shut down at 20°.
- **Acid–base balance:** Acidosis due to increased lactic acid production.
- **Endocrine:** Hyperglycemia.
- **Drug metabolism:** Markedly decreased and also the MAC requirement goes down as a consequence of hypothermia.
- **Wound healing:** Poor wound healing and increased risk of infections.

Overviewing the adverse effects of hypothermia, it is mandatory to do temperature monitoring in:

- All patients undergoing general anesthesia for more than 30 minutes, and in all patients where surgery lasts for more than 1 hour (irrespective of the mode of anesthesia).
- All cardiac surgeries.
- Infants and small children.
- Patients of burns, febrile patients.
- Patients at risk of malignant hyperthermia.

Treatment of intraoperative hypothermia includes warm IV fluid, increase ambient temperature, covering the patients with blankets, and the use of forced warm air.

The optimal operation theater temperature for an adult is 21°C and for the children is 28°C.

Neuromuscular Monitoring

Neuromuscular monitoring is used to evaluate the effect of a neuromuscular blocking agent for which muscle response after stimulation of its corresponding motor nerve is assessed. *Ulnar nerve and adductor pollicis are the most frequently used nerve-muscle unit for this purpose. The effects in corrugator supercilii and orbicularis oculi (supplied by facial nerve) parallels with the laryngeal muscles; they are the ideal muscles for monitoring.*

The most common indications of neuromuscular monitoring are:

- Duchenne muscular dystrophy.
- Myasthenia gravis.

The train of four (TOF) is the most useful pattern of stimulation for monitoring (**Fig. 6.3**); other patterns include:

- Single twitch.
- Tetanic stimulation.
- Posttetanic facilitation.
- Double burst stimulation.

The details of all these patterns and effects of nondepolarizing and depolarizing muscle relaxants on them have been described in detail in the chapter on neuromuscular blocking agents.

Conclusion

The practice of perioperative monitoring of patients is continuously evolving, with advancements in technology and equipment.

The level and type (invasive vs. noninvasive) of monitoring should be tailored, based on the patient's risk of perioperative morbidity and mortality. The standards of ASA monitoring must be in place and practiced in all cases to ensure the safety of patients.

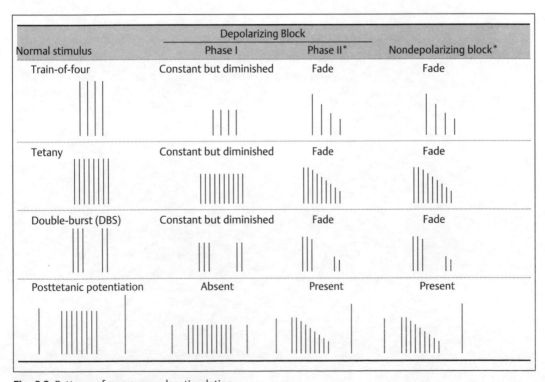

Fig. 6.3 Patterns of neuromuscular stimulation.

Note: *Fading is characteristic of phase II and nondepolarizing block.

Section II
General Anesthesia

CHAPTER 7

Glimpse of General Anesthesia

Heena Garg and Nishant Patel

Introduction

General anesthesia is a drug-induced, reversible condition, including specific behavioral and physiological components, with concomitant stability of the autonomic, cardiovascular, respiratory, and thermoregulatory system. It can also be perceived as a pharmacological intervention to prevent surgical trauma's psychological and somatic adverse effects and create favorable conditions for surgery. This chapter will discuss important aspects of general anesthesia under the following headings:

- Components of general anesthesia.
- Concept of preoxygenation and its techniques.
- Apnea safety margin and its implication.
- Guedel's stages of anesthesia.

Components of General Anesthesia

Oliver Wendell Holmes coined the term general anesthesia. In 1926, John Lundy described the concept of balanced anesthesia. Balanced anesthesia is achieved by using hypnotic agents, anxiolytics, muscle relaxants, and analgesics. The use of the specific drug helps in achieving the specific target with minimal side effects of each drug. The balanced anesthesia comprises the following:

- Unconsciousness.
- Amnesia.
- Antinociception.
- Immobility.
- Homeostasis.

Concept of Preoxygenation

Under the state of anesthesia, cessation of breathing leads to continuous oxygen uptake with no replenishment of the oxygen store in the lung, which puts the patient at risk of hypoxemia. Preoxygenation is essential to avoid hypoxemia and related end-organ damage. The functional residual capacity (FRC) works as an oxygen buffer, which gets filled during preoxygenation. Preoxygenation can also be considered as denitrogenation, as a high inspired oxygen concentration displaces the nitrogen in the lungs. *The aim is to increase the physiological reserve of oxygen to increase the time to desaturation during the apnea time, which can occur with the induction of anesthesia.* It is especially desirable if a rapid sequence induction (RSI) is planned, as positive pressure ventilation is avoided in RSI before tracheal intubation. The effectiveness of preoxygenation is assessed by its efficacy and efficiency.

- *Indices of efficacy* include increase in the fraction of alveolar O_2 (FaO$_2$), decrease in the fraction of alveolar nitrogen (FaN$_2$), and increase in arterial O_2 tension (PaO$_2$).

- *The efficiency of lung oxygen reserves* is a product of the fraction of oxygen within the alveoli (oxygen fraction in expired gas = FeO$_2$) and FRC.

Increased oxygen consumption and a decrease in oxygen reserve can lead to rapid desaturation despite adequate preoxygenation.

- Increased oxygen consumption is seen in growing adolescents, fever, sepsis, and pediatric population.

- Decreased oxygen reserve is seen in obesity, pregnancy, and patients with large abdominal mass/ascites.

Preoxygenation Techniques

Before initiating preoxygenation, the following prerequisites must be met:

- The tight-fitting facemask.
- 100% oxygen.

The inappropriate seal leads to inhalation of ambient air and can cause up to 20 to 40% dilution of the inspired oxygen. The preoxygenation can be done with any of the following techniques:

a. *Tidal volume breathing (TVB)*:

The traditional tidal volume breathing is an effective technique of preoxygenation. At FiO_2 of 1, 3 minutes of TVB ensures maximal preoxygenation in adults with normal lung function. The various anesthetic circuits (circle system, Mapleson A, and Mapleson D) with a flow rate ranging 5 to 35 L/min have been used successfully, but the circle system with flow rate 5 L/min remains the standard. The classic preoxygenation increases the apnea safety margin by up to 10 minutes.

b. *Deep breathing method*:

The deep breathing technique includes the following:

- Single vital capacity breath.
- Four deep breaths (four inspiratory capacity breath over 30 s).
- Eight deep breaths (eight inspiratory capacity breaths over 60 s).

Initial studies found deep breathing as effective as the tidal volume technique in terms of achieving preoxygenation goals. However, later on, it was found to be inferior because of the following reasons:

- If the ventilation during the short time (0.5–1.0 min) is higher than the oxygen flow rate, rebreathing is likely to occur

and hence lead to a decrease in the inspired concentration of oxygen.

- The FRC may get saturated within 0.5 minutes of ventilation, but the tissues and venous compartment need a longer duration to fill.

Since deep breathing techniques provide suboptimal oxygenation, these should be reserved for emergency scenarios where time is lacking, and the patient's cooperation is inadequate.

The anesthesiologist must target the endpoints of preoxygenation, irrespective of techniques, because the efficiency of preoxygenation gets reflected as the rate of decline in oxyhemoglobin saturation during apnea. The endpoints of preoxygenation are as follows:

- End-tidal oxygen concentration more than 90%.
- End-tidal nitrogen concentration less than 5%.

The standard technique of preoxygenation is not helpful in patients who require securing airway rapidly and at risk of aspiration. It also does not work in patients who cannot be preoxygenated because of agitation and uncooperativeness. Here, the techniques like RSI and delayed sequence intubation replace the standard technique of preoxygenation.

Rapid Sequence Induction

- It is the method of inducing anesthesia in patients who are at risk of aspiration.
- After adequate preoxygenation (patient is allowed to breathe spontaneously and no sedatives are given), while cricoid pressure is being applied, a predetermined dose of intravenous anesthetic agent and muscle relaxant is given to intubate the trachea, without attempts at positive pressure ventilation (PPV).
- The goal is to intubate the trachea as quickly and as safely as possible.

- The application of cricoid pressure requires a force of 10 Newton while the patient is awake and a force of 30 Newton once the patient is induced.

- The cricoid pressure occludes the upper esophagus, preventing the regurgitation of gastric content into the pharynx. However, some studies suggest that cricoid pressure lowers the lower esophageal sphincter tone, leading to increased risk of aspiration.

- In addition, the application of cricoid pressure may make the visualization of glottis difficult during direct laryngoscopy.

- The indications of RSI are as follows:

  ▸ Full stomach patients.

  ▸ Diabetes mellitus with autonomic neuropathy.

  ▸ Hiatus hernia.

  ▸ Bowel obstruction.

  ▸ Pregnancy.

  ▸ Altered consciousness with loss of airway reflexes.

Delayed Sequence Induction (DSI)

- DSI is used for preoxygenation and induction of patients when preoxygenation is ineffective due to agitation (hypoxia, hypercapnia).

- The steps of DSI are as follows:

  ▸ Identify the agitated patients requiring intubation.

  ▸ Keep the patient head up at 30 degrees.

  ▸ Administer induction agent (ideal agent is ketamine because of its ability to keep airway reflexes preserved).

  ▸ Give ketamine 1 mg/kg as an intravenous push over 15 to 30 seconds and apply nonrebreathing mask at an oxygen flow of 15 L/min (ensuring the patency of airway).

  ▸ If the airway gets obstructed, use the bag and mask ventilation with the application of positive end-expiratory pressure (PEEP).

  ▸ Preoxygenate for 3 minutes.

  ▸ Administer neuromuscular agent (succinylcholine—1.5 mg//kg OR rocuronium—1.2 mg/kg) and intubate the trachea after 45 to 60 seconds.

Stages of Anesthesia

Anesthesia continually moves from one phase to another, and there exists no single anesthetic state. John Snow divided the effects of ether into five stages, progressing from consciousness to deep coma, muscle flaccidity, and respiratory paralysis.

Guedel extended these observations, and during World War I, he developed a scheme that took account of patient responses to determine the degree of anesthesia present (**Table 7.1**).

To summarize:

- Stage 3 plane III is best for surgical anesthesia as loss of laryngeal reflex facilitates endotracheal intubation.

- The first reflex to go is eyelash, and the last to go is carinal reflex. *The recovery of reflexes occurs in the opposite direction.*

General Anesthesia: Principles of Induction and Maintenance (AS4.3)

Provision of general anesthesia to a patient starts from preoperative evaluation, goes through intraoperative preparation, induction, maintenance, and emergence from anesthesia.

Once a patient is found to be fit to undergo surgery, based on preoperative assessment and optimization, the operating room is prepared with adequate equipment and drugs.

The patient's records and nil per mouth status are reviewed before proceeding further. Standards

Table 7.1 Guedel's stages of anesthesia

Stage	Definition	Reflexes abolished
Stage I (stage of analgesia or disorientation)	From the beginning of induction of general anesthesia to loss of consciousness	Nil
Stage II (stage of excitement or delirium)	From loss of consciousness to onset of automatic breathing Coughing, vomiting, and struggling may occur; respiration can be irregular with breath-holding	Eyelash reflex
Stage III (stage of surgical anesthesia)		
• Plane I	From the onset of automatic respiration to cessation of eyeball movements	Eyelid reflex, swallowing reflex, conjunctival reflex
• Plane II	From the cessation of eyeball movements to the beginning of paralysis of intercostal muscles	Corneal reflex
• Plane III	From beginning to completion of intercostal muscle paralysis. Diaphragmatic respiration persists	Laryngeal reflex
• Plane IV	From complete intercostal paralysis to diaphragmatic paralysis (apnea)	Carinal reflex, anal sphincter
Stage IV (medullary paralysis)	From stoppage of respiration till death	

ASA monitors are applied, and the patient is preoxygenated with techniques and principles described earlier in this chapter. Following adequate preoxygenation, the patient is induced with intravenous agents (propofol, thiopentone, ketamine, or etomidate) OR inhaled anesthetic agents, and the trachea is intubated by paralyzing the patient, taking care of hemodynamic consequences that these agents could have.

Once the patient gets induced, anesthesia is maintained (intravenous or inhaled agents) for the duration of surgery, targeting the goals of:

- Amnesia.
- Analgesia.
- Muscle relaxation.

The patient is continuously monitored for the duration of surgery, with all efforts to keep vitals stable and ensure smooth emergence from anesthesia at the end of surgery.

Near the end of the surgery, delivery of anesthetic agents is stopped, and neuromuscular blockade is reversed with a reversal agent (neostigmine/physostigmine) to facilitate extubation.

The patient is shifted to the recovery area for further monitoring and care till he or she is shifted to ward or home.

Conclusion

A patient needs to be unconscious, relaxed, and hemodynamically stable throughout the surgery. Induction agents, sedatives, and muscle relaxants in appropriate dosage achieve optimal surgical condition with minimal side effects. Preoxygenation increases the apnea safety margin and must be practiced in all cases. The techniques like RSI and DSI become helpful in patients at risk of aspiration and agitated patients, respectively.

CHAPTER 8

Inhalational Anesthetics (AS4.1)

Tanvir Samra

Introduction

Any chemical agent with general anesthetic properties and the ability to be delivered via inhalation is labeled as an "inhalational anesthetic agent."

Characteristics of an ideal inhalation anesthetic used for induction and maintenance of general anesthesia in the operating room are as follows:

- Nonflammable.
- Molecular stability.
- Ability to be obtained in pure form with low cost of production.
- High potency.
- Safe when used for long durations.
- No acute cardiovascular or respiratory side effects.
- Low blood: Gas solubility ensuring rapid induction and elimination.

The use of inhalational anesthetic agents has been extended to the intensive care units (ICUs) where they have been administered for *sedation*, for the management of *refractory bronchospasm*, and for the *control of status epilepticus*, which are unresponsive to conventional anticonvulsant medications.

History

The concept of inhalational anesthesia dates back to the 11th century when the Arab physicians used a sponge soaked in a narcotic drug on a patient's face.

Table 8.1 summarizes the milestones in the history of inhalational anesthesia.

Classification

The inhalational anesthetics can be either volatile anesthetic agents or nonvolatile anesthetic gases.

Volatile Anesthetic Agents

- These agents are liquid at room temperature and require a specialized device called a vaporizer for inhalational administration.
- A vaporizer accurately varies the amount of anesthetic vapor added to the total gas mixture and in turn the concentration of vapor in the alveoli.
- Volatility is the tendency of a liquid to vaporize, and the pressure developed by the evaporation of the liquid volatile agent is called the *vapor pressure*, which is dependent on the surrounding temperature and the physical properties of the liquid.
- The most commonly used volatile anesthetic agents are summarized below:
  ▸ Sevoflurane.
  ▸ Isoflurane.
  ▸ Desflurane.
  ▸ Methoxyflurane.
  ▸ Enflurane.
  ▸ Halothane.
  ▸ Ether.

Nonvolatile Anesthetic Gases

- These are gases at room temperature and are thus stored in gas cylinders and administered using flow meters, rather than vaporizers.

Table 8.1 Historical milestones of inhalational anesthesia

Agent	Year of discovery
Nitrous oxide	1772
Ether	Produced by Cordius in 1540; used as anesthetic in 1842
Chloroform	Used by Simpson in 1847, discontinued due to severe cardiovascular collapse and hepatotoxicity
Cyclopropane	Discovered in 1929, low potency and inflammability
Halothane	1956
Isoflurane	1981
Desflurane	1992
Sevoflurane	1994
Xenon	1997

- The predominant nonvolatile anesthetic agents are:
  - ► Cyclopropane.
  - ► Nitrous oxide.
  - ► Xenon.

Delivery of Inhalational Anesthetics

They can be administered using:
- A facemask.
- A supraglottic device.
- An endotracheal tube.
- A tracheostomy tube.

Mechanism of Action

It is still largely unknown, and the action of the agents on multiple targets contributes to the anesthetic effect.

The site of action for the immobilizing effect is in the *spinal cord*. In contrast, the supraspinal sites, namely, the amygdala, hippocampus, and cortex, are the targets for sedation, hypnosis, and amnesia. The hypothesis behind the action of inhaled anesthetics is still an area of ongoing research. However, the common hypotheses are as follows:

A. **Lipid-based theories**

Lipid solubility theory: It states that the movement of gas into the lipid membrane disrupts the ion channels and the propagation of the action potential. Lipid solubility forms the basis of the Meyer–Overton hypothesis.

Meyer–Overton theory:

- It is suggested that when a sufficient number of inhalational anesthetic molecules bind to target sites in the brain cells and dissolve in the lipid cell membrane, they produce an anesthetized state.

- It postulated that the *number of molecules dissolved in the lipid cell membrane* and not the type of inhalational agent is important to cause anesthesia. It thus supports the additive nature of anesthetic agents.

- This concept was supported by the fact that there existed a direct correlation between lipid solubility of inhaled anesthetics and the potency expressed as minimum alveolar concentration (MAC). Potency increased as oil:gas solubility increased.

Lipid bilayer expansion theory: Binding of anesthetic agents can modify the lipid bilayer by changing its curvature/elasticity, by causing changes in phase separation, and by creating changes in bilayer thickness. Lipid bilayer expansion is the basis of the critical volume hypothesis by Mullins.

Critical Volume Hypothesis by Mullins: It stated that the absorption of bulky and hydrophobic anesthetic molecules into the hydrophobic region within the cell membrane causes its distortion due to volume displacement. Expansion beyond a "critical volume" distorts channels necessary for sodium-ion flux and the development of action potentials essential for synaptic transmission.

B. Protein-based theory

These theories were introduced to overcome the weakness of the lipid-based theories (stereoisomers of an anesthetic agent have variable potency but same oil:gas partition coefficient).

It states that the anesthetics bind to the hydrophobic portion of the ion channels/proteins and can either induce/prevent or alter the kinetics of the conformational change or compete with various ligands. Some examples are:

- Action at the molecular level: Two-pore domain potassium channels contribute to potassium membrane conductance and are widely distributed in the central nervous system (CNS) both pre- and postsynaptically. Halothane, isoflurane, sevoflurane, and desflurane enhance the activity of these channels, leading to hyperpolarization of the plasma membrane and potentially explaining their anesthetic effects.
- Neuromodulator theory states that the anesthetics bind to cell surface receptors and increase the flux of chloride ions.

Pharmacokinetics of Inhalational Agents

Pharmacokinetics involves the uptake and elimination of inhalational agents. Several partial pressure gradients exist between the anesthetic machine and the final target organ, that is, the brain. Thus, we can alter the brain concentration indirectly by in-depth knowledge of pharmacokinetics. The factors which account for the difference in gradients are further classified as inflow and outflow factors:

1. Inflow factors: The inflow factors determine the concentration of inhaled anesthetics in the alveoli. These are as follows:

   a. **Vaporizer setting/inspired concentration of agent (Fi):** The greater the inspired concentration, the faster the induction of anesthesia. The inspired concentration can be achieved by either increasing the higher dial setting of the vaporizer or by increasing the amount of fresh gas flow.

   b. **Breathing system**: Lower volume of breathing system with lower circuit absorption leads to higher inspired concentration.

   c. **Effective alveolar ventilation:** Increased and effective alveolar ventilation results in a faster increase in alveolar partial pressure.

   The factors which govern it are as follows:

   o Functional residual capacity (FRC): A larger FRC leads to a decrease in alveolar partial pressure because of dilution of inspired gases and, consequently, slower onset of anesthesia.

   o The time constant: It is an important concept to be understood. The time constant for the circuit is the total volume of circuit divided by the fresh gas flow rate, while that for lungs, it is the volume of FRC divided by minute ventilation.

It takes three time constants for 95% of a concentration change to be achieved.

d. **Second gas effect:** The coadministration of an anesthetic agent with nitrous oxide results in the increased partial pressure of inhaled anesthetic agents. This occurs due to the rapid uptake of nitrous oxide by the lungs. This phenomenon is termed as the second gas effect.

2. Outflow factors: These factors are the determinant of uptake of inhaled anesthetics from the lungs. The uptake of the inhaled anesthetic agent can be calculated using the formula:

    Uptake = $\lambda_{B/G} \times Q \times (P_A-P_V)$ divided by barometric pressure, where

    $\lambda_{B/G}$ = blood-gas partition coefficient;

    Q = cardiac output, and

    (P_A-P_V) = difference between alveolar partial pressure and mixed venous pressure.

    The factors governing the uptake are:

    a. **Solubility:** It is defined as the ratio of its concentration in the blood to alveolar gas when there is no difference in their partial pressures. The blood solubility of an inhalational agent is expressed as a blood/gas partition coefficient ($\lambda_{B/G}$).

        The agents with a higher blood–gas partition coefficient (*chloroform, ether*) have a greater uptake in the pulmonary circulation, a slower increase in alveolar partial (FA/Fi ratio), and therefore prolonged induction.

    b. **Cardiac output (Q):** Increase in cardiac output means a greater uptake, that is, amount of agent removed from the alveolus increases leading to a fall in alveolar concentration.

    b. **Alveolar venous partial pressure gradient (PA–PV):** The value of this gradient depends on the tissue uptake. The tissue uptake, in turn, depends on:

        o   Tissue solubility.

        o   Tissue blood flow.

        o   The partial pressure difference between the arterial blood and tissue.

        Out of all, *blood flow is the most important factor,* and based on it, the tissues have been classified into:

        o   Vessel rich group (brain, heart, kidney, liver, etc.).

        o   Muscle group.

        o   Fat group.

        o   The poor vessel group.

High absorption and slow release of anesthetic agents from fat tissues result in more delayed induction and emergence in obese.

Lower albumin and cholesterol levels also account for rapid onset of anesthesia.

Minimum Alveolar Concentration

MAC is the minimum end-tidal concentration of inhaled anesthetic at 1 atm pressure in 100% oxygen at equilibrium, which produces immobility in 50% of subjects in response to a standard surgical midline incision. *It reflects the actions of an inhalation agent on spinal cord-mediated reflexes. It is equivalent to the ED50 expressed for intravenous (IV) agents.* The MAC value of commonly used anesthetic agents is listed in **Table 8.2**.

MAC is a useful measure because it mirrors the brain's partial pressure of the anesthetic agent.

Some of the properties of MAC are:

- Each additional 0.1 above or below a MAC of 1.0 corresponds to a one standard deviation (SD) increase or decrease in dose, that is, 50% of patients will not move at 1.0 MAC, 68% at 1.1 MAC, 95% at 1.2 MAC, and 99.7% at 1.3 MAC.

- MAC values are roughly additive.

- MAC can be used clinically to assess unconsciousness, amnesia, eye-opening, and autonomic response.

  ▶ **MAC-awake:** Anesthetic concentration needed to suppress a voluntary response to verbal command (i.e., eye-opening) in 50% of patients. *Value is* approximately one-third of MAC for the inhaled anesthetic being used.

  ▶ **MAC-amnesia:** Anesthetic concentration required to suppress recollection or explicit memory of a noxious stimulus. Anterograde amnesia is achieved at roughly 0.25 MAC, while unconsciousness is generally achieved at 0.5 MAC.

  ▶ **MAC-bar:** Anesthetic concentration that blocks autonomic responses (changes in pupil dilation, heart rate, and blood pressure) to surgical incision in 50% of patients. The value of the MAC-bar is determined by measuring the level of catecholamine in venous blood and is roughly 1.5 MAC.

Standard MAC values assume the absence of all other potentially sedative or hypnotic drugs.

Numerous physiological and pharmacological factors affect the MAC. The factors affecting MAC are enlisted in **Table 8.3**.

Table 8.2 MAC values of inhaled anesthetic agents

Agent	MAC value
Nitrous oxide	104
Desflurane	6.0
Sevoflurane	2.2
Isoflurane	1.2
Halothane	0.75

Abbreviation: MAC, minimum alveolar concentration.

Pharmacodynamics of Inhalation Agents

The presence of the "therapeutic concentration" of the anesthetic agent in the brain leads to the

Table 8.3 Factors affecting MAC

Factors which increase MAC	Factors which decrease MAC
• Ephedrine, MAO inhibitors, acute amphetamine intoxication • Hyperthyroidism (15%) • Hypernatremia • Hyperthermia • Chronic ethanol abuse	• Increasing age • Hyponatremia, hypercalcemia • Hypothermia, hypo-osmolality • Anemia (Hgb < 5 g/dL) • Hypercarbia, metabolic acidosis • Hypoxia (< 40 mm Hg) • Pregnancy • Opioids, diazepam, clonidine, reserpine, alpha methyldopa • Acute ethanol consumption

Abbreviations: MAC, minimum alveolar concentration; MAO, monoamine oxidase.
Note: Obesity and gender do not affect MAC values.

clinical effects of the inhalation anesthetic; however, they are known to affect all the organ systems of the body.

Effects on the Respiratory System

- All halogenated agents depress medullary respiratory centers and affect ventilation by reducing tidal volume; consequently, $PaCO_2$ increases. An increase in frequency counteracts the decrease in tidal volume, so that the amount of change in minute volume is minimized.

- All inhalation agents, when present in sufficient concentration, *raise the threshold (i.e., decrease the sensitivity) of the respiratory center to CO_2 and hypoxia.* Chemical control of breathing is hampered. The margin between MAC and concentration producing apnea (*respiratory anesthetic index*) is an indicator of the anesthetics margin of safety for breathing.

- Isoflurane and sevoflurane decrease airway resistance partly due to bronchodilation. Desflurane does not produce any significant change in bronchial tone.

- Chemically induced tracheal contractions are inhibited by inhalational agents in the order:
  Halothane > enflurane ≥ isoflurane > sevoflurane.

- Hypoxic pulmonary vasoconstriction: Inhaled anesthetics inhibit the diversion of blood from the atelectatic lung and cause hypoxia.

- Tracheal mucociliary flow is inhibited by inhaled anesthetics.

- Concentration effect: The increased inspired concentration of nitrous oxide leads to rise in its alveolar concentration, which is termed as concentration effect. It occurs due to rapid transfer of nitrous oxide from alveoli to blood, causing volume loss and consequently increased gas flow to alveoli to make up for the lost volume.

- Second gas effect: The administration of inhalational agent (e.g., halothane) along with nitrous oxide leads to augmented alveolar flow and concentration of inhaled agent, due to alveolar volume loss, owing to rapid transfer of nitrous oxide to pulmonary blood.

Effects on the Cardiovascular System

- Blood pressure:

  All halogenated agents cause a dose-related reduction in mean arterial pressure (MAP). The causes of the decrease are:

  ▶ Reduction in systemic vascular resistance (desflurane, isoflurane, and sevoflurane).

  ▶ Decreases cardiac output and increases venous compliance (e.g., halothane).

- Oxygen consumption:

  There is a decrease of 10 to 15% below awake values.

- Pulmonary vascular effects of nitrous oxide:

  Elevated pulmonary artery pressure may be further increased by nitrous oxide.

- Myocardial protection from ischemia-reperfusion injury:

  Ischemic preconditioning with inhalation anesthetics (isoflurane, desflurane, and sevoflurane) reduces perioperative myocardial injury.

- Distribution of cardiac output:

  Blood flow to the liver, kidney, and gut is decreased. Blood flow to the brain, muscle, and skin is increased. *Isoflurane causes hepatic arterial vasodilation; thus, although total hepatic blood flow decreases, oxygen delivery is preserved better with isoflurane.*

- Cardiac dysrhythmia:

  Isoflurane is more arrhythmogenic than desflurane and sevoflurane.

Heart rate changes least with halothane and increases most with desflurane. Sevoflurane can prolong the QT interval; to be administered with caution in patients with long QT interval syndrome.

Susceptibility of the heart to the dysrhythmic effects of epinephrine differs among anesthetics. The cardiac dysrhythmia dose of epinephrine for anesthesia with inhalational agents is shown in **Table 8.4**.

Table 8.4 Arrhythmogenic dose of epinephrine

Agent	Arrhythmogenic dose
Desflurane	
0.8 MAC	6.9 ± 0.7 µg/kg/min
1.2 MAC	6.6 ± 0.9 µg/kg/min
Isoflurane	
0.7 MAC	5.7 ± 1.1 µg/kg/min
1.1 MAC	6.0 ± 1.0 µg/kg/min
Halothane	
0.7 MAC	1.3 ± 0.2 µg/kg/min
1.3 MAC	1.1 ± 0.3 µg/kg/min
Sevoflurane	
1.3 MAC	8.8 ± 1.18 µg/kg/min

Abbreviation: MAC, minimum alveolar concentration.

From **Table 8.4**, it is evident that the dose of epinephrine required for arrhythmia is minimum with halothane.

The cardiovascular effects of inhalational agents are summarized in **Table 8.5**.

Effects on the CNS

- CNS electrophysiology:
  - ▶ Anesthetic doses producing surgical anesthesia decrease the frequency with a corresponding increase in amplitude towards the θ- and δ-range.
  - ▶ Higher concentrations of some inhalation anesthetics induce burst suppression.
  - ▶ Preconditioning agents in ischemic brains: Volatile anesthetics have been shown to initiate early ischemic tolerance (preconditioning) in neurons.
- $CMRO_2$: All inhalation agents decrease cerebral metabolic rate and oxygen consumption. They also partially uncouple the reactivity of cerebral blood flow to CO_2. Order of effect from greatest to least is *isoflurane > enflurane ≥ halothane*.
- Cerebral vasodilation: It has the potential to increase intracranial pressure. Inhalational

Table 8.5 Cardiovascular effects of inhalational agents

Agents/effects	Cardiac output	SVR	MAP	HR
Halothane	↓	↔	↓	↓↓
Enflurane	↓↓	↓	↓↓	↑
Isoflurane	↓	↓	↓	↑
Desflurane	↔	↓	↓	↑
Sevoflurane	↔	↓	↓	↔
Nitrous oxide	↓	↑	↔	↑
Xenon	↔	↔	↔	↑

Abbreviations: HR, heart rate; MAP, mean arterial pressure; SVR, systemic vascular resistance.
Notes: ↔, no effect; ↓, decrease; ↑, increase; ↓↓, marked reduction.

agents reduce MAP, and the combined effect results in decreased cerebral perfusion pressure. Halothane causes maximum dilatation of the cerebral vessels.

- Production and reabsorption of cerebrospinal fluid (CSF): Enflurane is the least favorable drug, as it increases CSF production and increases the resistance to reabsorption. *Isoflurane has a minimum effect on CSF production and reabsorption.*

- Sensory-evoked potentials (SEP): Dose-related decrease in the amplitude and an increase in the latency of cortical components of SEP by inhalational anesthetics (N_2O included) is seen. A similar effect is seen on visual- and auditory-evoked potentials.

Effects on the Liver

They affect the liver in two ways:
- All inhaled anesthetics reduce hepatic blood flow.
- The extent of hepatic toxicity correlates with the degree to which metabolism by cytochrome enzymes occurs, as the intact molecule is nontoxic.

The percentage values of inhaled anesthetics metabolized are 20 to 30% for halothane, 2% for enflurane, 1% for sevoflurane, 0.2% for isoflurane, and 0.02% for desflurane.

Hepatotoxicity of halothane is predominantly due to its metabolism. Trifluoroacetic acid (TFA) is the major protein-bound metabolite that induces a T-cell-mediated immune response, resulting in mild transaminitis to fulminant hepatic necrosis. The estimated risk of fatal hepatic necrosis is approximately 1:10,000 anesthetics. Adult females and repeated exposures increase the risk.

Effects on the Kidneys

Renal blood flow is preserved as a decrease in blood pressure is attenuated by renal autoregulation.

Glomerular filtration rate (GFR) and urine output decrease but is not a cause for concern, as urine flow is reestablished when blood pressure is normalized.

Production of inorganic fluoride by the metabolism of halogenated agents causes direct nephrotoxicity:

- The serum fluoride level of >50 mmol/L with methoxyflurane cause polyuric renal failure.

- The less nephrotoxic potential of enflurane is due to an earlier peak and rapid decrease of serum fluoride levels.

- Isoflurane does not cause significant increases in serum fluoride levels, as it is resistant to defluorination.

- Sevoflurane undergoes significant defluorination, and fluoride levels exceed 50 µmol/L. *But evidence of renal dysfunction lacks as defluorination is not intrarenal.*

- Halothane and desflurane are not significantly defluorinated.

Uterine and Fetal Effects

- Cause myometrial relaxation and greater blood loss during the termination of pregnancy.
- Cross the placenta and affect the fetus.

Neuromuscular Effects

- Potentiate the action of neuromuscular blocking agents.
- Inherent muscle relaxant properties due to postsynaptic action on neuromuscular (NM) junction.

Physical Properties of Inhalational Agents

The comparative features of inhalational agents are summarized in **Table 8.6**.

Table 8.6 Physical properties of inhalational agents

Agent	Blood/gas coefficient	MAC (%) at 1 atm	Boiling point	Vapor pressure	Special features
Nitrous oxide	0.47	104	−89		• Causes expansion of gases trapped in a cavity (nitrous oxide is 30 times more soluble than nitrogen. It quickly diffuses into closed spaces) • Rapid onset and recovery • Analgesic property
Xenon	0.115	63–71	−107		• Rapid induction and recovery • Depresses postsynaptic excitatory transmission via NMDA receptor block • Minimal cardiovascular side effects • Anesthetic-induced preconditioning of the heart and brain against ischaemic damage • Nonirritant to the airway, suited for smooth induction • Decreases respiratory rate and increases tidal volume • Increases pulmonary resistance • Caution in patients with severe chronic obstructive pulmonary disease and premature infants • Not metabolized in liver/kidneys • Does not trigger malignant hyperpyrexia • Potent intraoperative analgesic • Nonflammable and does not cause ozone depletion or environmental pollution
Desflurane	0.42	6	23	664	• Very rapid onset and recovery • Airway irritation due to pungent odor; avoided for induction
Sevoflurane	0.69	2	58	160	• Rapid onset and recovery • Nonpungent, odor suitable for induction • Most commonly used inhalational anesthetic agent
Isoflurane	1.40	1.4	48	238	• Most potent flurane • Pungent odor; avoided for induction • Relatively slow onset and recovery
Enflurane	1.80	1.7	56	175	• Proconvulsive • Medium speed of onset and recovery
Halothane	2.30	0.75	50	243	• Medium speed of onset and recovery • Hepatotoxicity

Abbreviations: MAC, minimum alveolar concentration; NMDA, N-methyl-D-aspartate.

Contraindication for the Volatile Anesthetic Agents

- Genetic disorders:

  The volatile anesthetics can cause malignant hyperthermia in susceptible individuals. So, individuals with positive family history for malignant hyperthermia must be evaluated prior to surgery, and volatile anesthetics should be avoided.

- Relative contraindications:

  ► Severe hypovolemia.

  ► Severe intracranial hypertension.

Contraindication for the Use of Nitrous Oxide

- Patients undergoing open brain surgeries, bowel surgery, intraocular and middle ear surgeries.

- Patients with pneumothorax or pulmonary hypertension.

Precautions to be Taken with the Use of Halothane

Although it has been replaced with the newer inhalational agents in major operating theaters, certain precautions need to be highlighted with its use in rural/undeveloped hospitals:

- Unexplained pyrexial illness, unexpected liver damage after halothane anesthesia, or exposure within the last 3 months contraindicates a second exposure.

- Avoid heavy sedation with morphine.

- Administer atropine before induction with halothane.

- Epinephrine dose to be monitored and administered only when there is no hypoxia/hypercapnia. *Dose not to exceed 20 mL of 1:2,00,000 in 10 minutes or 30 mL in an hour.*

Adverse Effects of Inhalational Agents

- **Acute toxicities**

  ► Carbon monoxide (CO) toxicity:

    The propensity of volatile anesthetic agents to form CO in contact with anhydrous soda-lime or baralyme is potentially life-threatening. *Desflurane is the largest producer of CO,* followed by enflurane and isoflurane.

    Carbon monoxide toxicity was reported during the first case of anesthesia on Monday (Monday morning phenomenon), on account of the gas flows in anesthesia machines being left open after the last case on Saturday. The continuous flows of gas through carbon dioxide absorbent leads to desiccation of soda lime, resulting in decreased absorption of CO_2 and formation of carbon monoxide on exposure to inhaled anesthetics. So, switching off the gas flow when the machine is not in use and changing the carbon dioxide absorbent (in case of uncertainty about the duration of exposure to gas flows) should be practiced to avoid carbon monoxide toxicity.

    Modern carbon dioxide (CO_2) absorbents do not contain potassium and sodium hydroxide. They contain calcium and lithium hydroxide and generate one-tenth of the CO produced by the traditional absorbers.

  ► Nephrotoxicity:

    It occurs most commonly with sevoflurane. Its metabolism leads to high levels of inorganic fluoride. Levels of fluoride correlate with the degree of renal impairment.

The interaction of sevoflurane with CO_2 absorbents leads to the formation of products like trifluoromethyl vinyl ether; also known as Compound A. The levels of compound A in the range of 25 to 50 ppm or greater in rodent models has shown to cause renal injury.

- **Diffusion hypoxia**

The gases entering into alveoli from the bloodstream at the end of the surgery, particularly nitrous oxide, can displace oxygen and lead to diffusion hypoxia. This effect can be minimized by diluting the alveolar nitrous oxide with supplemental oxygen.

- **Overdose**

It may lead to cardiovascular and respiratory depression. There is no pharmacological intervention for an overdose of inhaled anesthetics. The treatment involves supportive care with optimal ventilator settings and alveolar clearance.

- **Chronic toxicities of inhalational anesthetics**

These include hematotoxicity, teratogenic effects, and carcinogenic toxicities.

Hematotoxicity with prolonged exposure to nitrous oxide is due to a reduction in the recycling of vitamin B12, which can cause megaloblastic anemia and peripheral neuropathies.

- **Postoperative nausea and vomiting (PONV)**

All the volatile anesthetics have the potential to cause nausea and vomiting. Therefore, prophylactic antiemetics should be administered in patients receiving inhalational agents for anesthesia.

- **Environmental pollution**

Greenhouse effect–waste anesthetic gases (WAG) contain nitrous oxide. Only 0.004% of nitrous oxide is metabolized and is thus exhaled unchanged into the atmosphere. It accounts for 6% of the total thermal effect of all the greenhouse gases (GHG) emitted in the atmosphere. Halogenated anesthetics like isoflurane, sevoflurane, and desflurane are also included in the category of "greenhouse gases."

Ozone depletion: Nitrous oxide and halogenated chlorofluorocarbons (halothane, enflurane, isoflurane) cause depletion of the earth's ozone layer. Fluorinated hydrocarbons (sevoflurane and desflurane) have little effect on ozone.

Conclusion

The use of inhaled anesthetics has been continuously evolving since the introduction of ether and chloroform. The delivery of inhaled anesthetic requires vaporizers and appropriate dial concentration, while fresh gas flows achieve adequate concentration in the alveoli. Each inhaled anesthetic has specific pharmacokinetic and pharmacodynamic properties which anesthesia providers must be aware of. The inhaled anesthetic agents are not without adverse effects. The byproducts of halothane can cause hepatotoxicity, while that of sevoflurane can cause nephrotoxicity.

CHAPTER 9

Intravenous Anesthetic Agents (AS4.1)

Tanvir Samra

Introduction

Intravenous (IV) anesthetic agents are the most common drugs used in day-to-day anesthesia practice. It encompasses agents like sedative-hypnotics, anxiolytics, opioids, and muscle relaxants. The combination of all these agents is used to achieve the desired level of anesthesia and analgesia with minimal side effects collectively known as "balanced anesthesia."

Classification

The IV anesthetic agents can be classified, as shown in the schematic flowchart below (**Flowchart 9.1**).

The sedatives and hypnotics can be further categorized into barbiturates and nonbarbiturates:

- Barbiturates, for example, thiopentone, methohexitone.
- Nonbarbiturates, for example, propofol, ketamine, etomidate.

Nonopioid IV Anesthetic Agents

Barbiturates

Thiopentone: Thiopentone is a barbiturate, and its introduction in 1934 by Water and Lundy has changed the face of modern anesthesia practice.

Physicochemical Properties

- A rapid-acting barbiturate derived from barbituric acid. The substitution with a particular chemical group in barbituric acid imparts characteristic property to the parent compound:
  - Sulfur at second position—increases lipid solubility.
  - Aryl/alkyl group at fifth position—has hypnotic and sedative effects.
  - Increase in length of alkyl chain at fifth position—increases potency.

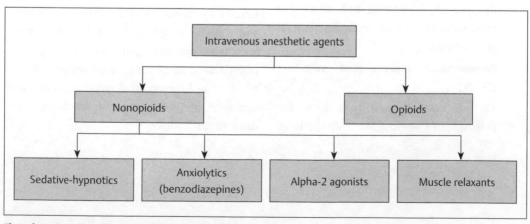

Flowchart 9.1 Classification of intravenous anesthetic agents.

▶ Phenyl group at fifth position—increases anticonvulsant activity (but no effect on hypnotic activity).

▶ Methyl group on nitrogen—increases hypnotic potency but lowers the seizure threshold.

- Preparation: Yellow amorphous powder (500- and 1,000-mg vial) prepared in the atmosphere of nitrogen and 6% anhydrous sodium carbonate is added to prevent precipitation of free acid by carbon dioxide from the atmosphere.

- The powder is diluted to prepare a 2.5% solution (*acidic pH of Ringer lactate can precipitate thiopentone; so it should not be used for dilution*).

- The 2.5% solution is highly alkaline with a pH of 10.4 and pKa of 7.6.

- The freshly prepared solution should be used within 48 hours; however, it can be used for 1 week if refrigerated.

Mechanism of Action

- It acts on GABA$_A$ receptors in the central nervous system (CNS) and causes the opening of chloride channels, leading to CNS depression through hyperpolarization of neurons.

- At low-dose, *it is GABA-facilitatory, while at higher doses, it acts as GABA-mimetic.*

- It also acts on glutamate, adenosine, and neuronal nicotinic acetylcholine receptors.

Pharmacokinetics

- It has rapid uptake and rapid distribution out of the brain into inactive tissues, leading to unconsciousness in one brain-arm circulation time (i.e., 15 s) after an IV dose.

- 80 to 90% is bound to plasma proteins (mainly albumin).

- 99% of thiopentone is metabolized by the liver (*low-hepatic extraction ratio and capacity-dependent elimination*) and excreted through the kidney.

- The prolonged infusion or repeated doses of thiopentone leads to its accumulation in muscle and fat. The thiopentone is released into circulation after stopping the infusion and causes delayed awakening.

- With usual induction doses (4–5 mg/kg), it follows first-order kinetics (i.e., a constant fraction is cleared per unit time), while at higher doses (200–300 mg/kg), it follows zero-order kinetics (a constant amount is cleared per unit time).

- The children and adults are similar in terms of protein binding and volume of distribution.

- Increased protein binding in pregnant patients leads to longer elimination half-life.

Pharmacodynamics and Clinical Applications

CNS

- It produces unconsciousness in 15 seconds after an IV dose.

- It causes a dose-dependent decrement in cerebral metabolic rate, cerebral oxygen consumption, and intracranial pressure (ICP) and thus provides neuroprotection against partial cerebral ischemia (however, there is no neuroprotection in global ischemia).

- At lower doses, barbiturates decrease pain threshold.

- There is dose-related suppression of EEG.

- There is a lower degree of amnesia compared to benzodiazepines.

Respiratory system

- Dose-related central respiratory depression with increased susceptibility in patients with chronic lung diseases.

- Respiratory depression correlates with EEG suppression and minute ventilation.

- The peak respiratory depression occurs at 1 to 1.5 minutes of drug administration and returns to baseline within 15 minutes.

- Thiopental causes "double apnea" in 20% of cases, which can be described as apnea of few seconds succeeded by few breaths of normal tidal volume, with subsequent prolonged apnea (25 s).

Cardiovascular system

- It causes hypotension by the following mechanisms:

  ▶ Negative inotropic effect.

  ▶ Decreased ventricular filling (venous pooling).

  ▶ Reduced sympathetic outflow from CNS.

- There is baroreceptor reflex-mediated tachycardia (avoid in patients with coronary artery disease [CAD]).

- Prolongation of QT interval and flattening of T wave (so, it is not good for patients at risk of QT prolongation and ventricular arrhythmias).

- Significant reduction in cardiac output (not good for hypovolemic patients).

Complications

The IV use of thiopentone can sometime result in local complications such as thrombophlebitis, tissue necrosis due to intramuscular (IM)/subcutaneous (SC) injection, but the most dreadful is an intra-arterial injection which needs special attention here.

Intra-arterial injection: The inadvertent intra-arterial injection (commonly happen when thiopentone is injected in antecubital fossa) can cause gangrene and loss of limb if timely diagnosis and intervention are not instituted. The high alkalinity and pH of blood lead to precipitation and crystal formation which, in turn, leads to vasospasm and thrombus formation with consequent ischemia. Utmost precautions should be taken to prevent such incidents, and these are as follows:

- Always use a 2.5% solution.

- Slow injection in incremental doses.

- Avoid injection in the antecubital fossa.

Once the intra-arterial injection has happened, the definitive measures include:

- Leave the needle at its site and use it for all therapeutic injections.

- Dilution with normal saline.

- Inject heparin to prevent thrombus formation.

- Papaverine or 1% lignocaine to cause local vasodilation.

- Relieve vasospasm with stellate ganglion block if the above measures do not work.

- Defer the elective surgery.

- Prescribe oral anticoagulants and follow-up in consultation with the vascular surgeon.

Dosing

Induction dose is 3 to 4 mg/kg.

Uses

- Induction and maintenance of anesthesia.

- Electroconvulsive therapy (ECT).

- Cerebral protection.

Side Effects

- Hypotension.

- Coughing and laryngospasm.

- Apnoea at induction.

- Allergic reactions.

Contraindications

- Absolute:

  ▶ Porphyria (except porphyria cutanea tarda).

  ▶ History of allergy.

- Relative:
  - ▶ Hypovolemia, fixed cardiac output lesions, CAD.
  - ▶ Asthmatics (risk of asthma precipitation).
  - ▶ Severe hepatic dysfunction (decreased metabolism).
  - ▶ Renal dysfunction (dose reduction required).

> Endpoint of induction with thiopentone = loss of eyelash reflex

Methohexitone

It is an ultrashort-acting barbiturate with an anesthetic effect lasting for 2 to 5 minutes. It is twice as potent as thiopentone. The epileptogenic potential of methohexitone makes it an attractive choice for ECT.

The solution is stable for 6 weeks at 25°C.

Nonbarbiturates

Propofol: Propofol is popularly known as "milk of anesthesia" among anesthesia providers. It was discovered in 1970 by John B. Glenn and approved by the Food and Drug Administration (FDA) in 1989 for clinical use.

Physicochemical Properties

- It is an alkylphenol, and its chemical name is *2,6-diisopropyl phenol.*
- It is milky white in appearance due to scattering of light by the lipid droplets.
- pH = 6 to 8.5.
- Protein-binding: 97 to 99%.
- Constituents of 1% propofol preparation are as follows:
  - ▶ 1% propofol.
  - ▶ 10% soyabean oil (emulsifier).
  - ▶ 1.2% purified egg phospholipid (emulsifier).
  - ▶ 2.25% glycerol (to maintain tonicity).
  - ▶ NaOH (to maintain the pH of the solution).
- Caloric value = 1 kcal/mL.

> Because of the risk of bacterial contamination, EDTA/sodium metabisulphite is added as a bacteriostatic agent, and it is recommended to discard the propofol vial after 6 hours of opening it.

- The propofol causes pain at the injection site due to soyabean oil. The fospropofol, a water-soluble preparation of propofol, introduced in 2008 by FDA does not cause pain on injection; however, perineal paresthesias and pruritus have been reported after bolus injection.

Mechanism of Action

The main site of action is the beta-subunit of $GABA_A$ receptors. It is GABA-facilitatory in a lower dose and GABA-mimetic with higher doses. The other receptors are:

- Potentiation of glycine receptors in the spinal cord.
- Serotonergic receptors in area postrema (antiemetic action).
- Inhibition of NMDA/glutamate receptors.
- Increase in dopamine in nucleus accumbens (possible role in pleasure-seeking behavior and abuse potential).

Pharmacokinetics

- It is oxidized to 1,4-diisopropylquinol in the liver, followed by conjugation with glucuronic acid and consequent excretion through kidneys.
- The major site of metabolism is the liver (high-hepatic extraction ratio, so the metabolism is hepatic blood flow-dependent). The other sites are kidneys and lungs.

- The context-sensitive half-life is 40 minutes after 8 hours of infusion.

- The dose requirement decreases with age.

- The children require a higher dose than adults because of the larger volume of distribution and rapid clearance of the drug.

- Elimination half-life: 4 to 7 hours.

Pharmacodynamics

CNS

- The hypnosis onset occurs in one brain-arm circulation time (30 s), with peak effect at 90 to 100 seconds.

- Effect on EEG shows an initial rise in alpha rhythm, followed by a shift to gamma and theta rhythm.

- It causes a dose-dependent decrease in cerebral metabolic oxygen consumption, cerebral blood flow, and ICP; however, its role in neuroprotection is controversial.

- It is a dose-dependent anticonvulsant; grand mal seizures have been described in the literature.

- It has abuse potential; however, the evidence for it among the general public is scarce.

- It causes a remarkable decrease in intra-ocular pressure (30–40%).

The awakening and orientation occurs at a plasma concentration of 1.6 and 1.2 µg/mL, respectively.

The endpoint of induction is the loss of response to verbal commands, and it correlates with the plasma level of 2.3 to 3.5 µg/mL (propofol alone).

Respiratory system

- An induction dose of propofol cause apnea in 25 to 30% of the subjects.

- Infusion of propofol decreases hypoxic drive through its action on carotid body chemoreceptors.

- A good bronchodilator in chronic obstructive pulmonary disorder (COPD) patients.

- It potentiates hypoxic pulmonary vasoconstriction.

- It blunts airway reflexes better than thiopentone.

Cardiovascular system

- It causes significant hypotension by decreasing systolic, diastolic, and mean arterial pressure. It occurs through the following mechanisms:

  ▶ Direct myocardial depression (controversial).

  ▶ Venous pooling because of vasodilation.

  ▶ Decreased sympathetic drive to the heart.

- *It blunts baroreceptor reflex* (so no significant tachycardia in response to hypotension).

- The hemodynamic response to propofol lags behind the hypnotic effect.

Gastrointestinal tract

- It is a potent antiemetic.

Other effects

- It does not enhance neuromuscular blockade produced by muscle relaxants.

- No effect on evoked responses.

- Does not trigger malignant hyperthermia.

- No effect on corticosteroid synthesis or adrenocorticotropic hormone (ACTH) stimulation.

- It decreases chemotaxis of neutrophils but has no effect on phagocytosis and killing.

Uses

- Induction of anesthesia: 1 to 2.5 mg/kg (adults), 2 to 3 mg/kg (children), 1 to 1.75 mg/kg (>60 years).

- Maintenance of anesthesia: Dose (50–150 µg/kg/min with opiates or nitrous oxide).

- For sedation in intensive care units: Dose (25–75 µg/kg/min).

- In combination with remifentanil for total intravenous anesthesia (TIVA).

- As an antiemetic: 10 to 20 mg IV can be repeated every 5 to 10 minutes or infusion of 10 µg/kg/min.

Side Effects

- Pain at injection site is quite common, and the following measures can decrease it:
  ▶ Use a large vein.
  ▶ Use of water-soluble preparation (e.g., fospropofol).
  ▶ Addition of lidocaine to the syringe of propofol.
  ▶ Use of opiates/nonsteroidal anti-inflammatory drugs (NSAIDs)/ketamine/esmolol/clonidine/dexamethasone.
  ▶ Use of Valsalva maneuver.
- Apnea.
- Hypotension.
- Thrombophlebitis.
- Risk of bacterial contamination and sepsis.
- Propofol-infusion syndrome:
  ▶ A rare lethal syndrome which occurs mostly in critically ill patients who receive it for sedation at doses 4 mg/kg/hr for more than 48 hours.
  ▶ Clinical manifestations:
    ○ Acute refractory bradycardia.
    ○ Metabolic acidosis.
    ○ Rhabdomyolysis.
    ○ Cardiac arrhythmias.
    ○ Hyperlipidemia.
    ○ Fatty liver.
    ○ Cardiomyopathy/skeletal myopathy.
    ○ Increased hepatic transaminases.
    ○ A rise in serum creatinine.

The risk factors for propofol infusion syndrome are:

▶ Sepsis.
▶ Significant brain injury.
▶ Larger propofol dose.
▶ Genetic disorders involving the metabolism of fatty acids.

Treatment of propofol infusion syndrome includes:

- Discontinue propofol infusion immediately.
- Supportive care with:
  ▶ Hemodialysis.
  ▶ Hemodynamic support (with fluids and vasopressors/inotropes).
  ▶ Extracorporeal membrane oxygenation (ECMO) in refractory cases.

Contraindications

- Known hypersensitivity or allergy to propofol.
- Fat metabolism disorder.

> The egg allergy occurs due to proteins in egg white not due to egg lecithin. So, patients who are allergic to egg proteins can safely receive propofol (as preparation contains egg lecithin and not the egg white).
>
> Propofol is safe in pregnancy and lactating mothers.

Etomidate

It was first manufactured by Janssen Chemicals in 1965 as an antifungal agent.

Physicochemical Properties

- It is an imidazole derivative.
- It is a R-enantiomer, which is five times more potent than S-enantiomer.

- Preparation: 0.2% solution (either in lipid emulsion or 35% propylene glycol).
- pKa = 4.2.

Mechanism of Action

- It acts on $GABA_A$ receptor and produces hypnosis.

Pharmacokinetics

- It can be given through IV/per oral/ rectal route.
- Context-sensitive half-life is less than propofol.
- Protein binding: 75%.
- It is metabolized into carboxylic acid and ethanol in the liver through ester hydrolysis and excreted in urine and bile.
- Use of continuous infusion is limited by adrenal suppression caused by etomidate.

Pharmacodynamics

CNS

- Hypnosis occurs in one brain-arm circulation time.
- Similar to thiopentone and propofol, it is GABA-facilitatory in low dose and GABA-mimetic in a higher dose.
- It decreases cerebral blood flow, cerebral oxygen consumption, and ICP (the neuroprotective effect is controversial).
- It has epileptogenic potential.
- It produces a dose-related increase in latency and decrease in amplitude of the auditory-evoked response.

Respiratory system

- It does not cause histamine release.
- It depresses ventilatory response to rising arterial carbon dioxide.

Cardiovascular system

- The lack of effect on the sympathetic system and baroreceptor makes etomidate a cardiostable agent (agent of choice in hemorrhagic patients).
- It maintains the myocardial oxygen demand–supply ratio.

Endocrine effects

- It causes dose-related, reversible inhibition of *11-betahydroxylase* enzyme, which is required for the synthesis of cortisol and aldosterone.
- The dose required to cause adrenal suppression is almost 20 times less than that required for the hypnotic effect. The adrenal suppression can persist for 72 hours.
- The recent literature suggests that the single-dose etomidate does not increase mortality in critically ill patients.

Uses

- Induction of anesthesia, as it is a popular agent for induction in patients with:
  ▶ Hemorrhagic shock.
  ▶ Traumatic brain injury with raised ICP.
  ▶ Unstable angina.
  ▶ Unstable CAD.
    Dose: 0.2 to 0.6 mg/kg.
- Short-term sedation for cardioversion.
- Acute hypercortisolism to decrease cortisol level.
- Etomidate speech and memory test to localize speech area before lobectomies.
- Localize epileptogenic foci before surgery.

Side Effects

- Hypocortisolism.
- Pain on IV injection.
- Myoclonus.
- Hiccups.
- Thrombophlebitis.
- Nausea and vomiting.
- Emergence delirium.

Ketamine

The use of ketamine dates back to 1956 when Corssen and Domino used it for the first time in humans.

Physicochemical Properties

- It is a phencyclidine derivative and consists of R(−) ketamine and S(+) ketamine.
- The S(+) form is a more potent analgesic with faster clearance and fewer psychomimetic effects.
- Partially water-soluble and 12% protein-bound.
- Molecular weight: 238 kilodalton.

Mechanism of Action

It antagonizes NMDA receptors and produces dissociative anesthesia rather than general anesthesia. Ketamine inhibits cortex (unconsciousness) and thalamus (analgesia) and stimulates the limbic system (emergence reaction and hallucinations).

Pharmacokinetics

- The major pathway of metabolism is through hepatic microsomal enzymes. The final product of metabolism is norketamine, which is conjugated with glucuronic acid and excreted in urine.
- It has high-lipid solubility and results in a larger volume of distribution.
- The onset of action occurs in 30 to 60 seconds, and the effect lasts for 10 to 15 minutes after an IV dose.
- It attenuates acute tolerance to opioids.

Pharmacodynamics

CNS

- It produces dose-dependent analgesia and unconsciousness.

- It produces the classic "dissociative anesthesia."
- It has profound analgesic potential.
- It increases cerebral blood flow, cerebral metabolism, and ICP.
- Emergency reactions: It is characterized by vivid dreams, extracorporeal experience, illusions which occur within 1 hour of awakening, and disappear within the next few hours. It occurs due to the inhibition of auditory and visual stimuli nuclei.
- Auditory and visual hallucinations are common (auditory > visual), with an incidence of 30 to 40%.

Respiratory system

- It has minimal effect on central respiratory drive.
- It is a potent bronchial smooth muscle relaxant.
- It increases tracheobronchial and salivary secretions, mandating the use of atropine/glycopyrrolate with ketamine.
- Although pharyngeal and laryngeal reflexes are preserved with ketamine, the possibility of silent aspirations cannot be ignored.

Cardiovascular system

- It increases cardiac output, causes hypertension and tachycardia by inhibition of vagal output, and decreases uptake of catecholamines.
- It has direct myocardial depressant action, which can lead to profound hypotension in debilitated patients (e.g., sepsis).

Other Effects

- It increases intraocular pressure.
- It increases intragastric pressure.
- It increases muscle tone, and the patient may show nonpurposeful movement.

Dosing

It can be through IV, IM, per oral, rectal, and intrathecal routes.

- Induction dose:
  - ▸ IV: 0.5 to 2.0 mg/kg.
  - ▸ IM: 4 to 6 mg/kg.
- Maintenance dose:
  - ▸ 0.5 to 1.0 mg/kg IV with 50% nitrous oxide.
  - ▸ 15 to 45 µg/kg/min with 50 to 70% nitrous oxide.
  - ▸ 30 to 90 µg/kg/min without nitrous oxide.
- Sedation:
  - ▸ 0.2 to 0.8 mg/kg (IV).
  - ▸ 2 to 4 mg/kg (IM).

Uses

- It is the induction agent of choice in:
  - ▸ Asthmatics (potent bronchodilation).
  - ▸ Shock (sympathetic stimulation and preservation or augmentation of blood pressure).
  - ▸ Low-cardiac output state (sympathetic stimulation).
  - ▸ Right-to-left shunt (Tetralogy of Fallot [TOF]); increasing systemic vascular resistance (SVR) decreases right-to-left shunt.
  - ▸ Full stomach patients (preserved laryngeal and pharyngeal reflexes).
- Pain management: Postoperative pain in chronic pain conditions like cancer pain and phantom limb pain.
- Sedation: Ketamine in combination with benzodiazepines and antisialologues can be used in pediatric patients for sedation.

Side Effects

- Hallucinations and emergency reactions.
- Potential for laryngospasm and bronchospasm (increase in pharyngeal and respiratory secretions).
- Increase in intracranial, intraocular, and intragastric pressure.

Contraindications

- Head injury with raised ICP.
- Ischemic heart disease.
- Glaucoma.
- Vascular aneurysm.
- Patients with psychiatric illness.
- Hypertension.
- Pheochromocytoma.
- Hyperthyroidism.

Benzodiazepines

Since the discovery of benzodiazepines (BDZs) in 1954, their use as anxiolytics and sedatives is well recognized in modern anesthesia practice. These can be short-acting (midazolam), intermediate-acting (lorazepam, temazepam), and long-acting (diazepam).

Physicochemical Properties

- The basic chemical structure is an imidazole ring, which opens up in the case of midazolam at pH of 3.5 and makes midazolam stable and lipophilic. This ring closes at physiological pH.
- They have a rapid onset of action due to high lipophilicity.

Pharmacokinetics

- The pharmacokinetic properties of benzodiazepines are summarized in **Table 9.1**.

Mechanism of Action

The benzodiazepines act on $GABA_A$ receptors and increases the frequency of opening of chloride channels, leading to repolarization and

Table 9.1 Pharmacokinetics of BDZs

Properties	Midazolam	Diazepam	Lorazepam	Remimazolam
Route of administration	Oral, IV, IM, nasal, rectal	Oral, IV, IM	Oral, IV, IM	IV
Protein binding (%)	94–98	98–99	88–92	Not applicable
Metabolism	Hepatic	Hepatic	Hepatic	Plasma esterases
Elimination half-life (h)	1.7–3.5	20–50	11–22	0.4

Abbreviations: BDZ, benzodiazepine; IM, intramuscular; IV, intravenous.

consequently decreased transmission of action potential along the neurons.

Pharmacodynamics

- **CNS**
  - ▶ The interaction of benzodiazepines with GABA receptors is complex. The interaction with a specific subunit produces a specific effect. For example, interaction with the alpha-1 subunit produces sedation, amnesia, and anti-epileptic effect, while that with the alpha-2 subunit produces anxiolysis and muscle relaxation.
  - ▶ They cause a dose-related decrease in cerebral oxygen consumption.
  - ▶ Midazolam has neuroprotective effect.
- **Respiratory system**
  - ▶ They cause dose-related respiratory depression. Old age and use of other sedatives further increase the risk.
  - ▶ They heighten the risk of upper airway obstruction due to a decrease in the tone of upper airway muscles.
  - ▶ They also decrease the respiratory drive in response to rising carbon dioxide in the blood.
- **Cardiovascular system**
  - ▶ BDZs decrease SVR, leading to a modest fall in blood pressure, with no effect on hemodynamic reflexes.

Uses

- **Premedication**
  - ▶ These are the most common drugs for premedication, with midazolam being the preferred agent.
  - ▶ The dose of midazolam is 7.5 to 10 mg in adults and 0.025 mg/kg in children.
- **Sedation**
  - ▶ Sedation reduces anxiety and enhances the patient's satisfaction. The dose for midazolam is 0.5 to 1.0 mg and can be repeated.
- **Induction and maintenance of anesthesia**
  - ▶ Midazolam is the agent of choice among all benzodiazepines. The dose for induction is 0.1 to 0.2 mg/kg in premedicated patients, and 0.3 mg/kg in unpremedicated patients. The onset of action is 3 to 5 minutes.
  - ▶ The elderly patients require a smaller dose than the adults.

Side Effects and Contraindications

- The most significant is the risk of respiratory depression.
- Pain on injection with water-insoluble preparations (lorazepam, diazepam).
- They can also cause prolonged amnesia, sedation, and respiratory depression in the postoperative period.

Advantages of Midazolam over Lorazepam and Diazepam

- Water-soluble preparation of midazolam causes less pain on injection compared to oily preparations of lorazepam and diazepam.
- Short elimination half-life of midazolam leads to lesser risk of respiratory depression and can therefore be used for ambulatory surgeries.
- The reversal with flumazenil is complete.

Flumazenil

It is the first antagonist for BDZs, causing reversible, competitive antagonism at BDZ receptors. It has high affinity and specificity, with minimal intrinsic effects on BDZ receptors. The risk of rebound sedation and respiratory depression is quite high (especially with lorazepam) because of rapid metabolism, rapid kinetics of binding as well as unbinding to BDZ receptors.

Doses

Reversal of BDZs: 0.2 mg repeated up to 3 mg.

Diagnosis in coma: 0.5 mg repeated up to 1 mg.

Alpha-2 Adrenergic Agonists

Alpha-2 adrenergic agonists were recognized to have hypnotic, sedative, anxiolytic, analgesic, and sympatholytic properties after using clonidine in patients. Dexmedetomidine is more selective for alpha-2 receptor compared to clonidine with alpha-2 to alpha-1 ratio of 1600:1 (220:1 for clonidine).

Dexmedetomidine was introduced in 1999 for short-term sedation (<24 h) in intensive care.

Dexmedetomidine

Physicochemical Properties

- S-enantiomer of medetomidine.
- It is an alpha-2 adrenergic agonist with pKa = 7.1.
- It is water-soluble.

Mechanism of Action

It acts on alpha-2 receptors. The action on presynaptic alpha-2 receptors inhibits the release of norepinephrine and attenuate vasoconstriction, while that on postsynaptic alpha-2 receptor causes peripheral vasoconstriction.

Pharmacokinetics

- The major pathway of metabolism is hepatic glucuronidation, followed by renal excretion.
- It is 94% protein-bound.
- Elimination half-life is 2 to 3 hours.

Pharmacodynamics

CNS

- The sedative-hypnotic effect is due to action on an alpha-2 receptor on locus ceruleus.
- The analgesic action is due to action on alpha-2 receptors on locus ceruleus and spinal cord.
- The cerebral blood flow decreases with increasing dose, with no effect on cerebral oxygen consumption.
- Minimal effect on amplitude and latency of evoked potentials.

Respiratory system

- It decreases minute ventilation, with no change in arterial oxygenation, pH, and slope of CO_2 ventilatory response.

Cardiovascular system

- There is initial hypertension due to alpha-1 mediated vasoconstriction.
- It causes hypotension, bradycardia, and consequent decrease in cardiac output.
- It reduces perioperative oxygen consumption and blunts sympathetic response to surgery.

Uses

- As premedication (0.33–0.67 µg/kg, 15 min before surgery).

- Sedation (for awake craniotomy, deep brain stimulation, surgical procedure near speech area, awake carotid endarterectomy, and sedation in intensive care).

- Treatment of addiction (cocaine withdrawal, rapid opioid detoxification).

- As an adjuvant to peripheral and central neuraxial blocks.

- To attenuate cardiovascular response to intubation.

Side Effects

- Initial hypertension.

- Hypotension (most common side effect).

- Bradycardia.

The adverse effects of dexmedetomidine can be reversed with atipamezole. However, it is not approved for use in humans.

Opioids

The origin of the term opioids lies in the word "opium (poppy juice)." The poppy juice is extracted from papaver somniferum. A few important terminologies related to opioids are as follows:

- **Opiates:** It includes all the drugs derived from opium.

- **Narcotic:** It is a drug with morphine-like analgesic activity and the potential to produce physical dependence.

- **Opioids:** All the exogenous substances (natural or synthetic) that bind to opioid receptors and produce agonist-like activity.

The opioids can be classified on the basis of their source/preparation (**Table 9.2**) and their interaction with the opioid receptors (**Table 9.3**).

Mechanism of Action

The opioids bind to opioid receptors (G-protein coupled) and alter the second messenger pathways as well as expression of genes, leading to:

- Increase in K+ efflux that leads to hyperpolarization of the cell membrane and consequent decrease in nerve transmission.

- A decrease in substance P release.

- NMDA antagonism in high concentration.

The most important sites of opioid action are:

- Periaqueductal gray matter.

- Ventral medulla.

Table 9.2 Classification of opioids based on source/preparation

Natural	Semisynthetic	Synthetic
• Morphine • Codeine • Thebaine • Papaverine	• Heroin • Dihydromorphone • Morphinone • Thebaine derivatives	• Morphinan series (levorphanol, butorphanol) • Benzomorphan (pentazocine) • Phenypiperidine (fentanyl, sufentanil, remifentanil) • Diphenylpropylamine (methadone)

Table 9.3 Classification of opioids based on receptor interaction

Agonists	Agonist-antagonists	Antagonists
• Morphine • Morphine-6-glucornide • Meperidine • Fentanyl/sufentanil/remifenatanil • Codeine • Tramadol	• Pentazocine • Butorphanol • Nalbuphine • Buprenorphine • Nalorphine • Dezocine	• Naloxone • Naltrexone • Nalmefene • Methylnaltrexone • Alvimopan

- Locus ceruleus.

- Substantia gelatinosa (spinal cord).

The opioid receptor types are described in **Table 9.4**.

Pharmacodynamics

CNS

- Analgesia: Opioids produce analgesia at both spinal as well as supraspinal levels, with no effect on consciousness. There is no effect on other sensory modalities, and when morphine is given to a pain-free individual, it produces unpleasant sensation.

- Consciousness: Opioids decrease the minimum alveolar concentration (MAC) requirement of volatile anesthetics and enhance the hypnotic effect of propofol.

- EEG: Opioids induce sleep-like pattern, with the replacement of alpha waves by delta waves.

- Evoked response: Opioids have minimal effect on latency and amplitude of somatosensory-evoked potentials (SSEPs).

- Cerebral blood flow (CBF)/cerebral metabolic rate (CMR): There is a modest decrease in CBF/CMR and ICP.

- Pupils: Opioids cause miosis through their action on Edinger–Westphal nucleus. *No tolerance is seen with miosis.*

- Stimulation of the chemoreceptor trigger zone lead to nausea and vomiting.

Respiratory system

- Opioids inhibit respiratory center in the brainstem and result in hypoventilation; the decrease in respiratory activity is more compared to the tidal volume.

- The effect on ventilation and analgesia happens through similar mechanisms; therefore, the reversal of respiratory depression with antagonists leads to the reversal of analgesia.

- There is a decrease in ventilatory drive in response to a rise in arterial carbon dioxide tension.

- They act as a cough suppressant.

- Opioids can increase airway resistance with the release of histamine.

- Delayed and recurring respiratory depression—delayed respiratory depression occurs due to:

  ▶ Sequestration of opioids in stomach and reabsorption in blood.

  ▶ Deposition of opioids in skeletal muscle and later released into circulation.

Cardiovascular system

- There is no hypotension in normovolemic patients in the supine position. However, hypotension does occur in susceptible individuals due to venous pooling and a decrease in central sympathetic tone.

- They cause bradycardia due to direct depressant action on the sinoatrial (SA)

Table 9.4 Types of opioid receptors

	μ Receptor (type 1)	μ Receptor (type 2)	Kappa	Delta
Effects	• Analgesia (spinal and supraspinal) • Euphoria • Miosis • Low abuse potential • Urinary retention	• Spinal analgesia • Physical dependence • Constipation	• Spinal and supraspinal analgesia • Dysphoria • Sedation • Miosis • Diuresis	• Suppression of ventilation • Physical dependence • Constipation • Urinary retention

node and increase in vagal tone (pethidine causes tachycardia).

- Opioids do not sensitize the heart to catecholamines.
- Opioids (especially morphine) can shift blood from pulmonary circulation to systemic circulation; hence, it can be used in pulmonary edema.

Muscular system

- The opioids can cause stiff chest syndrome or wooden chest syndrome due to an increase in the tone of intercostal muscles. Muscle rigidity is the most common with alfentanil. Hoarseness is the presenting feature in the awake patient, while the difficult bag and mask ventilation are seen after induction (due to rigidity of laryngeal musculature).
- The nondepolarizing muscle relaxants, thiopentone, and midazolam can be used to relieve muscular rigidity.

Gastrointestinal tract

- Opioids decrease gut motility and prolong the gastric emptying, leading to constipation.

Endocrine system

- There is a decrease in levels of ACTH, luteinizing hormone (LH), follicle-stimulating hormone (FSH), and cortisol, while an increase in the level of antidiuretic hormone (ADH), thyroid-stimulating hormone (TSH), growth hormone (GH), and prolactin.

Biliary tract

- Opioids increase the tone of sphincter of Oddi (maximum with fentanyl) and lead to difficulty in the interpretation of cholangiogram. They also cause an increase in contraction of the smooth muscle of pancreatic duct, with a resultant rise in lipase and amylase level, mimicking acute pancreatitis. Opioids should be avoided in case of biliary colic.

Genitourinary tract

- Opioids increase the tone and peristalsis of the ureter in addition to urinary urgency. They relax the bladder and can cause urinary retention.

Cutaneous

- Dilation of cutaneous blood vessels (of face, neck and upper torso) due to histamine release.

Immune effects

- Opioids suppress both innate and adaptive immunity.

Malignancy progression: Opioids, when given for general anesthesia, can lead to cancer recurrence as suggested by epidemiological studies.

Tolerance: Tolerance is mainly pharmacodynamic and is seen with all actions except constipation and miosis. There is cross-tolerance among all the opioids.

Placental transfer: Opioids cross the placenta and cause neonatal respiratory depression.

Salient Features of Individual Opioids

Opioid Agonists

- Morphine:
  ▶ Morphine can be given through IV, IM, oral, rectal, SC, intrathecal, and epidural routes.
  ▶ Dose (IV): 0.1 to 0.2 mg/kg.
  ▶ The onset after IV administration is at 10 to 15 minutes, with a peak effect at 45-90 minutes.
  ▶ The metabolism occurs in liver and kidney with morphine-3-glucuronide (inactive) and morphine-6-glucuronide (active) as metabolites.
  ▶ The metabolism and excretion may be impaired significantly in patients with hepatic and renal dysfunction, respectively; hence, dosing should be

adjusted based on hepatic and renal function.

► The elimination half-life is 2 to 4 hours.

► It has poor CNS penetrations because of:

  ○ Poor lipophilicity.

  ○ A higher degree of ionization at physiological pH.

  ○ Rapid conjugation with glucuronic acid.

• Pethidine:

  ► It has local anesthetic action.

  ► It is chemically related to atropine and hence has side effects like dry mouth, tachycardia, and blurred vision.

  ► It can be given through oral, IV, IM, SC, and epidural routes.

  ► It can be used in biliary colic patients, as it causes less marked smooth muscle contraction.

  ► It is the drug of choice for shivering.

  ► Pethidine is absolutely contraindicated in patients receiving MAO inhibitors.

  ► Pethidine is a myocardial suppressant which causes tachycardia. Therefore, it should be avoided in patients at risk of myocardial ischemia.

  ► The metabolite norpethidine has potential to cause myoclonus and seizures.

• Fentanyl:

  ► It can be given through IV, IM, transmucosal, transdermal, intrathecal, and epidural routes.

  ► It is the most common opioid to be used.

  ► It has the advantage of rapid onset (4–6 mins) and speedy recovery (1–2 h).

  ► Dose: 1 to 2 µg/kg IV for analgesia.

• Sufentanil:

  ► It is the thienyl analog of fentanyl.

► It is 10 times more potent than fentanyl.

► The analgesic dose is 0.1 to 0.4 µg/kg.

► It maximally inhibits airway reflexes and therefore is used to suppress stress response to laryngoscopy and intubation.

► It can cause bradycardia and chest wall rigidity.

• Alfentanil:

  ► It is one-fifth to one-tenth as potent as fentanyl.

  ► The blood–brain barrier (BBB) penetration is faster because of the higher unionized fraction.

  ► It is used to prevent stress response to laryngoscopy and intubation.

  ► It is associated with chest wall rigidity and acute dystonia in Parkinson patients.

• Remifentanil:

  ► It is 15 to 20 times more potent than alfentanil.

  ► It has a rapid onset of action (1 min) and fast recovery (5–10 mins) due to metabolism by plasma esterases.

  ► Because of its short duration of action, a longer-acting opioid must be given before stopping the infusion for maintaining the level of analgesia.

  ► It is used to prevent laryngoscopy, intubation stress response, and response to retrobulbar block.

  ► It is associated with nausea, vomiting, respiratory depression, and seizure-like activity.

• Tramadol:

  ► It is a derivative of codeine with properties of local anesthetics and antibacterial actions.

  ► It is 5 to 10 times less potent than morphine.

- It produces centrally mediated analgesia. It is helpful in chronic pain management due to inhibition of uptake of serotonin and norepinephrine in the spinal cord.

- The respiratory rate and minute ventilation remain unchanged after tramadol administration.

- It produces nausea, dizziness, and has seizure potential. The potential for tolerance and dependence appears to be low.

- It is not licensed for intraoperative use, as it can cause recall with enflurane and nitrous oxide anesthesia.

- Dose: 50 to 100 mg every 4 to 6 hours (IV/IM).

Agonists-Antagonists

These agents have less potential for abuse and have a ceiling effect on respiratory depression.

- Pentazocine:
  - It is a buprenorphine derivative and can be given through oral, IV, and epidural routes.
  - It has agonistic action at kappa and delta receptors, while antagonist action at μ receptors.
  - Its potency as an antagonist is one-fifth of nalbuphine.
  - Half-life = 2 to 3 hours.
  - It causes hypertension and tachycardia due to stimulation of the sympathetic system.
  - It is effective in the treatment of pruritus after cesarean under subarachnoid block.
  - Nausea and vomiting are less than the morphine.
  - Ceiling effects on analgesia and respiratory depression occur at doses of 30 and 70 mg, respectively.

- Buprenorphine:
  - It is a thebaine derivative with partial agonism at μ receptor and antagonism at kappa receptor.
  - Its potency is almost 33 times of morphine.
  - Slower onset of action, with a peak effect around 3 hours of administration.

Opioid Antagonists

- Naloxone:
  - It was introduced in clinical practice in the late 1960s. It antagonizes the effects of opioids at all receptors, with the maximum propensity for the μ receptors.
  - The onset occurs within 1 to 2 minutes of IV administration, and the duration of action lasts for 30 to 60 minutes.
  - The short duration of action of naloxone necessitates continuous infusion after bolus dose to prevent renarcotization.
  - It can also be given through intrathecal route if the IV access is not available.
  - The reversal of buprenorphine is partial because of high affinity and slow dissociation from the receptors.
  - The administration naloxone can result in a rise in blood pressure and heart rate through the following mechanisms:
    - Pain.
    - Rapid awakening.
    - Sympathetic activation.
  - The oxygen consumption can increase markedly after naloxone administration in hypothermic patients.
  - The pheochromocytoma patients may be at higher risk of hypertension and tachycardia after naloxone administration. However, the studies do not support a significant rise in plasma

catecholamine concentration and rise in blood pressure up to 10 mg of naloxone.

▸ Dose: Opioid overdose—0.4 to 2 mg IV/SC/IM, repeat every 2 to 3 minutes, not to exceed 10 mg.

Other uses of naloxone:

o Prevention of acute opioid tolerance.

o Reversal of effects of alcohol, barbiturates, and benzodiazepine.

o Septic shock—naloxone increases mean arterial pressure.

o Therapeutic role in heatstroke disorders.

• Naltrexone and nalmefene:

Naltrexone and nalmefene are longer acting (8–12 h) and effective when taken per orally.

• Methylnaltrexone and alvimopan:

These are quaternary ammonium compounds with no ability to cross the BBB.

Therefore, they do not affect centrally mediated analgesia.

They can be used to treat opioid-related constipation and have found to be effective in postoperative ileus.

• Naloxegol:

It is an oral, peripherally acting μ receptor antagonist. A daily dose of 12.5 to 25 mg has been found to improve bowel movement without affecting the pain score.

Conclusion

IV anesthetic agents play an important role in day-to-day anesthesia practice. Sedation and analgesia are induced by these agents for the benefit of patients. The specific pharmacokinetic and pharmacodynamic properties make them unique for a given patient's profile and clinical scenario. The appropriate dosing achieves optimal anesthetic goals with minimum side effects.

CHAPTER 10

Muscle Relaxants (AS4.1)

Shashikant Sharma and Puneet Khanna

Introduction

Discovery and use of muscle relaxants in anesthesia practice dates back to 1942, when Griffith and Johnson used d-tubocurarine to provide muscle relaxation during surgery. Since then, a number of muscle relaxants have been discovered, and their use has not only revolutionized the practice of anesthesia but also made possible the development of cardiothoracic, neurologic, and organ transplant surgeries. Muscle relaxants can be categorized into different groups, based on their chemical structure, site of action, and their duration of action.

History

Curare (also known as d-tubocurare), prototype of muscle relaxant used in anesthesia practice, was discovered in South America and was used for hunting. Its use in anesthesia was first described in 1940. In 1954, Beecher and Todd reported increased mortality with use of muscle relaxants. This was probably because of inadequate knowledge of pharmacology of muscle relaxants, suboptimal use of artificial ventilation, and unavailability of reversal agents and neuromuscular monitoring. With growing knowledge of pharmacology of muscle relaxants, reversal agents and advancement in neuromuscular monitoring has improved safety profile of these agents in the modern era of anesthesia practice.

1942: Griffith and Johnson described d-tubocurarine.

1952: Thesleff and Foldes introduced succinylcholine (SCh), the first used clinically by Bovet (for which he got Nobel prize).

1967: Baird and Reid used the first synthetic aminosteroid, pancuronium.

Classification

There are three types of neuromuscular blocking agents:

- Directly acting (dantrolene, quinine).
- Blockers of neuromuscular junction (**Table 10.1**).
- Centrally acting (benzodiazepines, mephensin, baclofen).

Table 10.1 Clinical duration of blockers of NM junction

	Long acting (>50 mins)	Intermediate acting (20–50 mins)[a]	Short acting (10–20 mins)	Ultrashort acting (<10 mins)
Steroidal compounds	Pancuronium	Vecuronium Rocuronium		
Bezylisoquinolinium compounds	d-Tubocurarine	Atracurium Cisatracurium	Mivacurium	
Asymmetric mixed-onium fumarates		CW002		Gantacurium

Abbreviation: NM, neuromuscular.
Notes: [a] Neuromuscular blocking agents (intermediate acting) are most commonly used muscle relaxants in anesthesia practice.

Neuromuscular Physiology and Mechanism of Action of Neuromuscular Blocking Agents

It is imperative to have the knowledge of transmission of signal across neuromuscular junction, and the events occurring during transmission, in order to understand the mechanism through which muscle relaxants act.

During neuromuscular transmission, as soon as an action potential reaches presynaptic nerve terminal, it leads to opening of voltage-gated calcium channels. Calcium enters the presynaptic nerve terminal and binds to acetylcholine (ACh) vesicles. Calcium-bound ACh vesicles move near the presynaptic membrane, bind to it and release ACh into synapse. ACh binds to ACh receptors on postsynaptic muscle end plate and causes opening of Na channel. Opening of Na channel results in depolarization of muscle end plate.

SCh (depolarizing muscle relaxant) acts as an agonist at ACh receptor and causes depolarization of muscle membrane, while nondepolarizing muscle relaxants act as antagonists at ACh receptor and compete with ACh for binding sites (**Table 10.2**).

ACh receptors at neuromuscular junction are of nicotinic type (**Table 10.3**). It is a ligand-gated ion channel composed of five subunits: Two α and single β, δ, and ε subunits, which are all arranged around a central pore. When a molecule of ACh binds to each of the α subunits, the receptor undergoes conformational change, which results in opening of the central pore. *In case of nondepolarizing muscle relaxant, if one molecule binds to α subunit; two agonist molecules cannot bind, and neuromuscular transmission is inhibited.* This pore is a nonspecific ion channel, through with Na^+, K^+ and Ca^{2+} ions can flow, causing miniature end-plate potentials. When the threshold level of depolarization is reached, voltage-gated Na^+ channels open and the action potential is propagated across the muscle.

Sequence of Blockade

Central muscles (facial muscles, pharynx, larynx, diaphragm, abdominal muscles) are blocked earlier than peripheral muscles. Recovery follows the an identical pattern. Central muscles recover faster than peripheral muscles.

Factors responsible for it are:

- Muscle blood flow.
- Drug potency.
- Higher receptor density.
- Greater release of acetylcholine.
- Less acetylcholinesterase activity.

Table 10.2 Difference between depolarizing and nondepolarizing block

Depolarizing block	Nondepolarizing block
Also called as *phase 1 block*	-
Block preceded by muscle fasciculations	No fasciculations
No fading is seen (fading occurs only at higher doses, i.e., phase 2 block)	Shows fading
No posttetanic facilitations	Posttetanic facilitation present
Does not require reversal rather cholinesterase inhibitors (neostigmine) can prolong depolarizing block by inhibiting pseudocholinesterase	Require reversal agents like neostigmine
Rapid recovery of neuromuscular functions after blockade	Recovery depends on duration of action of relaxant used
Also called as *leptocurare*	Also called *pachycurare*

Table 10.3 Types of acetylcholine receptors

	Mature	Fetal	α7 type
Composition	α(2), β, δ, ε	α(2), β, δ, γ	Only alpha subunits
Properties	Fast conductance, short duration	Slow conductance, long duration: • Resistant to NDMR • Sensitive to succinylcholine	• Stimulated by both ACh and choline • Does not go under desensitization • Not antagonized by acetylcholinesterase inhibitors

Note: Both fetal and α7 type ACh receptors appear in burs and during immobilization.

Box 10.1 Factors that lower butyrylcholinesterase activity include:			
Liver disease	Malnutrition	Pregnancy	Burns
Oral contraceptives	MAO inhibitors	Neoplastic disease	Metoclopramide
Esmolol	Anticholinesterases	Cytotoxic drugs	Echothiophate

Abbreviations: MAO, monoamine oxidase.

Diaphragm in isolation is most resistant muscle to block and recovers the fastest. Respiratory muscles more resistant than muscles of upper airway. So, if extubated without proper recovery of these muscles, upper airway obstruction may occur.

Monitoring Neuromuscular Blockade

Adductor pollicis muscle is commonly used to monitor neuromuscular blockade. Orbicularis oculi can also be used and is better indicator.

Individual Neuromuscular Blocking Drugs

Succinylcholine

Physicochemical properties: Chemically, it is dicholine ester of succinic acid, that is, 2 ACh molecules linked back-to-back through acetate methyl group. It is stored at 4 degrees to prevent hydrolysis.

Dose: 1 to 2 mg/kg used to provide ideal intubating conditions for rapid sequence intubation and induction.

Onset of action: 30 to 60 seconds; duration of action: 3 to 9 minutes.

Metabolism: Hydrolyzed by butyrylcholinesterase (pseudocholinesterase) in plasma to succinylmonocholine and choline and ultimately to succinic acid and choline. Butyrylcholine esterase is present in plasma and not in neuromuscular junction. *Only 10% of administered drug reaches the site of action, due to metabolism by butyrlcholinesterase; so it should be given at a faster rate. The plasma levels of butyrlcholinesterase can alter the duration of action of SCh, with decreased levels prolong the duration of action.*

In addition to SCh, mivacurium is also metabolized by butyrylcholinesterase. Therefore, caution should pe paid while using both these agents in conditions listed in **Box 10.1**.

SCh produces prolonged depolarization of the end-plate region by binding to the 2 alpha subunits of the ACh receptor. As pseudocholinesterase is absent from neuromuscular junction, SCh causes repeated depolarization and contraction making the membrane refractory, which results in relaxation (phase 1 block).

Higher doses or repeated dosing can cause desensitization of the nicotine acetylcholine receptors (nAChR), inactivation of voltage-gated Na$^+$ channels, and increased permeability of K$^+$, which results in failure of action potential generation and neuromuscular blockade (phase 2 block). Patients with phase 2 block require respiratory support with positive pressure ventilation till SCh is metabolized and return of spontaneous respiration.

Prolonged duration of action is seen with atypical or deficient pseudocholinesterase or phase 2 block. Atypical butyrylcholinesterase can be assessed by dibucaine number and fluoride number (**Table 10.4**).

Dibucaine number: Dibucaine (a local anesthetic) inhibits activity of normal pseudocholinesterase by 80% and abnormal enzyme by 20%. Dibucaine number suggests the percentage of normal enzyme inhibited by it. Although the dibucaine number indicates the genetic makeup of an individual with respect to pseudocholinesterase, *it does not measure the concentration of the enzyme in the plasma*. Patients with atypical pseudocholinesterase have prolonged action of SCh due to its inadequate metabolism.

Fluoride number: It is the percent (%) inhibition of butyrylcholinesterase by 5×10^{-5} M (molar solution) of sodium fluoride (NaF) and can be used to assess atypical butyrylcholinesterase.

Side effects

- Muscle fasciculations.
- Myalgia: Commonly seen in neck, back, and abdominal muscles.
- Masseter spasm.
- Hyperkalemia: *Due to repeated fasciculations and rise in K$^+$ by 0.5 meq/L (in normal*

individuals). The hyperkalemic response does not change in patients with end-stage renal disease. However, the response gets exaggerated in patients with metabolic acidosis and hypovolemia (*the extra potassium comes from gastrointestinal [GI] tract not the muscles*).

- Increased intracranial pressure, intraocular pressure, intragastric pressure can be prevented by pretreatment with nondepolarizing neuromuscular blocking drugs (NMBDs).
- Malignant hyperthermia.
- Dysarrythmias: Sinus bradycardia, junctional rhythms, and ventricular dysrhythmias.
- Anaphylaxis.

Causes of anaphylaxis in operation theater (decreasing order)

Muscle relaxant > latex > antibiotics

Contraindications:

- Hyperkalemia.
- Head injury.
- Spinal cord injury.
- Neuromuscular diseases.
- Muscle trauma (up to 60 days).
- Burns: avoided after first 48 hours to 1 year after burns due to risk of hyperkalemia.

Hyperkalemia is due to proliferation of extrajunctional ACh receptors (fetal type). These are seen in denervated nerves and neonates and infants. These receptors are sensitive to depolarizing and resistant to nondepolarizing neuromuscular drugs. The various disease conditions which can alter

Table 10.4 Relationship between dibucaine number and duration of succinylcholine or mivacurium blockade

Type of butyrylcholinesterase	Incidence	Dibucaine number	Duration of blockade
Homozygous typical	Normal	70–80	Normal
Heterozygous atypical	1/480	50–60	Lengthened by 50–100%
Homozygous atypical	1/3200	20–30	Prolonged to 4–8 h

the expression of fetal type ACh receptors are tabulated in **Table 10.5**.

Nondepolarizing Muscle Relaxants

Quarternary ammonium compounds: These are hydrophilic; therefore, their volumes of distribution are small and not significantly redistributed.

Onset of action: 3 to 4 minutes, high dose–rapid onset of action within 30 to 60 seconds.

Mechanism of action involves competitive antagonism; binds to alpha subunit of nAChR and prevents binding of ACh to its receptor, in order to generate action potential. *The drug needs to occupy only one of the α subunits but must occupy at least 70% of all receptors before any effect is clinically evident* (**Table 10.6**).

Availability of newer muscle relaxants with better safety profile has replaced older agents. A summary of these old agents is tabulated in **Table 10.7**.

Potency of neuromuscular blocking agents is expressed as ED50, ED90 or ED95 (the dose required to cause 50, 90, and 95% suppression of twitch height, respectively).

Intubation dose = 2 × ED95

Potency is inversely related to ED95 while directly related to onset of action (more potent is the neuromuscular blocker; a smaller number of molecules are available at neuromuscular junction, resulting in delayed onset).

Factors Affecting Recovery from Neuromuscular Blockade

Some of the important factors which affect the recovery from neuromuscular blockade are:

- **Initial dose:** Higher dose leads to longer duration of action.
- **Drug metabolism:** Decreased metabolism of NMBDs (hepatic or renal dysfunction or deficiency of butyrylcholinesterase) results in prolonged blockade.
- **Anesthetic agents:**

  Volatile anesthetic agents: Potentiate neuromuscular blockade.

  Des > sevo > iso > halo > nitrous + barbiturates/opioids > propofol.

  Local anesthetics: Potentiate neuromuscular blockade.
- **Drug interactions:** Aminoglycosides, polymyxins, lincomycin, clindamycin, tetracyclines, magnesium, lithium, steroids, and dantrolene potentiate neuromuscular blockade, while phenytoin and other enzyme inducers can decrease the effect of neuromuscular blockers.
- **Diuretics:** No effect.
- **Administration of reversal agents:** Anticholinesterases (like neostigmine and pyridostigmine inhibit butyrylcholinesterase and can prolong the duration of blockade by SCh).

Table 10.5 Disease conditions that alter expression of fetal type ACh receptors

nAChR upregulation	nAChR downregulation
Spinal cord injury	Myasthenia gravis
Stroke	Anticholinesterase poisoning
Burns	Organophosphate poisoning
Prolonged immobility	
Prolonged exposure to neuromuscular blockers	
Multiple sclerosis	
Guillain–Barré syndrome	

Abbreviation: nAChR, nicotine acetylcholine receptors.

Table 10.6 Comparison of nondepolarizing muscle relaxants

Vecuronium	Rocuronium
• Most cardiostable muscle relaxant • Intubation dose: 0.1 mg/kg (IV) • Onset of action is 3–4 mins • Duration of action: 30–40 mins • Metabolized by liver and excreted through bile (60%) and kidney (40%)	• It is derivative of vecuronium with less potency • Intubation dose: 0.6 mg/kg • RSI: 1–1.2 mg/kg • Metabolized in liver and excreted mainly through bile • Potency less than vecuronium, so given in higher dose and hence faster onset of action. Action is reversed by neostigmine, can also be terminated by Sugammadex at any point of time in case of emergency • It is preferred relaxant for prolonged use in ICU as it does not produce any active metabolite • *It is only nondepolarizing muscle relaxant which can be given by intramuscular route*
Atracurium	**Cisatracurium**
• Intubation dose: 0.5 mg/kg • Metabolized by Hoffman elimination (*organ independent spontaneous degradation*)– temperature and pH dependent metabolism. Partly metabolized by nonspecific esterases. Spontaneous recovery occurs reliably from atracurium neuromuscular blockade • Safe in renal and hepatic diseases • Causes dose dependent histamine release, *thus transient hypotension and tachycardia can occur due to vasodilation* • 4–5 times more laudanosine is produced in its metabolism than cis atracurium, which has seizure potential	• Isomer of atracurium • Intubation dose: 0.1 mg/kg • 4 times more potent than atracurium • It has slower onset and longer duration of action compared to atracurium due to its high potency • 77% is metabolized by Hoffman elimination and there is no ester hydrolysis • 23% is eliminated from kidneys unchanged • No histamine release and decreased Laudanosine production compared to atacurium

Abbreviation: RSI, rapid sequence intubation.

Table 10.7 Drugs that are rarely or no longer used

Drugs	Properties
Pancuronium	• Vagolytic properties—tachycardia and hypertension • Releases noradrenaline • Excreted mainly by kidneys
Pipercuronium	• No vagolytic property
Rapacuronium	• Very high incidence of bronchospasm (M2 affinity 15 times more than M3 receptors) • Taken out of market
d-Tubocurarine	• Maximum histamine release (bronchospasm) • Maximum ganglion blockade (hypotension)
Mivacurium	• Short-acting, metabolized by plasma pseudocholinesterase • Causes histamine release
Gallamine	• Maximum vagal blockade • Crosses placenta

- **Acid–base status:** Respiratory acidosis and metabolic alkalosis prolong the duration of neuromuscular blockade.

> Long-term use of neuromuscular blockers in intensive care can cause critical illness myopathy and polyneuropathy.

Reversal of Neuromuscular Blockade

Residual neuromuscular blockade can lead to delayed extubation, hypoxemia, and need of reintubation in postoperative period. Therefore, adequate recovery from neuromuscular blockade must be ensured prior to extubation.

Anticholinesterases like neostigmine and pyridostigmine reverse the effects of non-depolarizing neuromuscular blockers. They act by increasing the concentration of ACh at the neuromuscular junction by preventing their degradation by acetylcholinesterases.

Increased ACh will act on both nicotinic and muscarinic receptors, thus producing side effects like *bradycardia, bronchospasm, and increased secretions.* To prevent these side effects, anticholinergic drugs like atropine and glycopyrrolate are often combined with them.

No attempt should be made to reverse neuro-muscular block unless there is some spontaneous recovery (sugammadex: An exception).

Neuromuscular monitoring (although not a recommended standard of American Society of Anesthesiologists [ASA] monitoring) is not only helpful in assessing depth of blockade but also to rule out residual paralysis. The various patterns of stimulation used in neuromuscular monitoring, depths of neuromuscular blockade, and their features are listed in **Tables 10.8** to **10.10**.

Fading and posttetanic facilitation are the features of nondepolarizing and phase 2 block.

Table 10.8 Patterns of stimulation

Criteria	Pattern
Single twitch	One stimulus at 1.0 Hz or 0.1 Hz
TOF	Four supramaximal stimuli at 2.0 Hz, repeated every 10–20 s
Tetanic stimulation	Multiple stimuli at 50 Hz for 5 s
PTS	Tetanic stimulation followed by single twitch at 1 Hz after 3 s
DBS	Two bursts of tetanic stimulation, separated by 750 ms

Abbreviations: DBS, double burst stimulation; PTS, posttetanic stimulation; TOF, train of four.

Table 10.9 Stages of anesthesia and pattern of stimulation (in terms of accuracy)

Stages of anesthesia	Pattern of stimulation
Induction and intubation	Single twitch
Intense and deep neuromuscular blockade	PTS
Moderate or surgical blockade	TOF
Reversal	TOF
Recovery/postanesthesia care unit (to detect residual neuromuscular blockade)	DBS

Abbreviations: DBS, double burst stimulation; PTS, posttetanic stimulation; TOF, train of four.

Table 10.10 Levels of neuromuscular blockade

Level of block	Properties	Reversal
Intense	Occurs during 3–6 mins of intubating dose of NDMR TOF = 0, PTC = 0	Cannot be reversed with anticholinesterases *Sugammadex (16 mg/kg) can reverse it*
Deep	TOF = 0, PTC ≥ 1	Cannot be reversed with anticholinesterases *Sugammadex (4 mg/kg) can reverse it*
Moderate/surgical	TOF ≥ 1	Can be reversed with anticholinesterases Sugammadex (2 mg/kg) can reverse it
Recovery	TOF ratio = 1	

Abbreviations: NDMR, nondepolarizing muscle relaxant; PTC, posttetanic count; TOF, train of four.
Note: Reversal with neostigmine should be done when TOF count > 2, and TOF ratio > 0.9 should be achieved prior to tracheal extubation.

Sugammadex (Org 25969)

It is also known as selective relaxant binding agent (SRBA).

Mechanism of action: It is a γ-cyclodextrin which works by completely enveloping the aminosteroid (rocuronium and vecuronium). Once it binds to rocuronium or vecuronium in plasma, the concentration of muscle relaxant decreases and therefore a gradient is created between neuromuscular junction and the plasma. This results in movement of muscle relaxant from neuromuscular junction to plasma and termination of effect.

The affinity of sugammadex for rocuronium is 2.5 times higher than that for vecuronium. The whole complex is then excreted in urine.

Use: Rapid sequence induction.

Dose: 4 to 16 mg/kg.

Side effects: These include allergic reactions, coughing and parasomnia.

Conclusion

Muscle relaxants not only facilitate tracheal intubation but also provide the surgeon with a relaxed patient. Muscle relaxants can be either depolarizing or nondepolarizing types, with unique properties and adverse effect profiles. The monitoring of neuromuscular blockade avoids overdosing, ensures timely reversal, and minimizes perioperative respiratory complications.

Section III
Regional Anesthesia

CHAPTER 11

Local Anesthetics

Richa Saroa, Sanjeev Palta, and Arushi Goyal

Introduction

Local anesthetics (LAs) form the subset of drugs that provide analgesia and anesthesia by reversible conduction blockade of autonomic, sensory, and motor nerve impulses. The earliest description of "coca leaves" consumption, the derivative of cocaine, dates back to the 16th century when nobles and higher officials primarily used it for recreational purposes. The LAs were used initially by the dentists for a dental procedure and later altered the entire concept of anesthetic as well as surgical practices.

History

Milestones reached in the history of LAs are listed below:

Year	Milestones
1860	Cocaine isolated from leaves of erythroxylon coca by Albert Niemann at Freidrich Wohler Laboratory in Gottingen
1884	Cocaine used as LA in ophthalmology by Karl Koller Dr Nash used cocaine for infraorbital block Dr William Steward Halstead performed inferior dental block with cocaine
1898	Cocaine was used for spinal anesthesia by Bier
1905	Procaine, first synthetic LA, was used by Einhorn
1943	Lignocaine synthesized by Nilis Lofgren and Bendt Lundquist
1949	Lignocaine was first used clinically
1957	Bupivacaine and mepivacaine synthesized by Bo Af Ekenstam
1963	Bupivacaine was first used clinically
1972	Prilocaine synthesized by Nilis Lofgren and Claes Tegner Etidocaine was developed by Adam
1983	Ropivacaine was studied by Roseberg and Einhurn
1997	Ropivacaine and lignocaine were clinically used

Classification

LAs consist of a hydrophilic amine group and a lipophilic aromatic ring that connect through an intermediate chain. *The structural bond in the intermediate chain determines whether the LA belongs to the ester or amide group.* LAs may be classified based on the chemical structure, duration of action, or the potency as explained in **Tables 11.1 to 11.3**.

Anatomy and Physiology of the Peripheral Nerve

Since LAs exert their action by inhibiting the nerve impulses, it is essential to revise the anatomy and physiology related to peripheral nerves.

Table 11.1 Classification of LAs (based on the chemical structure)

Aminoesters	Aminoamides
Cocaine	Lidocaine
Procaine	Mepivacaine
Chloroprocaine	Prilocaine
Tetracaine	Etidocaine
	Bupivacaine
	Ropivacaine

Abbreviation: LAs, local anesthetics.

Table 11.2 Classification of local anesthetics (based on duration)

Drugs	Concentration (%)	Duration (min) (plain solution)	Duration (min) (with epinephrine)
Short duration			
Procaine	1–2	20–30	30–45
Chloroprocaine	1–2	15–30	30
Moderate duration			
Lidocaine	0.5–1	30–60	120
Mepivacaine	0.5–1	45–90	120
Prilocaine	0.5–1	30–90	120
Long duration			
Bupivacaine	0.25–0.5	120–240	180–240
Ropivacaine	0.25–0.5	120–240	180–40

Table 11.3 Classification of LA (based on potency)

Drugs	Relative conduction-blocking potency
Low potency	
Procaine	1
Intermediate potency	
Mepivacaine	1.5
Prilocaine	1.8
Lidocaine	2
Chloroprocaine	3
High potency	
Bupivacaine	8
Etidocaine	8
Tetracaine	8

Abbreviation: LA, local anesthetic.

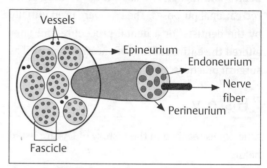

Fig. 11.1 Structure of a peripheral nerve.

A peripheral nerve usually comprises a bundle of neurons/axons that are generally arranged as one or more fascicles (**Fig. 11.1**). Each axon consists of an outer connective tissue layer known as endoneurium. The fascicles formed by many axons are surrounded by another connective tissue layer known as perineurium that is similar to the epithelium, and the entire nerve sheath is enclosed exteriorly in a loose sheath known as epineurium (**Fig. 11.1**). While nonmyelinated nerves have axons enveloped in a single Schwann cell sheath, myelinated nerves (large motor and sensory nerves) are usually encased in myelin, which is the specialized plasma membrane of the Schwann cells that wraps the axons during their growth with periodic interruptions at nodes of Ranvier that form the site for impulse generation. Myelin primarily increases the speed of conduction in the nerves by providing insulation from the exterior environment, thus creating a barrier to the action of various drugs acting on nerves, including LAs. The sodium channels that facilitate the generation as well as the initiation of the nerve impulse are present along the entire length of the nonmyelinated nerve but are concentrated at the nodes of Ranvier in myelinated nerves.

The normal resting potential of the membrane varies between –60 and –90 mV, and it is impermeable to sodium ions and selectively permeable to potassium ions at rest. Energy driven Na-K pump maintains the constant resting membrane potential by a continuous extrusion of the Na ions from the cell interior with the intrusion of K ions to maintain the electrical neutrality. During an action potential, the permeability to Na ions is increased, thus changing the membrane potential momentarily and conducting a unidirectional impulse in one direction. While Na channels open faster and cause further depolarization, it continues till K channels open to balance or inactivates Na channels that lead to repolarization.

Mechanism of Action

Many factors affect the activity of LAs:

- pKa: It is the pH at which the ionized and unionized fractions are equal. pKa near to the pH implies more unionized fraction for given pH and faster onset of action and vice versa.

- pH: Lower pH, that is, acidic medium, which means the predominance of an ionized fraction of drug and thus lower potency of the LA. *This explains the fact that LA has reduced efficacy in conditions like abscess or infection, owing to the acidic milieu.*

- Protein binding: LAs having higher protein binding have a longer duration of action.

- Intermediate chain: The longer the intermediate chain, higher is the potency of the LA; for example, *bupivacaine has a longer intermediate chain as compared to lignocaine and, thus, is four times more potent.*

The agents usually exert their action by blockade of intracellular fast voltage-gated sodium channels subsequent to the concentration-dependent action at the site of application, thereby interrupting the initiation and propagation of axonal impulses in the dermatomal distribution of the innervated area. *The unionized fraction of the drug crosses the lipid bilayer neuronal membrane and renders the sodium channels inactive and inhibits the conduction of impulse along the peripheral or central nerve.* The recovery is governed by the removal of the drug from the site by circulation, tissue binding, and the local hydrolysis of the LA as described under pharmacokinetics.

Factors Affecting Pharmacokinetics of Local Anesthetics

The concentration of LAs in the blood is multifactorial and is determined by:

- Rate of absorption from the site of injection.

- Rate of tissue distribution.

- Rate of biotransformation and excretion.

- Patient factors such as age, comorbidities, etc.

Absorption

Systemic absorption is determined by the:

- Site of injection: LA drug concentrations are higher with intravenous (IV) administration > intercostal nerve blockades > caudal epidural > lumbar epidural > brachial plexus > subarachnoid > subcutaneous tissue. *Greater rate of absorption is seen in an area with greater vascularity.*

- Volume and dosage: Higher the volume and concentration of LA, earlier is the nerve blockade and longer the duration of action.

- Use of an additional vasoconstrictor agent and carbonation: Epinephrine decreases the blood flow, slows down the rate of absorption, reduces plasma concentration, thereby increasing the duration of action of LA. *The addition of sodium bicarbonate leads to an increase in pH, resulting in a higher unionized fraction of LA and thus leading to the rapid onset of action.*

- Use of additives/adjuncts: Addition of agents like opioids (morphine, fentanyl, tramadol), benzodiazepines (midazolam), dexamethasone, α2 agonists (dexmedetomidine, clonidine) to LA have an advantage of reducing the dose of LA and prolong the action of the same. *Preservative-free preparations are utilized for neuraxial blocks.*

- Pharmacological nature of drugs: Intrinsic vasodilatory activity, degree of protein binding, and lipid solubility affect the rate of absorption and distribution of the drug.

Distribution

Some noteworthy points of consideration are:

- The plasma concentration of LA is determined by the rate of tissue distribution and clearance of the drug.

- Lipid solubility of LA is important in redistribution and is a primary determinant of intrinsic LA potency.

- Highly perfused tissues have a higher concentration of LA than less perfused tissues, including skeletal muscles and fat.

- The concentration of LA decreases as it passes through pulmonary vasculature due to rapid extraction by the lung tissue.

- Clinically significant amounts of transplacental transfer may be seen between the fetus and mother, depending upon the protein binding and hydrolysis of the drug.

Biotransformation and Excretion

Important points to be considered are:

- Esters undergo hydrolysis in plasma and, to a lesser extent, in the liver by enzyme pseudocholinesterase, forming benzoic acid and para-aminobenzoic acid (PABA). The enzymatic activity is low at birth and reaches the adult levels by 1 year of age. Cocaine, an ester by exception, undergoes metabolism predominantly by hepatic carboxylesterase.

- Amides undergo enzymatic degradation in the liver by oxidative dealkylation with some extrahepatic degradation in the kidney. *Articaine, LA, that is widely used in dentistry is an exception to this rule and is inactivated by plasma carboxylesterase-induced cleavage of a methyl ester on the aromatic ring.*

- Renal clearance of drugs is inversely proportional to protein binding and pH of urine.

- More water-soluble ester metabolites such as PABA are excreted in the urine, whereas less than 5% amides appear in the urine unchanged.

Patient Factors

Important patient factors to be borne in mind while administering LAs are:

- The patient's age influences the distribution of LA; newborns have prolonged elimination due to immature hepatic enzymatic biotransformation and decreased alpha-1 acid glycoprotein.

- Pregnancy: Increased sensitivity to LA, faster onset, and longer duration of action may be present during pregnancy. Altered protein binding in parturients predisposes them to side effects and toxicity at lower levels, thereby increasing the toxicity potential. The LAs having pKa close to the physiological pH exhibit greater placental transfer. In fetal acidosis, LA becomes ionized after the placental transfer and is unable to reach the maternal circulation, leading to "ion trapping" that may jeopardize fetal well-being.

- Higher LA plasma concentration may be encountered in patients with congestive heart failure, hepatic, or renal failure.

Techniques of Administering Local Anesthesia

Topical/Surface Anesthesia

When applied topically, LAs provide an effective but relatively shorter duration of analgesia, which may be increased by longer duration of application. Commonly employed LAs for topical anesthesia are lidocaine, tetracaine, dibucaine and benzocaine (5/10% cream/ointment), eutectic mixture of LAs with 2.5% lidocaine, 2.5% prilocaine (EMLA); tetracaine 0.5%, epinephrine 1:200,000, cocaine 11.8% (TAC); lidocaine 4%, epinephrine 1:20,000, tetracaine 0.5% (LET).

Infiltration Anesthesia

LA is injected directly into the extravascular space in the intradermal or subcutaneous tissues, with immediate onset of action but varying duration of analgesia. The dosage of LA depends on the extent of the surface area to be anesthetized and the duration of the procedure to be performed, for example, lidocaine, bupivacaine, ropivacaine, mepivacaine, prilocaine (**Tables 11.1** and **11.2**).

Peripheral and Truncal Nerve Blockade

Minor blocks involve single nerve blockade, whereas major blocks may include two or more distinct nerves or nerve plexus. The concentration and volume of the LA depend upon the type and duration of the surgical procedure. The property of differential blockade of sensory and motor fibers at lower and higher concentrations, respectively, has a role in postoperative pain relief and ambulatory surgeries, where the rapid return of functions is deemed necessary.

Intravenous Regional Anesthesia (IVRA)/Bier Block

LA is directly administered into the peripheral vascular bed in a tourniquet applied limb from where the drugs diffuse around axons and nerve endings to provide anesthesia. It is commonly used for upper limb procedures. Lignocaine is the most frequently employed LA for Bier's block, as the safety profile of the block is entirely dependent on the occlusion of the blood supply. Other LAs have been used but with little success; for example, lidocaine and bupivacaine (with or without epinephrine).

Epidural and Spinal Anesthesia

Preservative-free preparations and hyperbaric preparations are utilized for epidural and subarachnoid blocks. The hyperbaric preparations for spinal anesthesia are commercially available as 0.75% or 0.5% bupivacaine with 8.25% dextrose.

Tumescent Anesthesia

Large volumes of the appropriate concentration of LA with vasoconstrictor and other adjuvants are injected into the subcutaneous tissue. It is *most commonly used in liposuction procedures.*

Individual Drugs

The drugs belonging to the amino amide and amino ester group are discussed in this chapter. Their physiochemical properties have been enlisted in **Tables 11.4** and **11.5**.

Aminoesters

The clinically used aminoesters include cocaine, procaine, chloroprocaine, and tetracaine.

Cocaine

It is the first local anesthetic to be discovered and is the only naturally occurring one. *Cocaine is the only local anesthetic that causes vasoconstriction at all concentrations* by its ability to inhibit the norepinephrine uptake at presynaptic neuronal areas. Earlier used for ophthalmic surgery, it is now usually employed in otorhinology to achieve nasal vasoconstriction and LA effect. It has been replaced by other agents, primarily a1-adrenergic agonists (oxymetazoline or phenylephrine),

Table 11.4 Pharmacokinetics and pharmacodynamics of LAs

Drugs	Lignocaine	Bupivacaine	Ropivacaine
Synthesis	Lofgren (1943) (used in 1948 by Gordh)	Ekenstam (1957) (used in 1963)	Roseberg (1983) (used in 1997)
Chemical name	Diethylamino 2, 6 acetoxylidide	1-N-butyl-OH-piperidine-2-carboxy acid 2,6 dimethylaniline HCl	S-propyl-pipecoloxylidide
Routes of administration	Topical, intravenous, intrathecal, epidural, infiltration, peripheral nerve block	Intrathecal, epidural, infiltration, peripheral nerve block	Intrathecal, epidural, infiltration, peripheral nerve block
Pharmacokinetics plasma protein binding	64%	70–90% (alpha-1 acid glycoprotein)	94%
Metabolism	Microsomal enzymatic activity in liver, 73% excreted in urine (monoethyl-glycine-xylidide [MEGX] has antiarrhythmic activity)	Aromatic hydroxylation, n-dealkylation, amide hydrolysis, conjugation	Hepatic biotransformation by Cyt P450
Solubility	Soluble in water, pH: 5–7, stable, highly concentrated in kidneys, lungs, spleen, heart and brain, fat	Soluble in water	Less lipid-soluble, a smaller volume of distribution, short elimination half-life
Pharmacodynamics dose	IV: 1–1.5 mg/kg (preservative-free)	IV: 2.5–3 mg/kg	IV: 2.5 mg/kg
Onset of action	5–10 mins	15–20 mins	15–20 mins
Duration of action	60 mins 100 mins (with vasoconstrictor)	180–350 mins	180–350 mins
Toxic dose	3 mg/kg (plain) 7 mg/kg (with vasoconstrictor)	2–3 mg/kg (with or without vasoconstrictor)	3 mg/kg with/without vasoconstrictor
Preparations	2–4% nebulized solution for nose, throat and tracheobronchial tree, 2.5–5% ointment for skin and mucous membrane, 2% jelly for urethra, 7% patch, 10% rectal suppositories, 10% aerosol for gingival mucosa (0.5–1%) for infiltration, 1–2% for neuraxial block, EMLA, TAC, LET	0.2–0.5% for infiltration, 0.25–0.5%, 0.5% isobaric/0.75% hyperbaric (levobupivacaine: 0.25–0.75%, 0.5% isobaric/0.75% hyperbaric) for neuraxial block	0.2%, 0.5%, 0.75%, and 1.0% preservative-free preparations
Side effects	Tachyphylaxis, convulsions, hypotension	Cardiotoxicity, Convulsions, hypotension, bradycardia, seizures	Lower systemic toxicity than bupivacaine

Abbreviations: EMLA, eutectic mixture of local anesthetics with 2.5% lidocaine, 2.5% prilocaine; IV, intravenous; LA, local anesthetic; LET, lidocaine 4%, epinephrine 1:20,000, tetracaine 0.5%; TAC, tetracaine 0.5%, epinephrine 1:200,000, cocaine 11.8%.

Table 11.5 Concentrations and preparations of LAs available/used clinically

Drug	Preparations
Procaine	• 0.25–0.5% for infiltrative anesthesia • 1%/2% for peripheral nerve blocks • 10% (hyperbaric) for neuraxial block
Chloroprocaine	• 2–3% for neuraxial block
Tetracaine	• 4% gel for venous cannulation • 0.5–15% ointment/cream for skin, rectum, mucous membrane • 0.25–1.0% Hyperbaric/ 0.25% Hypobaric/ 1.0% Isobaric- for neuraxial block
Prilocaine	• 0.5–0.1% for infiltration • 1–3% for neuraxial block
Mepivacaine	• 0.5–0.1% for infiltration 1%, 2%, 4% (hyperbaric) for neuraxial block

Abbreviation: LA, local anesthetic.

owing to the abuse potential and toxicity at lower levels.

Procaine

Procaine is a short-acting amino ester, which was synthesized by Alfred Einhorn, under the trade name "novocaine." It has been utilized for regional as well as neuraxial anesthesia. However, with the availability of newer LAs, it is used only in certain procedures sparingly such as dental anesthesia, coadministration with intramuscular penicillin, or in patients allergic to the amide group of LA.

Chloroprocaine

It is an ultrashort-acting ester LA that is metabolized by pseudocholinesterases but *went into disrepute owing to reports of neurological injury due to the bisulfite preservative in the commercial preparations*. However, recently its use has resurfaced in ambulatory surgeries, using preservative-free preparations with rapid onset and shorter duration of action.

Tetracaine

It is an ester LA employed for perineal or abdominal surgeries, although the extent of the block may be unreliable. Since it has a potential for systemic toxicity, it is not used for clinical practices.

Aminoamides

The clinically used aminoamides include lidocaine/lignocaine, prilocaine, bupivacaine, levobupivacaine, and ropivacaine.

Lidocaine/Lignocaine

It is the most commonly used LA that features on the WHO essential drug list and is available in many preparations in hydrochloride form as enumerated in **Table 11.4**. It can be administered intravenously, in epidural space, intrathecal/subarachnoid space, and is a class Ib antiarrhythmic too. It possesses anti-inflammatory, antinociceptive, and immune-modulating properties along with antibacterial effects. *It is the least toxic of all the LAs, owing to low-protein binding capacity.* While the safe dose of lignocaine is 3 mg/kg, it can be used in a dosage of 7 mg/kg with adrenaline in peripheral blocks. Adrenaline increases the duration of action and reduces the toxicity by vasoconstriction of the local blood vessels. The intrathecal preparation had gone into disrepute due to transient neurological symptoms and has been introduced without the preservative for short-duration procedures.

Prilocaine

Prilocaine is an amide LA that is pharmacologically similar to lignocaine, with an intermediate duration of action having more sensory blockade and duration than lignocaine. It causes less vasodilation than lidocaine and, therefore, does not require adrenaline for prolongation of the clinical effect. The LA has the propensity to cause methemoglobinemia due to the metabolite o-toluidine and, therefore, should be used with caution in children less than 3 months of age and in patients susceptible to develop the same. However, it causes less neurological and cardiac toxicity than other amide anesthetics. It is mostly employed for dental procedures.

Bupivacaine

Bupivacaine is a highly protein-bound, long-acting amide with a relatively slower onset of action, which provides excellent sensory as well as motor blockade, depending upon the concentration used. It exists as both levo and dextro forms, and a racemic mixture was introduced in 1963. It too features as an essential drug on the WHO list. It is widely used anesthetic for surgical procedures, ambulatory procedures, and postoperative or intraoperative analgesia in lower doses, owing to its property of differential blockade that makes it a popular choice for "walking epidurals" in parturients. It is available as isobaric as well as hyperbaric concentration, as mentioned in **Table 11.4**. It is slightly hypobaric in comparison to cerebrospinal fluid (CSF) at room temperature. It is contraindicated in any history of allergy to amide LAs and *has maximum cardiotoxic potential amongst all the amide anesthetics.* Liposomal bupivacaine preparations have been introduced that supposedly are less cardiotoxic and provide a longer duration of analgesia as compared to the standard preparations. *The maximum safe*

permissible dose of bupivacaine is 2 to 3 mg/kg with/ without adrenaline as the addition of the latter has no beneficial effect on the duration of action.

Levobupivacaine

It is an S enantiomer of bupivacaine. It has a similar clinical profile as that of bupivacaine in terms of onset, duration, and indications for use. It also possesses the differential blockade property similar to bupivacaine. However, its potency is little less than bupivacaine and is less cardiotoxic than bupivacaine, making it the LA of choice over bupivacaine in clinical settings.

Ropivacaine

Ropivacaine is levorotatory S(-) enantiomer of bupivacaine and has a structural similarity with the same in terms of similar slower onset and longer duration. It also possesses the property of differential blockade, has lesser toxicity potential than bupivacaine, and therefore has emerged as a popular choice for peripheral nerve blocks, neuraxial (epidural) block, and pain management.

Local Anesthetic Toxicity

LAs are relatively safe when administered with caution in correct calculated dosages at the site of action that may be peripheral nerve, epidural space, or intrathecal space. However, accidental transit into the bloodstream either by inadvertent arterial injection or higher than recommended dosages may lead to local or systemic side effects. Local effects may present as allergic reactions mostly following administration of ester group LAs and usually present as a rash or itching with redness at the site of administration, and therefore, it is important to ask for any history of allergies to LAs before injecting the same. However, if already developed, the patient needs to be observed and administered local or systemic antihistamines for symptomatic treatment. Other local symptoms may be encountered, depending upon the site of administration. Rarely, irreversible conduction blockade may be seen, but it is usually due to nerve damage secondary to the procedure than the LA itself.

The systemic toxicity: Local anesthetic systemic toxicity (LAST) usually presents with central nervous system (CNS) symptoms followed by the cardiovascular symptoms. Factors that affect the risk profile of LA for toxicity include:

- The dosage and class of LA.
- Site of administration (more vascular leads to more absorption).
- Associated comorbidities in patient.
- Age (more in children and elderly).
- Muscle mass (less muscle mass with the same dose predisposes to more toxicity).

The discussion of LA complications would be incomplete without highlighting the concept of the cardiac collapse (CC)/CNS ratio. It is defined as the ratio of dose, causing cardiovascular collapse to that of causing seizures/convulsions. The lower the ratio, the more cardiotoxic is the drug; for example, CC/CNS ratio for bupivacaine is 3 versus 7 for lignocaine. Therefore, bupivacaine is more cardiotoxic and has higher toxicity potential as compared to the other LAs, due to its lipophilic nature and higher affinity towards the voltage-gated sodium channels. The clinical symptoms of LAST may range from mild to severe, presenting as hypotension, seizures, arrhythmias, and death. The symptoms are tabulated in **Table 11.6**.

Treatment of Toxicity

In a conscious patient, the neurological or cardiovascular symptoms give warning signs of LAST. However, in patients undergoing procedures in general anesthesia (GA), the diagnosis of the same may be delayed as certain symptoms are masked and, usually, cardiovascular symptoms

provide a guide toward LAST. The management of LAST includes:

- Stop the administration of LA.
- Maintain airway, breathing, and circulation.
- Call for help.
- Start oxygenation through a face mask or perform endotracheal intubation if required.
- Support circulation with the help of IV fluids and vasopressor agents (norepinephrine, dopamine).
- Benzodiazepines, especially midazolam in titrated dosages, may be employed for seizure control. Thiopentone/propofol may also be utilized, but the potential to worsen hypotension should be kept in mind, and lower titrated doses should be employed.

Table 11.6 Manifestations of LAST

Central nervous system
- Lightheadedness
- Circumoral numbness
- Metallic taste
- Dizziness
- Visual/auditory disturbances
- Tinnitus
- Disorientation
- Drowsiness
- Tremors
- Seizures
Cardiovascular system
- Bradycardia
- Arrhythmia (lidocaine has antiarrhythmic activity)
- Hypotension
- Vasoconstriction/vasodilation
Respiratory system
- Hypercapnia/tachypnea/difficulty in breathing
- Acidosis
- Hypoxia

Abbreviation: LAST, local anesthetic systemic toxicity.

- Antiarrhythmic drug, amiodarone, is preferred to resolve arrhythmias.

- If epinephrine is used, small doses of < 1 µg/kg are preferred to avoid impaired pulmonary gas exchange and increased afterload.

- Bupivacaine toxicity/amides are cardiotoxic and warrant the use of IV lipid emulsion–*intralipid 20%, which is administered in a loading dose of 1.5 mL/kg over 1 minute, followed by infusion of 0.25 o 0.5 mL/kg/min. The boluses may be repeated twice for unrelenting cardiovascular collapse.*

- In the case of cardiac arrest, basic and advanced life support is provided as protocolized.

- It is important to obtain informed consent before administration of LA and, more importantly, to keep a verbal communication with the patient during the procedures being conducted under the peripheral/neuraxial blocks, in order to detect the warning signs at the earliest.

- If LAST does occur, it is important to document the kind of reaction, the type, and dose of LA that was used during the procedure.

Conclusion

LAs are one of the most commonly used agents through multiple routes for variety of procedures. The use of local anesthetics facilitates surgery on lower limbs, lower abdomen and upper limbs, and avoids the complications associated with GA. It is important to be well versed with pharmacokinetics as well as pharmacodynamics of these agents to use them safely and efficiently.

CHAPTER 12

Central Neuraxial Blocks

Richa Saroa, Sanjeev Palta, and Arush Singla

Introduction

Central neuraxial blocks (CNBs) collectively encompass the subarachnoid/spinal, epidural, caudal epidural, and combined spinal-epidural anesthesia. Before the advent of anesthesia, crude methods have been described in the literature to perform various surgical procedures. After that, with the introduction and discovery of anesthetics into clinical practice, the alleviation of pain and good working conditions by adequate muscle relaxation became widespread. However, the concerns of prolonged recovery after general anesthesia (GA) and certain other complications like postoperative nausea and vomiting (PONV) prompted the need for an anesthetic technique that provided the components of anesthesia while retaining the consciousness. This led to the introduction of CNBs, the first being spinal anesthesia by German surgeon Sir August Bier on August 16, 1898. After that, the use of CNBs expanded and laid the foundation of modern-day regional anesthetic practices.

Historical Perspective

Historical milestones in the field of CNBs are as follows:

- 200 AD: Neuraxial fluid presence demonstrated by Galen.
- 1891: Dural puncture described by Essex Wynter.
- August 16, 1898: First case of spinal anesthesia administered by German surgeon Sir August Bier using local anesthetic cocaine.
- 1901: First use of intrathecal morphine by Racoviceanu-Pitesti.

- 1901: The first description of caudal anesthesia was by Cathleen.
- 1905: Braun used procaine in spinal anesthesia.
- 1921: Fiedel Pages described the first lumbar epidural anesthesia in humans.
- 1930s: Dogliotti described the loss of resistance method for identification of epidural space (also known as Dogliotti's principle).
- 1935: Tetracaine used by Sise for spinal anesthesia.
- 1941: Robert Andrew Hingson (1913–1996), Waldo B. Edwards and James L. Southworth developed technique of continuous caudal anesthesia.
- 1947: First lumbar epidural catheterization for surgery was done by Manuel Martinez Curbelo.
- 1949: Lidocaine was used for spinal anesthesia by Gordh.
- 1952: Chloroprocaine was used in spinal anesthesia by Foldes and McNall.
- 1961: Mepivacaine was used in spinal anesthesia by Dhuner and Sternberg.
- 1966: Bupivacaine was used in spinal anesthesia by Emblem.
- 1979: First use of epidural morphine for analgesia by Behar.

The CNBs are the most commonly employed regional anesthetic or analgesic techniques for a plethora of surgical procedures. Conventionally, CNBs have been practiced, utilizing the anatomical landmark technique, tactile perception of the structures, and visible markers (free flow of cerebrospinal fluid [CSF] in spinal, loss of resistance in epidural). In the absence of any abnormal anatomy, these blocks can be performed with reliable accuracy and provide excellent sensory and motor blockade that wears off, depending upon the concentration and volume of the local anesthesia (LA) used.

Applied Anatomy and Physiology (AS5.1, AS5.2)

The recapitulation of the anatomy of the spinal cord and the surrounding structures is imperative for an insight into the physiological considerations of CNBs. The axis of the human body is formed by the vertebral column that extends from the base of the skull up to the pelvis and is integral for providing support to various organs and structures of the body, aid locomotion, and protect the spinal cord that is encased within the bony structures. The vertebral column has 33 vertebrae (cervical 7, thoracic 12, lumbar 5, sacral 5, and coccygeal 4). It has two primary curves (thoracic and lumbar) and two secondary curves (cervical and sacral) that aid in maintaining the posture and flexibility of the entire body.

A vertebra comprises an anterior body and a posterior vertebral arch (**Fig. 12.1**). A pedicle forms the vertebral arch on each side that arises from the posterolateral side to fuse with the lamina, in order to enclose the vertebral foramen.

The spinal cord, along with the structures and spinal nerves, runs in the vertebral canal that exits through the lateral space between the pedicles. The transverse process arises from the lamina that fuses in the midline, and a spinous process projects to form an important landmark for the CNBs, with intervertebral spaces that can be palpated through the entire length of the vertebral column. The line joining the highest point of the iliac bones (Tuffier's line) usually corresponds to L4–L5 intervertebral space.

Proximally, the spinal cord is continuous with the brainstem and terminates distally in

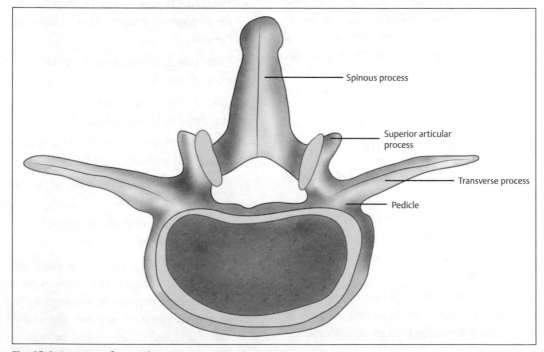

Fig. 12.1 Anatomy of a vertebra.

the conus medullaris as the filum terminale (fibrous extension) and cauda equina (neural extension). The distal termination of the spinal cord varies from L3 in infants to the lower border of L1 in adults because of differential growth rates between the bony vertebral canal and the central nervous system (CNS) during the growth.

The spinal cord is surrounded by three membranes centrifugally: The pia mater, the arachnoid mater, and the dura mater. The pia mater is a highly vascular membrane that encloses the spinal cord closely. The space between pia mater and arachnoid mater is called the subarachnoid or intrathecal space that is filled with CSF, which is produced by the choroid plexuses of the cerebral ventricles and spinal nerves traversing this space. Approximately 500 mL of CSF is produced daily, out of which 30 to 80 mL occupies the intrathecal space from T11–T12 downward. The arachnoid mater is a nonvascular membrane that acts as the principal barrier to the migration of drugs to CSF. Exterior to the arachnoid mater, between the arachnoid mater and outermost layer dura mater, lies the subdural space, which is a nonuniform space.

The epidural space surrounds the dura mater and extends from foramen magnum to the sacral hiatus. It is bound by posterior longitudinal ligament anteriorly, ligamentum flavum (yellow ligament) posteriorly, and pedicles and intervertebral foramina laterally. The contents of the epidural space include nerve roots with dural extensions, areolar tissue, fat, lymphatics, and blood vessels, including the Batson venous plexus.

Ligamentum flavum, also known as yellow ligament, forms the posterior boundary of the epidural space and extends from foramen magnum to sacral hiatus. It comprises a pair of ligaments (left and right) that fuse in the middle. The thickness of ligamentum flavum varies from 3 to 5 mm being thickest in the lumbar region, followed by thoracic and thinnest in the cervical region. Immediately posterior to ligamentum flavum lies the lamina, spinous process, and interspinous ligament. Further posterior to these structures lies the supraspinous ligament that joins the spinous processes together and runs from external occipital protuberance to the coccyx, which is covered by the skin and subcutaneous tissue (**Fig. 12.2**).

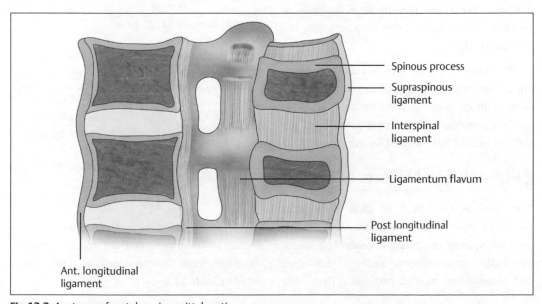

Fig.12.2 Anatomy of vertebrae in sagittal section.

The dural sac terminates in the sacral canal at S2 level (S3 in children). The volume of the caudal canal in adults, excluding the foramina and the dural sac, is about 10 to 27 mL. This wide variability of volume accounts for the variation in the height of the block in caudal anesthesia.

While spinal/subarachnoid block is performed in the lumbar region, epidural blocks can be performed in the epidural space, extending through the entire length of the vertebral canal, although lumbar and thoracic epidurals are the most frequently performed procedures.

Indications of CNBs (AS5.1)

CNBs are indicated in a variety of surgical procedures in obstetrics, acute, and postoperative pain management (**Box 12.1**). However, there are certain contradictions to the administration of CNBs as listed in **Box 12.2**.

A single shot spinal or epidural anesthesia is mainly employed for the lower abdominal or lower limb surgeries. Catheter-based techniques wherein a catheter is placed in the subarachnoid or epidural space are usually employed for perioperative (preoperative, intraoperative, postoperative period) or postoperative analgesia in thoracic, abdominal or lower limb surgeries and for labor analgesia.

The choice and type of CNBs are also dependent on nature and duration of surgery, associated comorbidities, ease of performance of block (patient position or underlying pathology), and the risk-benefit ratio tailored for every patient.

Physiological Effects of CNBs

The physiological effects of CNBs are due to the blockade of the sympathetic and somatic nervous system (including sensory and motor neurons), compensatory reflex mechanism, and unrestricted parasympathetic activity. The

Box 12.1 Indications of central neuraxial blocks

Surgical specialty

- Orthopedics:
  - Lower limb trauma.
  - Knee replacement surgeries.
  - Hip replacement surgeries.
  - Pelvic fractures.
  - Lumbar spine surgery.
- General surgery:
  - Appendectomy.
  - Laparoscopic cholecystectomy.
  - Diabetic foot debridement/amputation.
  - Anal canal surgeries.
  - Perineal surgeries.
  - Perioperative analgesia for major abdominal surgeries like Whipple's procedure, etc.
- Obstetrics and gynecology:
  - Lower (uterine) segment Caesarean section (LSCS).
  - Labor analgesia.
  - Laparoscopic/abdominal hysterectomy.
- Plastic surgery:
  - Lower limb flap cover.
- Urology:
  - Transurethral resection of prostate gland (TURP).
  - Orchidectomy.
  - Circumcision.
  - Penile surgery.
  - End assessment of the urinary bladder.

Other uses

- Thoracic epidural catheter placement—flail chest, severe trauma of chest (for pain relief).
- Lumbar epidural for perioperative analgesia in lower limb pathologies.
- Caudal/epidural injection: Management of chronic pain.

physiological effects of epidural anesthesia are similar to those of spinal anesthesia; however, the difference in the characteristics of the CNBs is listed in **Table 12.1**.

Box 12.2   Contraindications to central neuraxial blocks

Absolute

- Patient refusal.
- Localized sepsis.
- Allergy to any drug to be administered intrathecally or in epidural space.
- The inability to stay still during the needle placement: May cause inadvertent trauma to neural tissue.
- Increased intracranial pressure: May cause brainstem herniation.

Relative

- Neurologic:
  - Myelopathy: Preexisting neurologic deficit.
  - Spinal stenosis: Carries higher risk to neurological complications after neuraxial blockade.
  - Spine surgery: Previous spine surgery may alter spinal anatomy due to adhesions, scar tissue, hardware, and/or bone grafts; leads to difficult needle access in subarachnoid or epidural space; unpredictable and incomplete neuraxial blockade.
  - Multiple sclerosis: Increased sensitivity to LA; may prolong the duration of motor and sensory blockade.
  - Spina bifida: Traumatic injury to the spinal cord may occur due to neural tube defect, tethering of the spinal cord, and absence of ligamentum flavum or dura mater; unpredictable response to LA may be seen.
- Cardiac:
  - Aortic stenosis (AS): Hemodynamic instability or cardiac arrest in severe AS.
  - Hypovolemia: May lead to an exaggeration of hypotensive response.
- Hematological:
  - Thromboprophylaxis: Spinal hematoma formation leading to paraplegia with the use of low-molecular weight heparin (LMWH) and other antiplatelet drugs. All drugs need discontinuation as per the American Society of Regional Anesthesia (ASRA) guidelines before placing a block, and restarting the therapy is also guided by the coagulation profile and removal of an epidural catheter.
  - Inherited coagulopathy: Increased risk of bleeding and hematoma formation.
- Systemic infection:
  - Infection: Exaggerated hypotension due to systemic vasodilation; risk of iatrogenic meningitis; and epidural abscess.

The systemic effects of CNBs need to be understood for the safe conduct of the blocks as well as to detect and deal with any complications arising as a result of administration of the same.

1. Cardiovascular system

Blockade of the sympathetic activity leads to decreased peripheral vascular resistance with peripheral venous pooling of blood and a resultant decreased venous return to the central compartment, thereby leading to hypotension, which is the most common physiological side effect also encountered after administration of a CNB.

While the blockade of sympathetic fibers till T6 causes hypotension primarily, the cardio-accelerator sympathetic fiber blockade at T4 levels is associated with bradycardia and subsequent reduction in stroke volume. The preoperative intravascular volume may be contracted due to fasting in patients and, therefore, preloading or coloading with intravenous (IV) fluids is recommended to decrease the hypotension occurring due to spinal anesthesia. Similarly, the elderly are more prone to hypotension due to a higher resting sympathetic tone of the vessels along with decreased baroreceptor response.

Table 12.1 Differences in the characteristics of various CNBs

Type of block	Characteristics	Disadvantages
Spinal/subarachnoid block (drug administered in subarachnoid space)	• Can be performed quickly • Rapid onset • Bilateral sensory and motor blockade • Relative technical ease as compared to other CNBs	• Requires more time for placing a block and catheter • Limited duration • Cannot be extended if required • Cephalad
Epidural block (drug administered in epidural space)	• Slower onset of action • Anesthesia can be extended by insertion of a catheter in the epidural space • Usually utilized for postoperative analgesia and to decrease the opioid and muscle relaxant requirement in the intraoperative period	• Requires higher volume and concentration of drug for the sensory and motor effects • Have higher potential for the complications like dural puncture • More chances of local anesthetic systemic toxicity • More chances of post-dural puncture headache in case of accidental dural puncture • More probability of patchy block • The sacral block is relatively unreliable
Combined spinal-epidural block (drug administered in both subarachnoid and epidural space)	• Rapid onset and reliable bilateral motor and sensory blockade • Possible to extend the duration of the block through the epidural catheter • Can be kept in situ for around 96 h for postoperative analgesia/acute pain services	• Technically needs more expertise

Abbreviation: CNB, central neuraxial block.

Epidural anesthesia causes a gradual decrease in the blood pressure, and the magnitude of the same depends upon the number of segments involved during the epidural blockade. The small aliquots of local anesthetic administered in epidural space at spaced time intervals cause lesser hypotension, and thus graded epidural is one of the anesthetic choices in cardiac patients. Hypotension triggers the compensatory reflexes above the level of the block that usually include vasoconstriction and tachycardia. However, in a blockade at levels cephalad to T4, the decreased venous return may trigger bradycardia or even asystole, resulting from the unopposed parasympathetic activity and denervation of the sympathetic activity, especially in hypovolemic patients. The coronary blood flow decreases, myocardial oxygen demand increases, and myo-cardial work may increase with a reduction in the mean arterial pressure.

Hypotension usually responds to intravascular fluid administration, but exaggerated hypo-tension or that leading to nausea, vomiting and neurological symptoms like dizziness, loss of consciousness, may require treatment with vasopressors (both direct and indirect), alpha agonist with direct-acting (phenylephrine, epinephrine, norepinephrine) or indirect-acting vasoconstrictors (ephedrine, mephentermine).

2. Central nervous system

In the absence of severe hypotension, old age, or preexisting hypertension, the administration of CNBs usually does not affect the autoregulation and thus does not lead to alterations in the cerebral blood flow, which is usually maintained. However, with the loss of autoregulation at lower mean arterial pressures, the CNS may exhibit the signs of inadequate perfusion. This may lead to complaints of sedation, headache, altered respiratory pattern which, in turn, leads to unconsciousness; therefore, mandatory monitoring is recommended throughout the procedures under regional anesthetic techniques.

Higher blocks may be associated with rare complications like Horner's syndrome (miosis, anhidrosis, ptosis), cranial nerve palsies, and pupillary dilatation due to III cranial nerve blockade. The brainstem and the cortex may be affected due to the involvement of the thalamus or the reticular activating system.

3. Respiratory system

The paralysis of the lower abdominal muscle secondary to the motor block during CNBs affects the forced expiration and thus may be associated with decreased expiratory reserve volume and decreased vital capacity. However, the function of the diaphragm and other accessory muscles like sternocleidomastoid and scalene muscles is unaltered and compensates for the reduced volume. The respiratory rate is usually unchanged.

The block up to midthoracic level usually has no effect in the absence of any underlying pulmonary pathology. A, however, higher blockade may result in an ineffective cough in patients with underlying pulmonary pathology. Respiratory arrest, although rare, usually occurs due to hypoperfusion of the respiratory centers in the brainstem. Transient apnea may occur due to severe hypotension but usually resolves with the restoration of the hemodynamics and cardiac output. Obese patients are prone to exaggerated respiratory effects with more incidence of apnea and decreased vital capacity. Therefore, extreme caution must be exercised, and thorough monitoring must be ensured in obese individuals.

4. Gastrointestinal system

Neuraxial blockade involving the innervation from T6 to L1 hampers the splanchnic circulation and may lead to nausea, hyperperistalsis, or contracted gut, resulting from the unopposed parasympathetic activity. Atropine has been found to be effective for treating nausea during the CNBs.

5. Renal system

In healthy individuals, the transient decrease in renal blood flow that may occur with CNB has little clinical significance. Kidneys have large physiological reserves that are maintained if the blood pressure is maintained and adequate fluid resuscitation is performed. CNBs may lead to urinary retention and delay the discharge due to urinary catheterization, although the evidence is still not clear on the same.

Advantages of CNBs over General Anesthesia

CNBs carry some benefits over GA in certain procedures. They are also utilized for postoperative pain control as a part of multimodal anesthesia in addition to anesthesia. Some advantages of regional anesthesia over GA include the following:

- Avoidance of airway-related risks of GA (especially in patients with a high risk of aspiration and regurgitation).
- The patient remains awake during the surgical procedure.
- Minimal postoperative sedation as compared to GA.
- Shorter stay in the postoperative care unit (PACU).
- Early recovery and discharge.
- Beneficial modulation of the stress response.
- Reduced blood loss.

- Reduced incidence of thromboembolic events.
- Improved pulmonary function.
- Effective postoperative analgesia.
- May be used as an adjunct to GA, especially epidural anesthesia.
- CNBs in cardiac patients reduces the incidence of cardiac complications in the perioperative period.
- Blood loss is reduced when CNBs are administered.
- CNBs are associated with less incidence of nausea and vomiting as compared to GA.

Position for CNBs

Before performing any CNB, it is mandatory to prepare the anesthesia trolley with all emergency drugs and resuscitation equipment to tackle the complications, if any, and to administer GA in case the surgical procedure exceeds the stipulated time beyond the duration of the CNB. There are three primary positions in which neuraxial block may be performed, and relative merits and demerits of the same are enlisted in **Table 12.2**.

Level of Block Required for Common Surgeries

The dermatomal level required for various surgical procedures is several segments higher than the actual skin incision since the intra-abdominal structures like peritoneum (T4), bladder (T10), and uterus (T10) have innervation from spinal cord segment much more cephalad compared to that of the corresponding skin incision. Also, the sensory dermatomal level is two segments higher than the motor, and the sympathetic blockade is two dermatomal levels higher than the sensory level. The dermatomal levels for various procedures are enumerated in **Table 12.3**.

Table 12.2 Various positions for the administration of CNBs

	Advantages	Disadvantages
Lateral decubitus	• Facilitates sedative administration if required • More open intervertebral space achieved	• Faster onset of action
Sitting	• Faster needle placement • Easier identification of midline in cases of an anatomical anomaly	• Slow onset of drug • Hypotension is more common in sitting position
Prone (rarely used nowadays)	• Can be used for prone surgeries (rectal, perineal, and lumbar surgeries)	• Minimum CSF pressure hence may need to aspirate to confirm

Abbreviations: CNB, central neuraxial block; CSF, cerebrospinal fluid.

Table 12.3 Dermatomal level required for various surgical procedures

Type of surgery	Dermatomal level
Upper abdominal surgery	T4
Cesarean delivery	T4
Transurethral resection of the prostate	T10
Hip surgery	T10
Foot and ankle surgery	L2

The major landmarks that provide some information about the corresponding dermatomal levels and are commonly employed for clinical interpretation during CNBs include:

- Little finger—C8.
- Level of nipples—T4.
- The lower level of xiphoid—T6.
- Umbilicus—T10.
- Midpoint of inguinal line—T12.

This chapter discusses the individual CNBs under the headings of spinal, epidural, and caudal anesthesia.

Subarachnoid Block (Spinal Anesthesia) (AS5.1, AS5.2)

Subarachnoid block that involves the administration of local anesthetic with or without adjuvant in the subarachnoid space is variously termed as a spinal block, intrathecal or intradural block, and the subsequent anesthesia due to action on the spinal nerves is commonly termed as spinal anesthesia. The indications and contraindications of the procedure are the same as those mentioned in **Boxes 12.1** and **12.2**. It can be administered in sitting or lateral decubitus position and is usually performed in the lumbar region below the L1 level. Spinous processes form an important landmark to perform the procedure, and the puncture is generally achieved by the use of spinal needles ranging from 23G to 27G.

The block can be performed in the intervertebral space through either the midline or the paramedian approach. While all the structures mentioned in anatomy are pierced through the midline approach, the supraspinous and interspinous ligament are bypassed in the paramedian technique. The free flow of CSF after tactile perception of loss of resistance to the ligamentum flavum is the most confirmatory sign of the accurate needle placement.

The factors affecting as well as having no effect on the block height, that is, the difference in the cephalad spread of the drug with the same volume of the drug in different individuals are enumerated in **Table 12.4**, and the important ones are discussed hereby. When only sacral roots are anesthetized by the use of a hyperbaric local anesthetic solution, which is achieved in sitting position for a longer duration, the block is referred to as the "saddle block" that is mainly employed for daycare perineal surgeries.

Table 12.4 Factors affecting block height

	Major determinants	Minor determinants	No effect
Drug factors	• Dose • Baricity (relative density of the drug to that of CSF)	• Volume • Concentration • Temperature • Viscosity • Opioids as additive	Additives other than opioids
Patient factors	• CSF volume • Age • Pregnancy	• Weight • Height • Spinal anatomy • Intra-abdominal pressure	• Menopause • Gender • Coughing
Environment factors	• Patient position • Epidural injection post spinal	• Level of injection • Fluid currents • Needle orifice direction • Needle type	

Abbreviation: CSF, cerebrospinal fluid.

a. Drug factors

Baricity is the ratio of the density of the drug solution to the density of CSF and is defined as the mass per unit volume at a specific temperature. Local anesthetic solutions with a density similar to CSF are termed isobaric, while those with higher and lower baricity than CSF are known as hyperbaric and hypobaric, respectively. Dextrose and sterile water are commonly added to render local anesthetic solutions either hyperbaric or hypobaric. While hyperbaric solutions spread preferentially to the dependent regions, hypobaric solutions tend to spread to the nondependent areas. Isobaric solutions are usually unaffected by the gravitational forces, and the same concept is capitalized by anesthesiologist by alteration of the position of the patient during the subarachnoid block.

b. Patient factors

Patient characteristics that may influence block height include patient height, weight, age, sex, pregnancy, the anatomic configuration of the spine, and the CSF properties.

The CSF volume significantly influences the block height as well as the regression of sensory and motor blockade. Therefore, neonates and children who have higher CSF volumes (mg/kg BW) require higher doses of the local anesthetic in subarachnoid space as compared to adults.

Advanced age is associated with increased block height due to decreased CSF volumes and increased sensitivity of the neural structures to LAs.

Variation of spine and pelvis contributes to variation in block height in male or female gender.

Obesity also has an effect on the block, as the increased epidural fat content has an impinging impact on subarachnoid space, thereby resulting in more cephalad spread with the same volume and concentration of the drug.

Lumbar lordosis, as seen during pregnancy, leads to higher cephalad spread, and a similar effect is observed with twin pregnancies compared with a singleton pregnancy.

c. Procedure-related factors

Usually, intrathecal spread occurs up to 20 to 25 minutes of injection of the drug in the intrathecal space, and therefore positioning is an important determinant of block height initially. The thoracic curve of the spine usually limits the block height up to T4 until large volumes, as intended for the epidural block, are accidentally placed in subarachnoid space.

Higher intervertebral space injection results in greater cephalad spread with higher block height for the same volume and concentration of drugs. Higher injection rate and barbotage (repeated aspiration and reinjection of CSF) of hyperbaric solutions are associated with higher cephalad spread. Injecting local anesthetic or saline in epidural space also increases the block height after the subarachnoid block.

Local Anesthetics Used in Subarachnoid Block (AS5.4)

Only preservative-free preparations are recommended for use with CNBs, as the preservatives can cause permanent neurological damage. Hyperbaric bupivacaine (0.5%) is the most commonly preferred local anesthetic utilized for surgical procedure and is preferred because of the longer duration of action, though the onset of action is slow (5–7 mins).

The addition of adjuvants like fentanyl (20–25 µg) and sufentanil (2–10 µg) have the advantage of prolongation of the duration of the block and reduction of the dose of the local anesthetic drug and thus may be beneficial in patients with underlying cardiac and respiratory disorders. Opioids are the most commonly used adjuvants and have numerous mechanisms of action:

- Direct spinal cord dorsal horn opioid receptor activation.

- Cerebral opioid receptor activation after CSF transport.
- Peripheral and central systemic effects after vascular uptake.

However, the incidence of nausea and vomiting, pruritus, urinary retention, and delayed respiratory depression is more with the use of opioids. Morphine in the dose of 100 to 500 µg has also been utilized, but the use has decreased with the availability of short-acting opioids.

α_2-agonists (clonidine) act on prejunctional and postjunctional α_2-receptors in the dorsal horn of the spinal cord and are used (15–225 mg) to prolong the sensory and motor blockade as well as improve analgesia. However, it may lead to sedation, hypotension, and bradycardia and thus requires caution while using.

Lignocaine 5% (with 7.5% dextrose) has a rapid onset of action with an intermediate duration of action (60–90 mins) but was withdrawn due to side effects like transient neurological symptoms (TNS) and permanent nerve damage. It has recently been introduced again with a better safety profile. Other drugs that are used for spinal anesthesia are mentioned in **Table 12.5**.

Epidural Anesthesia (AS5.1)

Epidural anesthesia is multifaceted in anesthesia by the fact that apart from being employed in the perioperative period for anesthesia, it is utilized as pain control therapeutic measure in multivaried conditions like postoperative analgesia, labor analgesia, and multimodal analgesia in trauma.

It can be administered as a single shot or continuous technique by the placement of a catheter in the epidural space and provides all the benefits of CNBs as mentioned earlier. The onset of action is more in epidural anesthesia as the drug administered in the epidural space must diffuse through the dural cuffs to act on the spinal nerves and nerve roots. This also mandates higher amounts of drugs to achieve anesthesia, and therefore higher volumes are required to achieve the sensory and motor blockade.

Lumbar epidurals are employed for the abdominal and lower surgical procedures, while thoracic epidural placement is used for upper abdominal and thoracic procedures. Cervical epidural placement is usually performed for chronic pain syndromes and requires higher expertise for the procedure. The epidural anesthesia may be

Table 12.5 Drugs used for subarachnoid block

Drug	Composition and characteristic features
Chloroprocaine	• Preservative free formulation of chloroprocaine in doses of 30–60 mg to produce a reliable, short duration (40–90 mins) of anesthesia with a faster recovery time than procaine, lidocaine and bupivacaine • Has minimal systemic and fetal side effects • Ideal for ambulatory surgeries
Prilocaine	• 40–60 mg 2% hyperbaric prilocaine can provide long duration (100–130 mins) • Used for ambulatory arthroscopic knee surgery
Bupivacaine	• 0.25, 0.5, and 0.75% clear isobaric solutions and hyperbaric solution of 0.5 and 0.75% solution containing 80 mg/mL glucose
Tetracaine	• Hyperbaric 1% (with 10% glucose) • Onset (3–5 mins) with the duration of 80–120 mins with additives • Used for perineal and abdominal surgery • Incidence of TNS high

Abbreviation: TNS, transient neurological symptoms.
Note: Procaine, articaine, mepivacaine are not popular choices for subarachnoid block.

utilized in the intraoperative period for adequate muscle relaxation and opioid-sparing effects, and the postoperative analgesia can be extended through bolus or continuous infusions of low-dose LA with or without adjuvants.

Epidural space has lower pressures in comparison to the atmospheric pressure, and the same principle is applied to identify the same during the needle or catheter placement. It is usually identified with loss of resistance method by either saline or air in sitting or lateral decubitus position. Other methods like the hanging drop method, manometric methods, spring-loaded syringe, epiduroscopy, and ultrasound are seldom employed for its detection. Specially designed epidural needles (Touhy's needle) are used to place epidural blocks. The confirmation of the space occurs by the passage of catheter and ability to administer local anesthetic with a vasoconstrictor (usually epinephrine 15 μg) and without any adverse effects that rule out the subarachnoid and intravascular placement, respectively.

Factors Affecting Epidural Block Height

a. Drug factors
The dose and volume of injective are the most important drug-related factors responsible for block height. Larger volumes are required to achieve sensory and motor blockade.

b. Patient factors
Advancing age is associated with higher/more cephalad spread for the same volume of drugs due to decreased compliance of space and lesser exit of drugs through intervertebral foramina. Extremes of height also affect the block height as with spinal anesthesia. Engorgement of veins, as seen in pregnancy, decreases the requirement of LA to be administered in epidural space.

c. Procedural factors
For the same volume of drug injected in epidural space, the wider dermatomal spread is present in thoracic than the lumbar epidural. The epidural spread is more toward the dependent side, and

the fact may be utilized in patchy or inadequate blocks.

Preservative-free preparations of LAs with or without the adjuvants may be used in epidural space. While higher concentrations are required for the motor blockade, lower concentrations may be utilized for postoperative pain relief and labor analgesia. The LAs commonly employed are lignocaine (1–2%), bupivacaine (0.0625–0.5%), ropivacaine (0.1–0.75%), levobupivacaine (0.1–0.5%). Adjuvants (epinephrine, opioids, alpha 2 agonists, dexamethasone, midazolam) may be added to increase the duration as well as decrease the concentration of LA administered.

Combined Spinal Epidural (AS5.1)

Combined spinal-epidural anesthesia, first described in 1937, has undergone multiple modifications over the years. The rapid onset through spinal anesthesia allows early commencement of the surgical procedure, while the placement of the epidural catheter allows a prolongation of anesthesia and postoperative analgesia. Traditionally, it used to be administered by individual needles in either the same or different space. Over the years, needle through needle technique has become popular with availability of commercial combined spinal-epidural sets.

Epidural volume extension (EVE) is a technique used to extend the subarachnoid block by compression of the dural sac via saline injected into the epidural space to achieve sensory block by low volumes of LA given in subarachnoid space. It has shown advantages like greater hemodynamic stability, reduction in side effects, and faster recovery, leading to early discharge from the hospital.

Caudal Anesthesia (AS5.5)

Caudal anesthesia is a technique of injecting local anesthetic in the epidural space via the caudal canal. It is popular in pediatric anesthesia to provide analgesia and reduce the amount of volatile anesthetics necessary. It is, however, quite unpredictable in adults and is particularly useful where the sacral anesthetic spread is desired like in anal, rectal, or perineal surgeries and also useful for chronic pain management.

The local anesthetic used is similar to those described for epidural anesthesia and analgesia. However, the spread of drugs is unpredictable in adults, and twice the dose of the lumbar epidural is required. It is considered unreliable for procedures above the umbilicus.

Complications of CNBs

CNBs can lead to multiple side effects ranging from minor to major catastrophic events, resulting in death or neurological damage with resultant disability. Fortunately, the catastrophes are rare, although all the fatalities carry significant legal implications. The complications of CNBs are tabulated in **Table 12.6**. The incidence of complications secondary to CNBs is estimated to be between 1/1,000 and 1/10,00,000. However, the occurrence of major ones is relatively rare,

with others taking the predominance. The adverse effects secondary to CNBs are due to mechanical injury, inadvertent neural or vessel damage, misplacement of the catheters, or adverse effects of the LAs or other drugs administered.

Most of the minor effects after the block usually require reassurance and symptomatic treatment.

Postdural puncture headache is usually encountered in 30 to 50% patients after a spinal tap, 0 to 5% after spinal anesthesia, and in 81% of patients after an accidental dural puncture during epidural placement. The risk factors are:

• Young patients.

• Female sex.

• Larger needle size.

• Pregnancy.

• Multiple dural punctures.

• Cutting spinal needles as compared to non-cutting needles.

It presents with severe frontal headache usually after 24 hours of the block and can generally be managed by supine positioning and adequate hydration. Oral analgesics with caffeine can be prescribed for symptomatic relief. In severe

Table 12.6 Complications of CNBs

Minor	Moderate	Major
• Hypotension • Bradycardia • Nausea • Vomiting • Shivering • Dizziness • Transient hearing loss • Pruritus • Urinary retention • Backache	• PDPH • Transient neurological symptoms (recover over a week)	• Subdural injection (with an epidural) • High/total spinal (subarachnoid block) • Respiratory arrest • Cardiac arrest/death • LAST • Paraplegia • Cauda equina syndrome • Epidural hematoma • Direct nerve injuries (permanent neurological injury) • Arachnoiditis • Meningitis • Epidural abscess

Abbreviations: CNB, central neuraxial block; LAST, local anesthetic systemic toxicity; PDPH, postdural puncture headache.

unrelenting headaches, an epidural blood patch is performed in sterile conditions for optimal relief.

High spinal anesthesia refers to the spread of local anesthetics to the cervical region, following subarachnoid block or inadvertent intrathecal injection during epidural anesthesia—the patient complains of perioral paresthesia and difficulty in breathing due to involvement of phrenic nerve. The involvement of cardioaccelleratory fibers (T4-T6) results in hypotension, bradycardia, and cardiac arrest.

Total spinal anesthesia results from the spread of local anesthetics to cardiorespiratory center. The manifestations include loss of consciousness, apnea, hypotension, bradycardia, and cardiac arrest.

The management of total and high spinal anesthesia includes:

- *Airway:* 100% oxygen, bag and mask ventilation and intubation.
- *Circulation:* IV fluids, vasopressors (ephedrine 3–6 mg bolus, adrenaline 1:10000 [0.5-1 mL as required]).
- Continue mechanical ventilation till the effects of block wear off.

Major complications require immediate support of airway breathing and circulation in cases of respiratory arrest with advanced care.

Local anesthetic systemic toxicity (LAST) has been discussed in detail in chapter on local anesthetics. Infective causes mandate treatment with antibiotics, and the earliest surgical decompression needs to be performed in epidural hematoma, cauda equina, or abscess development. The permanent neurological sequelae need to be documented and carry high medicolegal implications.

Early recognition and detection with appropriate monitoring remain the mainstay to prevent the catastrophic complications, and therefore extreme vigilance is required throughout the conduct of the procedure until the block effect regresses completely.

Conclusion

CNBs are the most commonly performed procedure in the entire world. Although the learning curve for the same is small, they are associated with significant side effects and complications, even in experienced hands. Therefore, extreme caution and vigilance should be employed during their conduct with appropriate monitoring, and one should also anticipate the complications associated with it, and make the necessary preparation to handle them in the most effective manner.

CHAPTER 13

Peripheral Nerve Blocks (AS5.3)

Richa Saroa, Sanjeev Palta, and Aravind B. Guledagudd

Introduction

Daycare/ambulatory anesthesia, aiming at early discharge and resumption of daily activities, has prompted the anesthesiologists to mold the anesthetic techniques for the provision of the same. Therefore, the focus has been diverted to the use of regional anesthesia techniques that are minimally invasive and are utilized in the entire perioperative period. Peripheral nerve blocks (PNBs) have revolutionized the practice of anesthesia by the provision of adequate analgesia and muscle relaxation in the intraoperative period and extension of postoperative analgesia that aids in good quality of life with early functionality. The blocks are usually well-tolerated, minimally invasive, and safe when administered with all precautions. In PNBs, the local anesthetic (LA) is deposited near the nerve bundle/plexus or the individual nerve to achieve motor and sensory blockade from that part of the body. Traditionally performed through anatomical landmark techniques, the safety and efficacy have further been improved with the introduction of peripheral nerve stimulators and ultrasound (US) that helps in localizing the nerves and administration of drugs near the vicinity of desired structures while avoiding damage to other nearby structures.

Historical Perspective

Historical milestones in the field of peripheral nerve blocks are:

- 1564: Ambroise Pare administered LA by nerve compression.
- 1600: Val Verde performed regional anesthesia (RA) by compression of nerves and blood vessels supplying the operating area.
- 1646: Marco Aurelio Severino administered refrigeration anesthesia by use of freezing mixtures of snow and ice.
- 1784: James Moore administered LA of extremity by compression of nerve trunks.
- 1839: Taylor and Washington introduced hypodermic injection.
- 1843: Alexander Wood invented the first true hypodermic needle to administer morphine injection.
- 1855: Friedrich Georg Carl Gaedcke isolated the alkaloid from leaves of the coca plant.
- 1860: Albert Friedrich Emil Niemann was involved in the purification and naming of cocaine.
- 1873: Hughes Bennett discovered the anesthetic properties of cocaine.
- 1884: Carl Koller's first topical use of cocaine in eye surgery.

William Halsted and Richard John Hall (introduced brachial plexus blockade with cocaine).

William C. Burke (removed a bullet from finger under nerve block with cocaine).

- 1885: James Leonard Corning attempted spinal anesthesia.
- 1892: Karl Ludwig Schleich introduced infiltration anesthesia.

Francois-Frank coined the term nerve blocking.

- 1901: Cathelin and Sicard independently discovered caudal epidural block using cocaine.

- 1902: Heinrich F.W. Braun used epinephrine for nerve blockade and coined the term conduction anesthesia.

- 1908: George Washington Crile coined the term Anoci-association: regional block plus light general anesthesia (GA).

- 1922: Gaston Labat described the RA technique and clinical application.

- 1923: Gaston Labat founded the American Society of Regional Anesthesia (ASRA).

Indication and Applications (AS5.3)

PNBs may be used as a sole anesthetic technique for peripheral limb surgery or with GA for intraoperative and postoperative analgesia as well as reduction of the analgesic and anesthetic agents.

PNBs share advantages with the neuraxial anesthetic and analgesic techniques, the foremost being the lack of need for the airway instrumentation, especially in patients with underlying respiratory disorders or where the airway is deemed to be difficult and thus may be considered as the primary anesthetic choice in patients with underlying respiratory diseases or other comorbidities. However, the preoperative preparation for emergency airway management or for failed blocks is mandatory before the start of the procedure. The indications of PNBs are:

- For emergency surgeries where the patient presents with a full stomach.

- PNBs allow shorter time to discharge and are associated with lesser incidence of nausea and vomiting and thus is a choice of anesthetic technique in ambulatory surgeries, wherever feasible.

- A certain subset of patients may themselves opt for PNBs to be awake during the surgical procedure.

- PNBs may also be used for diagnostic, therapeutic, and prognostic purposes in the management of chronic pain syndromes.

- PNBs may diminish or prevent the development of chronic pain syndromes by a lack of central nervous system (CNS) sensitization that occurs after acute injury.

- Rarely, PNBs maybe opted as an anesthetic technique of the first choice in patients having allergies to multiple drugs, or patients wanting to avoid systemic drugs.

PNBs are also associated with decreased consumption of opioids, thus leading to reduced incidence of side effects of these drugs and therefore form the cornerstone of the multimodal analgesia and opioid-reducing approaches.

The contraindications to PNBs include:

- Patient refusal.

- Allergy to local anesthetics.

- Active infection at the site of injection.

- Pre-existing neural deficits along the distribution of nerve of interest.

- Patients with coagulopathy or receiving antithrombotic drugs.

PNBs are practiced by the anesthesiologists, surgeons, orthopedics, and emergency physicians. Irrespective of the specialty, PNBs require exemplary skill, mandatory monitoring, and preparation for all the resuscitative equipment before the conduct of the block.

Anatomy and Techniques (AS5.3)

The anatomy and landmarks relevant to the block to be performed depend upon the nerves required to be blocked for analgesia or anesthesia.

Techniques: The success of PNBs depends upon the accurate localization of nerve or plexus, and various techniques have been described and utilized for the same.

PNBs may be performed using the landmark technique with or without the peripheral nerve stimulator and the US-guided technology.

Landmark Technique

- Paresthesia technique: Traditionally, the technique of eliciting paresthesia by using the well-defined surface landmarks has been utilized to perform the PNBs. A short beveled needle is usually advanced toward the target nerve and plexus to elicit paresthesia in the sensory distribution of the nerve and thus recognize the proximity of the nerve before administering the LA solution. Although most frequently employed, it carries a significant potential for direct intraneuronal damage, thus causing permanent neurological sequelae.

- Nerve stimulation technique: The reports of neural damage with the paresthesia technique prompted the development of peripheral nerve stimulators. The target nerve or plexus is recognized by the help of electric current passed through an insulated plexus needle. The needle hub is attached to a wire that is further connected to a nerve stimulator that emits small pulses of electric current (0–0.5 mA, at a set frequency of usually 1–2 Hz), leading to depolarization and muscle contraction in the area of distribution of nerve supply. LA is deposited while the needle is in close proximity to the nerve, and the surety of the block can be determined by the rapid dissipation of the current density and elimination of the motor responses after the injection.

Ultrasound-Guided Technique

The capability to appreciate the neural and the associated delineation of the anatomy has popularized the use of US for performing the PNBs. The use of US also helps in reducing the complications related to drug, neural, and related structures and helps to deposit the LA at the intended place under direct visualization. The frequency of 1 to 20 MHz is employed for clinical imaging by ultrasonography with high-frequency probes for superficial structures and low frequency for the deeper structures.

Monitoring

All patients must receive premedication to alleviate anxiety. The procedure must be explained to the patient in his vernacular language, and informed consent sought before the block is administered. PNBs are conducted under aseptic conditions in the preoperative or the operative room with standard monitoring that includes ECG, noninvasive blood pressure, saturation, and respiratory pattern. An intravenous (IV) line must be secured before the block is performed, and the patient must receive oxygen supplementation if drapes are expected to cover the head and neck of the patient.

LAs that are utilized for anesthesia and analgesia have been discussed in Chapter 11 on LA, and the drugs may be administered with or without the adjuvants, depending upon the duration, nature, and extent of surgery.

The major peripheral blocks utilized for perioperative and postoperative pain have been discussed in the text.

Upper Limb Blocks

Brachial Plexus Anatomy (AS5.2, AS5.6)

The brachial plexus comprises the anterior primary divisions (ventral rami) of the fifth through the eighth cervical nerves and the first thoracic nerve. The nerve roots leave the intervertebral foramina and converge successively to form trunks, divisions, cords, branches, and finally, terminal nerves. The trunks are formed between the anterior and middle scalene muscles and are termed as superior, middle, and inferior trunk, based on their vertical orientation. As the trunks pass over the lateral border of the first rib and under the clavicle, each trunk divides into anterior and posterior divisions. As the brachial plexus emerges below the clavicle, the fibers combine again to form three cords that are named according to their relationship with the second part of the axillary artery, that is, lateral, medial, and posterior cord. The anterior division from the superior and middle trunks form the lateral cord, posterior divisions from all the trunks form the posterior cord, and the anterior division of the inferior trunk continues as medial cord. At the lateral border of the pectoralis minor muscle, each cord gives off a large branch before ending as a major terminal nerve. The lateral cord gives off the lateral branch of the median nerve and terminates as the musculocutaneous nerve. The medial cord gives off the medial branch of the median nerve and terminates as ulnar nerve. The posterior cord gives off the axillary nerve and terminates as a radial nerve (**Fig. 13.1**).

Brachial plexus blocks above the clavicle mainly target anesthetic placement near the ventral rami, trunks, and divisions. Blocks below the clavicle primarily target the cords and terminal nerves. Brachial plexus can be approached at many levels, as given in **Table 13.1** and described below.

1. Interscalene block

Interscalene block is indicated in surgeries involving shoulder and upper arm. While this approach densely blocks C5–7 roots, the ulnar nerve originating from C8 and T1 may get spared. Therefore, this approach of the block is not ideal for surgery at or distal to the elbow. Complete surgical anesthesia of the shoulder can be achieved by blocking the C3–4 cutaneous branches with a superficial cervical plexus block or local infiltration. In addition to the usual complications, the block should not be attempted in patients with phrenic nerve palsy and severe pulmonary disease.

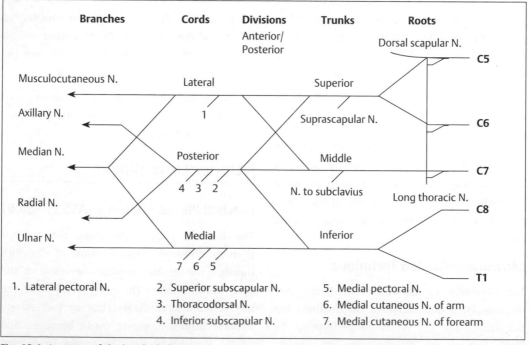

Fig. 13.1 Anatomy of the brachial plexus.

Table 13.1 Levels of brachial plexus block

S. no.	Block name	The level of brachial plexus block
1.	Interscalene block	At the level of C5–7 roots
2.	Supraclavicular block	At the level of brachial plexus trunks
3.	Infraclavicular block	At the level of cords around the axillary artery
4.	Axillary block	At the level of the axillary artery (axilla), blocks median, radial, and ulnar nerve
5.	Median nerve block	Median nerve block at the level of the wrist
6.	Ulnar nerve block	Ulnar nerve block at the level of the wrist
7.	Radial nerve block	Radial nerve block at the level of the wrist
8.	Intercostobrachial nerve block	Intercostobrachial nerve block at the level of medial aspect of the upper arm

Approach

The brachial plexus passes between the anterior and middle scalene muscles at the level of the cricoid cartilage or C6 vertebral body. The patient is placed in a supine or semi-sitting position with the head turned away from the side to be blocked. The interscalene groove is palpated by moving the fingers from the lateral border of sternocleidomastoid toward the anterior scalene muscle at the level of the cricoid cartilage. The external jugular vein usually crosses the interscalene groove at the level of the cricoid cartilage. A short beveled (5 cm) insulated needle is inserted medially at a caudal angle and advanced optimally to elicit a motor response of the deltoid or biceps muscles, suggesting superior trunk stimulation. Slow administration of LA is performed after negative aspiration of blood or cerebrospinal fluid (CSF).

The plexus can be identified as a traffic light sign (where) with the help of US, and the block may be performed using a high-frequency US probe.

Complications

- Horner syndrome.
- Spinal injection.
- Epidural injection.
- Vertebral artery or carotid artery puncture.

- IV injection.
- Pneumothorax.

2. Supraclavicular block

It is one of the most widely practiced approaches; it offers dense anesthesia for surgical procedures at or distal to the elbow.

Approach

It targets trunks of the brachial plexus superolateral to the subclavian artery. A short beveled, 5-cm needle is advanced lateral to the subclavian artery in the clavicular groove in a supine patient, with the head turned toward the opposite side and paresthesia, or muscle twitch is elicited along the arm or fingers. The brachial plexus gives a honeycomb appearance on US and carries an advantage of identification of pleura to avoid any damage to the same. The musculocutaneous nerve may be spared, and therefore it may need to be blocked in the arm for an adequate block or for tourniquet pain.

Complications

- Pneumothorax.
- Subclavian artery puncture.
- Ipsilateral phrenic nerve palsy.
- Horner's syndrome.

Since there is always a risk for a pleural puncture, caution should be exercised in patients with phrenic nerve palsy.

3. Infraclavicular block

The target nerves are arranged around the axillary artery as cords, and the approach offers dense anesthesia for procedures at or distal to the elbow. It is preferable to perform the landmark technique using a peripheral nerve stimulator.

Technique

It requires a longer, 10-cm needle that is inserted just medial to the coracoid process and directed posteriorly to elicit the motor response of finger flexion or extension, with a current intensity of less than 0.5 mA. Thereafter, the drug is deposited after negative aspiration of blood.

Technically, it is a difficult block when performed using US, and a low-frequency probe may be required to identify the cords around the artery.

Complications

- Vascular puncture.
- Pneumothorax.

4. Axillary block

This block reliably blocks the radial, ulnar, and median nerve that lie posterior, inferior, and superiorly, respectively, in relation to the axillary artery. The axillary, musculocutaneous, and medial brachial cutaneous nerves branch out from the brachial plexus block in the axilla, where they may also be individually blocked to provide anesthesia for procedures distal to the elbow.

Technique

A short beveled, 5-cm needle may be advanced with the axillary artery as a landmark through a transarterial technique, where the drug is deposited posterior as well anterior to the artery.

Complications

- Hematoma formation.
- Risk of accidental LA toxicity.

The use of US can help identify the nerves around the axillary artery and thus aid in performing the block without complications.

5. The rescue nerve blocks like that median nerve, ulnar and radial nerve may be performed at the level of the elbow, midarm, or the wrist for supplementation of inadequate blocks or procedure in the dermatomal distribution of these nerves.

Lower Limb Blocks (AS5.6)

Lumbar Plexus Anatomy

Lumbosacral plexus provides motor and sensory innervation to the lower limbs. It is formed by ventral rami of L1–4 innervating the anterior portion of the thigh and inner leg. It lies within the psoas muscle, with branches descending into the proximal thigh. Three major nerves arising from the lumbar plexus are femoral (L2–4), lateral femoral cutaneous (L1–3), and obturator (L2–4) nerve. Sacral plexus arises from L4–5 and S1–4 innervating posterior thigh (posterior femoral cutaneous nerve, S1-3), leg, and foot (**Fig. 13.2**). Individual nerve blocks and the indications are mentioned in **Table 13.2**.

- **Lumbar plexus block**

  It is usually employed for surgical procedures on knee, thigh, and hip along with GA to reduce intraoperative and postoperative analgesic consumption. It is generally performed in lateral decubitus position at a point that is midline between the two iliac crests, where a long needle is introduced, and the quadriceps muscle twitch recognizes the plexus with the help of a peripheral nerve stimulator. It can easily be recognized in the posterior part of the psoas muscle using US, where the drug is introduced for the desired effect.

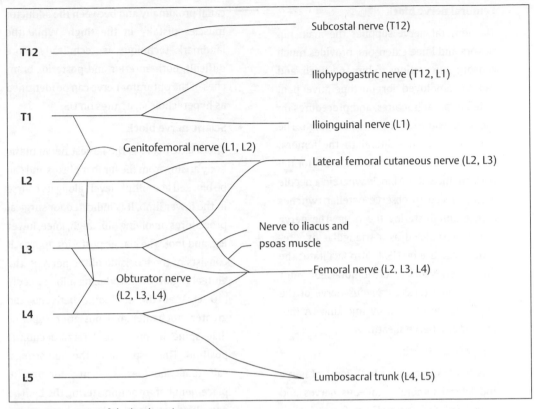

Fig. 13.2 Anatomy of the lumbar plexus.

Table 13.2 Indications of the lower limb blocks

Sl. no.	Block name	Indications
1	Lumbar plexus block	Combined with general anesthesia, it is used for surgery of knee, thigh or hip or with sciatic nerve block for most lower limb surgeries
2	Femoral nerve block	The femoral nerve supplies the main hip flexors and knee extensors and provides much sensory innervations to the hip and thigh
3	Fascia iliaca block	This block anesthetizes both femoral nerve and lateral femoral cutaneous nerves
4	Obturator nerve block	This block is done for complete anesthesia of the knee and is most often given along with femoral and sciatic nerve blocks
5	Popliteal nerve block	This block is ideal for surgeries of the lower leg, particularly leg and ankle
6	Sciatic nerve block	Blockade of the sciatic nerve may occur anywhere along its course, and it is indicated for surgical procedures involving hip and thigh, knee, lower leg, and foot
7	Adductor canal block	It is used for analgesia of the knee and medial aspect of the leg
8	Saphenous nerve block	They are mainly used in conjunction with a sciatic nerve block to provide complete analgesia/anesthesia below the knee

- **Femoral nerve block**

  The femoral nerve supplies the main hip flexors and knee extensors, provides much sensory innervations to hip and thigh, and can be employed for postoperative pain relief, femoral fractures, and procedures on the knee and medial side of the thigh. The femoral nerve lies lateral to the femoral artery that provides a true landmark for the performance of the block, wherein a needle is introduced to observe patellar twitches before administering the drug. The nerve can be visualized as a triangular hyperechoic structure on US. It also facilitates the three in one block where femoral, obturator nerve, and lateral cutaneous nerve of the thigh can be blocked by injecting LA into the femoral nerve sheath.

- **Fascia iliaca block**

  This block anesthetizes both femoral nerve and lateral femoral cutaneous nerves and is utilized for analgesia in femoral neck fractures and the application of plaster in children with femoral fractures. It is usually performed in supine patients by introducing a needle at a point between medial two-third and lateral one-third of the line joining the anterior superior iliac spine (ASIS) and pubic tubercle by the tactile feeling of the "pop" between the two planes. The use of US helps identify the fascia iliaca, fascia lata and iliacus muscle, and the drug is deposited beneath the fascia iliaca.

- **Obturator nerve block**

  The obturator nerve innervates the adductor muscles, hip joint, and provides cutaneous sensation on the medial side of the thigh. The block is usually performed with the femoral and sciatic nerve block to achieve complete anesthesia of the knee. The nerve can be blocked in the obturator canal proximally and between the adductor muscles distally in the thigh. While the landmark technique is technically more difficult, both anterior and posterior branches of the obturator nerve can be identified as hyperechoic structures on US.

- **Sciatic nerve block**

  The sciatic nerve is the largest nerve of the body arising from the lumbar plexus and can be blocked at multiple levels along its course in the lower limb. It is indicated for surgical procedures involving hip, thigh, knee, lower leg, and foot. The classic posterior approach consists of the blockade of the nerve in the gluteal region by introducing a long needle (10 cm) at the midpoint between the greater trochanter and posterior superior iliac spine in prone or lateral decubitus position. The response of the hamstrings, calf, foot, and toes is elicited for precise placement before administering the LA. The nerve can be visualized as a hyperechoic structure between the greater trochanter and ischial tuberosity on the US approach but may require the use of low-frequency probe, as the nerve is deep-seated and may be difficult to locate, especially in obese individuals. When used in combination with the femoral nerve block, anesthesia of lower limb till midthigh can be achieved.

- **Popliteal nerve block**

  The sciatic nerve can also be blocked at the popliteal fossa level before it bifurcates into the tibial and common peroneal nerve. This block is ideal for surgeries of the lower leg, particularly leg and ankle. It is performed in the supine or prone position most commonly through the intertendinous approach, where the needle is inserted at 7 cm above the popliteal fossa crease at the midpoint between the tendons to elicit dorsiflexion/plantarflexion of foot, in order to confirm the placement and subsequently inject the drug for the desired effect. The site of insertion usually corresponds to the bifurcation of the sciatic nerve, and therefore the LA is administered to block both the components of the sciatic nerve. Similarly, with the US technique, tibial and peroneal nerves are identified as superficial and lateral to the popliteal vessels and are blocked anterior to the same.

- **Adductor canal block**

The adductor canal is a fascial passage through which the femoral artery and vein enter the popliteal fossa in the knee. The saphenous nerve, posterior division of obturator nerve, and nerve to vastus medialis lie in the adductor canal and provide sensory innervation to the knee joint. The adductor canal offers an alternative to the femoral nerve block in surgical procedures involving the knee surgeries, lower limb, foot, and ankle surgery along with the sciatic nerve block. The block has an inherent advantage of the targeted sensory blockade and lesser quadriceps weakness, thus facilitating early ambulation and rehabilitation following the knee surgeries. In the landmark technique, the needle is inserted about 7 to 8 cm above the adductor tubercle to elicit the contractions of the vastus medialis muscle before the administration of the drug after negative aspiration for blood. Similarly, the femoral artery is identified deep to the sartorius muscle with US, and the drug is injected lateral to the artery for the requisite block.

- **Saphenous nerve block**

Saphenous nerve, the medial branch of femoral nerve, provides sensory innervation to the medial leg and ankle joint. It is mainly employed for complete anesthesia/analgesia below the knee in conjunction with the sciatic nerve block. It can be blocked above the level of the knee, at the level of the knee, below the knee, and at the level of the medial malleolus. While the femoral artery serves as a guide to block the nerve in the above-knee and at the level of knee approach, it may be difficult to locate it below knee, and infiltration around the saphenous vein usually provides reliable block. The nerve to vastus medialis is also utilized to locate the saphenous nerve, as it runs alongside the saphenous nerve.

- **Ankle block**

Ankle block is a complex block involving the blockade of five nerves at the ankle by separate injections. The five nerves include the superficial peroneal nerve, deep peroneal nerve, saphenous nerve, posterior tibia nerve, and the sural nerve. It is usually employed for surgeries on foot. While dorsalis pedis artery and posterior tibial artery serve as a guide for deep peroneal nerve, the posterior tibial nerve, medial and lateral malleolus serve as important guides for the performance of the other three blocks.

Truncal Nerve Blocks (AS5.6)

Most of the truncal blocks have traditionally been performed through the landmark technique. However, given improved and real-time view on US, which facilitates the correct localization of the interfascial planes and allows drug deposition appropriately with the advantage of reducing the injury to surrounding viscera and structures, the traditional approaches are seldom practiced. The main truncal blocks being performed with their innervation and indications are enlisted in **Table 13.3**.

Table 13.3 Truncal blocks

Name of the block	Dermatomal distribution	Indications	Interfascial plane for drug administration
TAP block	Anterior branches of T7–12 intercostal nerves and anterior rami of L1	Laparoscopic cholecystectomy, appendectomy, hernia repair, caesarean section, abdominal hysterectomy, prostatectomy	Between the internal oblique and transversus abdominis muscle through triangle of Petit
Rectus sheath block	T6–12 intercostal nerves	Postoperative pain relief in umbilical hernia and umbilical surgery, midline laparotomy	Between transversus abdominis and rectus abdominis muscle
Quadratus lumborum block	T4–L1 dermatomal distribution	Abdominal laparotomies, nephrectomy, caesarean section	• Transmuscular (between quadratus lumborum and psoas muscle) • Anterior approach (between anterior surface of quadratus lumborum muscle and thoracolumbar fascia)
Ilioinguinal/IH nerve block	Anterior ramus of L1–4 root of the lumbar plexus	Inguinal herniorrhaphy (especially in pediatric patients)	• IH between internal oblique and external oblique (at iliac crest) • *Ilioinguinal*—between internal oblique and transversus abdominis (at iliac crest)
PEC 1 block	Lateral (C5–7) and medial (C8–T11) pectoral nerve	Surgeries involving pectoralis major, breast expanders, chest trauma, pacemaker insertion	Between pectoralis major and pectoralis minor muscle
PEC 2 block	Both pectoral nerves T2–4	Extensive breast surgery, tumor resection, axillary clearance, tissue expanders	Between pectoralis minor and serratus anterior muscle
Serratus anterior muscle block	Long thoracic nerve C5–7, thoracic intercostal nerve, thoracodorsal nerve	Breast surgery, latissimus dorsi flap reconstruction	Between latissimus dorsi and serratus anterior muscle
Thoracic paravertebral block	Thoracic spinal nerves, sympathetic chain	Thoracic surgeries, liver surgeries, inguinal hernia repair, ambulatory surgery, cholecystectomy, rib fractures, breast surgery	Between pleura and superior costotransverse ligament
Erector spinae block	Dorsal and ventral rami of the thoracic and abdominal spinal nerves	Surgical procedures on anterior, posterior, lateral thoracic and abdominal parts, acute and chronic pain management, breast surgery, sternotomy, laparotomies	Below erector spinae muscle

Abbreviations: IH, iliohypogastric; TAP, transverse abdominis plane.

Complications of PNBs

Although rare, complications secondary to PNBs may range from minor to life-threatening, which mandates vigilance and prior preparation of all the anticipated problems that might occur either during the conduct or later in the intraoperative or postoperative period.

The following complications deserve special attention.

- **Nerve injury:** The transient nerve injury may occur in 8 to 10% of individuals who usually recover in 4 to 6 weeks. The permanent nerve injury has been reported in 0.01 to 0.09% of the patients receiving PNB. Nerve injury has traditionally been related to the direct neural damage by intraneuronal stimulation, needling, or drug administration. It is recommended to stop the drug administration if the patient complains of any pain while injecting the drug and if any resistance is encountered while injecting the drug. Patients with pre-existing neuropathies are more susceptible to nerve damage and therefore are a contraindication for the same. Also, short bevel needles are presumed to cause less damage and consequently utilized for most of the blocks. Transient or permanent nerve damage carries legal implications; therefore, necessitate prompt measures to diagnose and direct therapy, if any.

- **Formation of Hematoma:** Usually, all the nerves lie in the vicinity of major or minor blood vessels and always carry an inherent risk of hematoma formation. The hematoma may not be problematic in normal patients and may be controlled by pressure over the puncture site. However, in patients with underlying coagulation abnormalities or receiving thrombolytic therapy, it may cause perineural compression and thus may require surgical drainage if associated with overt symptoms.

- **Local anesthetic systemic toxicity (LAST):** Inadvertent intravascular administration of the LA may lead to devastating complications that have already been discussed in detail in the chapter dealing with LA.

- Catheter knotting, kinking, and accidental removal are frequent with continuous catheter techniques; therefore, appropriate fixation is recommended to avoid the same. The catheters introduced for any block need to be fixed up properly either by suturing or skin tunneling, in order to avoid the accidental removal or withdrawal from the stipulated site.

- **Infections:** The infections may range from localized inflammation and infection to abscess formation and even sepsis if appropriate aseptic measures are not undertaken at the time of the performance of the block.

- Allergic reactions to LA may occur; therefore, any history of drug allergies must be elicited in the preoperative period.

Conclusion

PNBs are the RA techniques that provide site-specific motor and sensory blockade, which provides excellent surgical anesthesia, postoperative pain relief, and facilitates early discharge and ambulation. In addition, the associated dense analgesia curtails the need for opioid analgesics and the side effects related to the same. The appropriate block selection and performance carry a favorable safety profile with fewer side effects, and the ability to prolong the duration of analgesia has several benefits to the patients. The disadvantage of longer time required to perform the block and slightly delayed onset may be mitigated by effective communication and dedicated preoperative block rooms to meet the clinician as well as patient's demands and safety.

Section IV
Anesthesia for Coexisting Diseases

CHAPTER 14

Anesthesia and Cardiac Disease

Rohan Magoon and Souvik Dey

Introduction

Heart, the pump of the cardiovascular system, often poses challenges to anesthetists during perioperative care when part of its functional capability is lost. Cardiac diseases can range from asymptomatic undiagnosed heart diseases to overtly symptomatic patients with heart failure (HF). So, understanding the pathophysiology of heart diseases and its anesthetic implications are of paramount importance for anesthetists.

Ischemic Heart Disease

A thorough preoperative checkup with possible optimization and an anesthetic management plan modified as per individual patient's need is critical.

Preoperative Evaluation

- **History:** This includes elicitation of the following:
  - History of the last episode of chest pain/myocardial infarction (MI).
  - History of treatment given:
    - Thrombolysis/percutaneous coronary intervention (PCI)/conservative management.
    - Time since the last PCI.
    - Type of stent (bare metal/drug-eluting), number of stents, location.
    - History of previous stent thrombosis.
    - History of adverse cardiac events.
  - Urgency of surgery.
  - Comorbidities: Diabetes/hypertension/congestive HF/renal failure.
  - Current drug regimen the patient is on and any history of irregularities.

Based on the history and presence of risk factors, the probability of major adverse cardiac events (MACE) is calculated as per Lee's revised cardiac risk index (**Box 14.1**).

The presence of two or more risk factors indicates an elevated risk of MACE (>1%).

- **Physical examination:**
  - Effort tolerance in terms of metabolic equivalents (METs).
  - General examination.
  - Systemic examination:
    - Respiratory (basal crepitations).
    - Cardiovascular: Murmur, S3 gallop, increased jugular venous pressure.
    - Neurological: Any sign of focal or generalized neurological deficit.
    - Abdomen: Enlarged +/– tender liver.

- **Investigations:**
  - Hematological: Complete hemogram, coagulation profile, blood sugar, urea, creatinine, serum electrolytes (if on diuretics) is needed.

Box 14.1 Lee's revised cardiac risk index

- High-risk surgery.
- Ischemic heart disease (IHD).
- Congestive heart failure (CHF).
- Cerebrovascular disease.
- Insulin-dependent diabetes mellitus.
- Preoperative serum creatinine concentration > 2 mg/dL.

- ► 12-lead ECG: The presence of q-wave, ST-T changes, obtain ST baseline.

- ► Chest X-ray: To rule out cardiomegaly, pulmonary edema.

- ► 2D echocardiography with color Doppler: Within last 1 year or since the clinical condition did not change.

- ► Exercise testing: Treadmill ECG/dobutamine stress echocardiography.

- ► Cardiac CT and MRI.

Other risk calculation scores available are as follows:

- • American College of Surgeons (ACS) National Surgical Quality Improvement Program Myocardial Infarction Cardiac Arrest (NSQIP MICA).

- • ACS NSQIP surgical risk calculator.

Flowchart 14.1 describes the management algorithm after risk stratification as per the 2014 American College of Cardiology (ACC)/American Heart Association (AHA) guidelines.

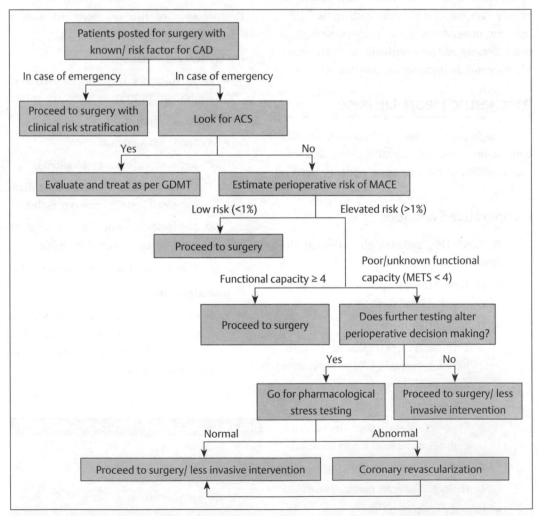

Flowchart 14.1 Management after risk stratification—stepwise approach as per 2014 American College of Cardiology (ACC)/American Heart Association (AHA) guidelines. Abbreviation: GMDT, goal directed medical therapy.

Management of Existing Drug Therapy

- β-blockers: Must not be stopped if already on it; any change in dose or commencement of β-blocker preoperatively should be done 24 hours before to look for the hemodynamic response.

- Antiplatelets: Aspirin should be continued except in cases of intraocular, intracranial, or spine surgeries; clopidogrel to be stopped 5 days before (however, central neuraxial block [CNB] can be given only after 7 days) and prasugrel to be stopped 7 days before surgery.

- The rest of the antianginal drugs (nitrates, calcium channel blockers, angiotensin-converting enzyme [ACE] inhibitors) should be continued. ACE inhibitors may be omitted on the morning of surgery to prevent vasoplegia.

Any discontinuation of antiplatelet drugs should be done after consultation with the cardiologist, keeping in mind the risk (stent thrombosis) versus benefit (intraoperative bleeding) ratio.

Monitoring

The American Society of Anesthesiologists (ASA) standard II monitoring includes:

- ECG: Lead II for arrhythmia and infarction and lead V5 for ST changes should be on display.

- Blood pressure (BP): Noninvasive BP (NIBP) and invasive BP may be useful in surgeries that require massive fluid shift, patients with an irregular rhythm, morbidly obese patients, reduced left ventricular (LV) function, and patients requiring frequent arterial blood gas (ABG) analysis for some other reason (e.g., chronic obstructive pulmonary disease [COPD]).

- Pulse oximetry.

- End-tidal CO_2 monitoring.

- Temperature monitoring: Prevent hypothermia as shivering can increase oxygen consumption manyfold.

Additional monitoring includes:

- Central venous pressure (CVP): To assess the preload.

- Pulmonary artery catheter (PAC): To evaluate the preload for cardiac output measurement and cardiac pacing.

- Transesophageal echocardiography (TOE): To assess LV function, detection of new regional wall motion abnormality, fluid status.

- Esophageal Doppler: Goal-directed fluid therapy via descending aorta flow Doppler analysis.

- Pulse Contour Cardiac Output (PiCCO): For continuous cardiac output measurement, extravascular lung water.

- Near-infrared spectroscopy (NIRS): For assessment of cerebral and tissue oxygenation.

- Blood gas analysis: Arterial and mixed venous blood.

Anesthetic Goals

The most important goal is to balance the myocardial oxygen demand and supply ratio.

Increased demand may be due to:

- *Tachycardia*: Pain, inadequate depth of anesthesia, arrythmia, withdrawal of β-blocker, hypotension, anemia, and shivering.

- *Increased wall stress*: Increased systemic vascular resistance (SVR), increased catecholamines, and increased end-diastolic volume due to bradycardia/fluid overload, aortic stenosis (AS), and concentric hypertrophy.

Decreased supply may be due to:

- *Decreased coronary perfusion pressure*: Hypotension, increased left ventricular end-diastolic pressure (LVEDP).

- *Decreased oxygen content of blood*: Anemia, hypoxia, hemoglobinopathy.

- *Decreased diastolic time*: Tachycardia, non-sinus rhythm.

- *Decreased cardiac output*: LV failure.

Other important anesthetic goals include the following:

- Heart rate (HR) to be kept between 10 and 20% of the baseline value. Tachycardia to be avoided. Bradycardia is dangerous as well.

- Maintain sinus rhythm. Check for serum electrolytes.

- Maintain BP between 10 and 20% of the baseline value. Diastolic BP (DBP) is more important in context to coronary perfusion pressure. *DBP < 40 mm Hg is poorly tolerated.*

- Adequate analgesia: Reduce catecholamine levels.

- Maintain an adequate depth of anesthesia.

- Blood transfusion: Anemia is poorly tolerated due to decreased oxygen-carrying capacity. Keep hemoglobin (Hb) > 10 g/dL.

- Coagulation: Prevent the hypercoagulable state from reducing stent thrombosis.

- Temperature: Maintain normothermia.

Anesthetic Management

Choice of Anesthesia

- Neuraxial block (spinal/epidural/para-vertebral block):

  ▶ Advantages: Adequate pain control, avoid stressful airway manipulation.

  ▶ Disadvantages: Hypotension challenging to manage, bleeding risk with antiplatelet agents.

- General anesthesia (GA):

  ▶ Advantages: Precise control on hemodynamics, no problem with antiplatelet drugs, better to handle emergencies.

  ▶ Disadvantages: Systemic analgesia needed, induction may cause profound hypotension, airway manipulation is associated with severe hemodynamic disturbances, strict vigilance is required.

Premedication

As stress can precipitate MI, premedication with anxiolytics like benzodiazepines is a must. Antisialagogue may be avoided.

Induction

Cardiovascular stability of etomidate makes it an induction agent of choice for cardiac patients. Other intravenous (IV) agents like thiopentone and propofol can be used if hypotension can be avoided. However, ketamine must be avoided due to its sympathomimetic effects. An opioid-based induction with fentanyl/sufentanil may be adopted for patients with compromised LV function. Sympathetic stimulation during laryngoscopy and intubation must be blunted by lignocaine, β-blockers, or opioids.

Neuromuscular Blockade

Vecuronium is ideal due to its cardiovascular stability. Rocuronium may be used for rapid sequence induction and intubation. Atracurium is to be avoided due to its histamine-releasing property. In the case of renal or hepatic failure patients, cisatracurium is the alternative. Succinylcholine should be avoided due to its arrhythmogenic propensity and muscle fasciculation.

Maintenance

- Nitrous oxide should be avoided for two reasons: It may cause mild sympathetic stimulation, and it is a pulmonary vasoconstrictor.

- FiO$_2$ should be adjusted to prevent hypoxia.
- Inhalational agents: All agents are myocardial depressants. Isoflurane causes vasodilation with a theoretical risk of coronary steal syndrome. Sevoflurane causes less hemodynamic perturbation, but cost restricts its widespread use. Desflurane causes cerebral vasodilation and increased sympathetic activity. All inhalational agents are well known for myocardial ischemic preconditioning.
- Etomidate cannot be used for its antisteroidogenesis effect. The propofol-fentanyl infusion may be an ideal choice. Patients with reduced LV function may be maintained on fentanyl alone.

Reversal

Only glycopyrrolate (no atropine) should be used along with neostigmine. Deep plane extubation is preferred to prevent hemodynamic derangements.

Postoperative Period

The majority of MI occurs in the postoperative period (within 48 h); therefore, all the events which can cause an imbalance between myocardial oxygen demand and supply (chiefly pain) should be avoided in the postoperative period.

Perioperative Myocardial Infarction

Characterized by a rise in troponin I level associated with either cardiac symptoms or ECG changes or supportive imaging.

Two types:

- Type I—Characterized by acute coronary syndrome (ACS) with sudden erosion of unstable coronary plaque and ECG depicts ST elevation with T inversion and "Q" wave.
- Type II—Characterized by myocardial demand—supply mismatch and ECG depicts persistent (>30 mins) ST depression.

Tachycardia (HR > 110/min) is the most crucial determinant of perioperative MI; mostly associated with ST-segment depression and are of the non-Q wave type.

If the patient is hemodynamically stable:

- IV nitroglycerine (the mainstay of treatment).
- β-blockers.

If the patient is hemodynamically unstable:

- Treat arrhythmia as per advanced cardiac life support (ACLS) protocol.
- Intra-aortic balloon pump.
- Inotrope for circulatory support.
- PCI angiography and/or angioplasty as early as possible in the postoperative period.

Valvular Heart Disease

The most crucial goal of preoperative assessment is to assess the severity of the valvular lesion. Invasive monitoring is reserved for severe cases of valvular lesions only.

Mitral Stenosis

The most common cause is rheumatic heart disease. The normal mitral valve area is 4 to 6 cm^2. **Table 14.1** depicts the assessment of severity of mitral stenosis (MS).

Table 14.1 Assessment of severity of MS

Severity	Mild	Moderate	Severe
Valve area (cm^2)	>1.5	1–1.5	<1
Mean gradient across the valve (mm Hg)	<5	5–10	>10
Pulmonary artery systolic pressure (mm Hg)	<30	30–50	>50

Abbreviation: MS, mitral stenosis.

Usually, 20% of diastolic filling occurs during atrial contraction. Being a fixed output disease, perseverance of sinus rhythm and avoidance of tachycardia are essential to maintain cardiac output.

Anesthetic Management

- Avoid tachycardia: Decreasing the diastole will decrease the LV filling and therefore stroke volume and cardiac output.
- Avoid hypotension: As these patients have already low cardiac output, hypotension can be detrimental.
- Avoid a sudden increase in blood volume: Sudden increase in preload with preexisting pulmonary hypertension may cause pulmonary edema and right ventricular (RV) failure.
- Maintain and avoid a decrease in SVR.
- Avoid hypoxia, hypercarbia: Hypoxia and hypercarbia by causing pulmonary vasoconstriction can worsen already existing pulmonary hypertension.

Choice of Anesthesia

CNBs should be avoided as hypotension is not acceptable in the already low cardiac output state, and the fluid infusion can precipitate pulmonary edema. However, CNB can be considered for mild-to-moderate lesions by ensuring that significant hypotension is avoided.

As atrial fibrillation is seen in one-third of the patients with MS, a significant number of MS patients will be on oral anticoagulants, contraindicating the use of CNB.

General Anesthesia

Induction: Etomidate, being the most cardiac stable, is the agent of choice.

Maintenance: Isoflurane, being the most cardiac stable, is most preferred; however, sevoflurane and desflurane in lower concentrations can

be safely used. Nitrous oxide can cause mild pulmonary vasoconstriction; therefore, it should be avoided.

Relaxant: Vecuronium is the muscle relaxant of choice.

Reversal: As tachycardia is not acceptable, atropine should not be used with neostigmine.

Mitral Regurgitation

Mitral regurgitation (MR) is defined as retrograde blood flow from LV to left atrium (LA) during systole due to multiple mechanisms. Carpentier classification is used for MR. Severe MR is characterized by a vena contracta width ≥ 0.7 and regurgitant volume of ≥ 60 mL/beat.

Anesthetic Management

MR is primarily a systolic event. The regurgitant volume will increase the back pressure in the pulmonary vascular system, causing pulmonary hypertension and also increase the preload of LV, causing volume overload, dilatation of LV, and decreased cardiac output.

- Avoid bradycardia: HR to be maintained at the normal upper limit (~90 beats/min). Maintain sinus rhythm.
- Decrease SVR: Increased afterload will increase the regurgitant fraction.
- Avoid an increase in pulmonary vascular resistance (PVR): Avoid hypoxia, hypercarbia, and acidosis. Avoid Trendelenburg position, check airway pressure during positive pressure ventilation.
- Contractility: To be maintained at pre-anesthetic level.
- Preload: Judicial fluid management to avoid pulmonary edema.

Choice of Anesthesia

As a decrease in afterload decreases the regurgitation, CNBs can be administered. However, excessive hypotension should be avoided.

General Anesthesia

Induction: Etomidate.

Maintenance: Isoflurane. Nitrous oxide is avoided due to pulmonary hypertension.

Muscle relaxant: Vecuronium.

Mitral Valve Prolapse

Generally, mitral valve prolapse (MVP) is a benign condition; however, it can become clinically significant if associated with MR. The hemodynamic principles of management of MVP without MR and with MR are substantially different, for example, increasing LV volume by giving fluids, or by causing bradycardia and hypertension to decrease the degree of prolapse in MVP. On the other hand, the same management strategies will worsen the degree of associated MR when present. Hence, preoperative echocardiography is very useful to identify the presence of associated MR in MVP.

The majority of the MVP cases have a normal ventricular function; therefore, it can be given GA. If GA is to be delivered, then cardiac stable (etomidate, isoflurane, and vecuronium) is preferred.

Aortic Stenosis

AS carries the most dangerous complications among all the valvular heart diseases (angina, syncope, and sudden cardiac death). As much as 75% symptomatic patients with severe AS may die within 3 years without replacement. The normal area of the aortic valve is 2.6 to 3.5 cm². The severity of AS can be classified as per **Table 14.2.**

Anesthetic Management

It is a fixed cardiac output disease. Cardiac output is preload dependent. An increase in contractility cannot increase cardiac output.

- Maintain normal sinus rhythm and HR: Bradycardia can cause overdistension of the already hypertrophied LV. Tachycardia, by decreasing the ventricular filling, can further reduce the cardiac output.

- Maintain normal BP: Decreasing SVR is not only ineffective but also detrimental by decreasing the DBP as well as the coronary perfusion. As phenylephrine does not cause tachycardia, it is the vasopressor of choice for patients with AS.

- LV preload is to be maintained at the higher side of the normal.

- Contractility and PVR to be maintained at a baseline level. The hypertrophied LV is prone to arrhythmia and ischemia. Hypotension to be managed aggressively.

Choice of Anesthesia

CNBs can cause hypotension. Therefore, the anesthetic technique of choice is GA.

General Anesthesia

Induction: Etomidate.

Maintenance: O_2 + N_2O and isoflurane if the LV function is not significantly compromised. However, if the LV function is compromised, then opioids are selected over the inhalational agent.

Muscle relaxant: Vecuronium is the choice.

Table 14.2 Assessment of severity of AS

Grade	Mild	Moderate	Severe
Aortic valve area (cm²)	>1.5	1–1.5	<1.0
Mean gradient (mm Hg)	<20	20–40	>40
Peak velocity of blood flow (m/s)	2.6–3	3–4	>4

Abbreviation: AS, aortic stenosis.

Aortic Regurgitation

It is a disease of the aortic valve itself, the dilation of the root, or a combination of both. The expected survival of a symptomatic patient of aortic regurgitation (AR) is only 5 to 10 years.

Anesthetic Management

AR is a diastolic event. Pulse pressure can reflect the severity of the disease.

- LV preload: Forward cardiac output is maintained by preload augmentation.
- HR: Reduced time spent in diastole will decrease the regurgitation fraction. HR is to be maintained at the normal upper side.
- Contractility: Must be maintained. The use of pure β agonists or phosphodiesterase inhibitors will increase the cardiac output by augmenting contractility and decreasing afterload.
- SVR: To be decreased and PVR to be maintained.

As a decrease in afterload decreases the regurgitation, CNB appears to be a good selection. However, excessive hypotension should be avoided.

General Anesthesia

Induction: Etomidate.

Maintenance: O_2 + N_2O and isoflurane if LV function is normal; otherwise, opioids.

Muscle relaxant: Vecuronium.

Prosthetic Heart Valves

Prosthetic heart valves may be mechanical (more prone for thromboembolism, long shelf-life of 20–30 years) or bioprosthetic (less likely for thromboembolism, shorter shelf-life of 10–15 years).

The two most important considerations for patients on prosthetic heart valves are as follows:

- *They are on oral anticoagulants*: Stop warfarin 5 days before the procedure and start unfractionated heparin, which is stopped 12 to 24 hours before surgery.
- *Antibiotic prophylaxis*: There has been a drastic change in guidelines for antibiotic prophylaxis for the patient with a prosthetic heart valve. Contrary to the previous recommendation of antibiotic prophylaxis to all patients undergoing any procedure, the new guidelines (2017 AHA update) recommend antibiotics prophylaxis only for the following conditions:

  ▶ Prosthetic cardiac valves, including transcatheter-implanted prostheses and homografts.

  ▶ Prosthetic materials used for cardiac valve repair, such as annuloplasty rings and chords.

  ▶ Previous IE.

  ▶ Unrepaired cyanotic congenital heart disease or repaired congenital heart disease, with residual shunts or valvular regurgitation at the site of or adjacent to the site of a prosthetic patch or prosthetic device.

  ▶ Cardiac transplant with valve regurgitation due to a structurally abnormal valve.

Congenital Heart Lesions

Congenital heart diseases (CHDs) could be classified as follows:

- Outflow tract obstruction:

  ▶ Left ventricular outflow tract (LVOT) obstruction: Coarctation of the aorta, AS.

  ▶ Right ventricular outflow tract (RVOT) obstruction: Pulmonary valve stenosis.

- Left-to-right shunting—atrial septal defect (ASD), ventricular septal defect (VSD), patent ductus arteriosus (PDA), endocardial cushion defect.

- Right-to-left shunting:
  - Increased pulmonary blood flow:
    - Transposition of great arteries (TGA).
    - Truncus arteriosus.
    - Total anomalous pulmonary venous return (TAPVR).
    - Single ventricle.
    - Double-outlet right ventricle (DORV).
    - Hypoplastic left heart syndrome.
  - Decreased pulmonary blood flow:
    - Tetralogy of Fallot (TOF).
    - Pulmonary atresia.
    - Tricuspid atresia.

Left-to-Right Shunts

This includes VSD, ASD, and PDA.

Anesthetic Management

Factors affecting left-to-right shunt like hematocrit, increased SVR, low PVR, hyperoxemia, hyperventilation, and negative airway pressure should be avoided. However, increased PVR can cause a reversal of left-to-right shunt and, therefore, should be avoided. Anesthetic consideration should be as follows:

- HR and rhythm: Should maintain age-appropriate rate and sinus rhythm.
- Preload: Avoid fluid overload, especially if congestive cardiac failure (CCF) is present.
- Afterload: Avoid an increase in SVR.
- Ventilation: Avoid hypoxia and hypercarbia, avoid hyperventilation and hyperinflation, and prevent atelectasis, as these can increase PVR.

Antibiotic prophylaxis to prevent infective endocarditis is recommended for VSD and PDA; however, for ASD, only if there is a concurrent valvular abnormality (MVPs may be associated with ASD).

Choice of Anesthesia

As CNB decreases afterload, therefore, it will be beneficial. However, excessive hypotension may not be acceptable in an already low-cardiac output state.

General Anesthesia

Induction: Propofol or thiopentone (causes hypotension). Increase in pulmonary blood flow causes dilution of IV agents and may result in delayed induction with IV anesthetics.

Maintenance: $O_2 + N_2O$ and isoflurane (sevoflurane, halothane, or desflurane < 6% can also be safely used) + intermittent positive pressure ventilation (IPPV). Inhalational agents are beneficial by decreasing SVR, while nitrous oxide and IPPV can potentially increase the PVR. In the case of poor LV function, opioids can supplement inhalational agents.

Muscle relaxant: Vecuronium is the choice.

Right-to-Left Shunts

This includes cyanotic heart diseases, TOF, Eisenmenger syndrome, and TGA.

Anesthetic Management

Factors increasing right-to-left shunt: Polycythemia, reduced SVR, increased PVR, positive end-expiratory pressure (PEEP).

Anesthetic considerations should be as follows:
- Maintain adequate preoperative hydration and sedation.
- Maintain SVR and intravascular volume.
- Minimize PVR: Avoid hypoxia, hypercarbia, and acidosis.
- Mild myocardial depression—this will reduce RVOT obstruction in TOF.
- Relatively slow HR is desirable.
- Maintain deep plane of anesthesia.

- Avoid histamine-releasing drugs—morphine, atracurium, pethidine.
- Avoid excessive PEEP: As it increases PVR.
- Paradoxical embolism can be catastrophic—avoid even minute volume of air in the IV line.
- Antibiotic prophylaxis is mandatory to prevent infective endocarditis (class IIa recommendation).
- Continue prostaglandin E1 (PGE1) infusion if already present.
- There are increased chances of coagulopathy and thromboembolism due to polycythemia.

Choice of Anesthesia

As CNB causes hypotension, it should be avoided; GA is the anesthetic technique of choice.

General Anesthesia

Premedication: With midazolam and ketamine; avoided in age < 6 months.

Induction: As ketamine increases the SVR, it is the agent of choice for induction in the right-to-left shunts. As pulmonary circulation is bypassed, the induction with IV agents will be rapid.

Maintenance: O_2 (50%) + N_2O (50%) + ketamine infusion (or desflurane > 6% if LV function is normal). Induction with inhalational agents is delayed due to the dilutional effect of shunted blood, which does not contain the inhalational agent. As high FiO_2 (delivered oxygen) decreases the PVR, the concentration of oxygen used is 50% (not 33%). Positive pressure ventilation and acidosis can increase PVR; therefore, avoid excessive airway pressure and treat acidosis promptly.

Muscle relaxant: As pancuronium causes hypertension, it is the muscle relaxant of choice. Nowadays, vecuronium is used in most of the centers.

Coarctation of Aorta

Classification of coarctation of aorta is as follows:

- Thoracic aortic coarctation:
  ▶ Preductal/infantile.
  ▶ Juxtaductal.
  ▶ Postductal/adult type.
- Lower thoracic coarctation.
- Abdominal aortic coarctation.

The majority of the coarctation is postductal (distal to the subclavian artery). The patient is at risk of ischemia to the spine, gut, kidney, and lower limbs; therefore, BP monitoring in lower limbs is a must in these patients to ensure that mean arterial pressure of lower limb remains at least > 40 mm Hg.

Hypercyanotic Tet Spells

This implies acute worsening of paroxysmal cyanotic episodes. Precipitating factors include increased sympathetic activity like crying, exercise, feeding, fear, anxiety, and defecation. Under anesthesia, fall in saturation corresponds to fall in diastolic blood pressure and tachycardia, and no improvement in oxygen saturation with increasing FiO_2 suggests tet spell.

Treatment

Treatment includes the following:

- Increase SVR:
  ▶ Squatting position, flex the legs over abdomen in knee-chest position.
  ▶ Correction of Hb.
  ▶ Drugs such as phenylephrine, norepinephrine, calcium.
  ▶ Consider emergency surgery if not responsive.
  ▶ If sternum is open, pinch the aorta or abdominal aorta in case of open abdomen.

- Reduce PVR:
  - ▶ Hyperventilate with 100% oxygen.
  - ▶ Correct acidosis with sodium bicarbonate.
- Reduce RVOT obstruction:
  - ▶ Deepen the anesthetic plane.
  - ▶ β-blockers such as propranolol/esmolol.
  - ▶ Volume administration.

Heart Failure

HF is a complex pathophysiologic state characterized by the inability of the heart to fill with or to eject blood as per the requirement of the body.

Patients afflicted with HF carry a very high risk of perioperative morbidity and mortality. Therefore, elective surgery is contraindicated in patients with acute HF.

The most common etiologies of HF are as follows:

- Impaired contractility due to myocardial ischemia or cardiomyopathy.
- Valvular heart disease.
- Systemic hypertension.
- Pericardial diseases.
- Cor pulmonale.

Types of Heart Failure

- The phase of the cardiac cycle:
  - ▶ Systolic failure is characterized by a low ejection fraction or impaired systolic function of the heart. Its causes are coronary artery disease (CAD), valvular heart disease, AS, systemic hypertension, etc.
  - ▶ Diastolic HF is characterized by impaired relaxation of the heart. It can coexist with systolic failure. Class I diastolic failure is characterized by normal left atrial (LA) pressure. Classes II, III, and IV are characterized by increased LA pressure. Its causes are myocardial edema, hypertrophy, fibrosis, aging, and pressure overload.
- Time of onset:
  - ▶ Acute HF occurs when signs and symptoms require emergency medical or surgical treatment. They are of three types: Acute on chronic HF, new-onset HF, and terminal HF refractory to therapy.
  - ▶ Chronic HF.
- Side of heart chamber: Left- and right-sided HF.
- On cardiac index: Normal cardiac index is 2.2 to 3.5 L/min/m².
  - ▶ Low output failure wherein cardiac index may be normal at rest but does not increase with exercise/stress. The most common cause is CAD.
  - ▶ High output failure occurs in the form of anemia, pregnancy, arteriovenous fistulas, severe hyperthyroidism, beriberi, and Paget's disease.

Diagnosis of Heart Failure

It is diagnosed by Framingham criteria which includes the following:

- *Major criteria*: Orthopnea/paroxysmal nocturnal dyspnea (PND), neck vein distension, rales, cardiomegaly, acute pulmonary edema, third heart sound, circulation time > 25 seconds, weight loss > 4.5 kg in 5 days with treatment, hepatojugular reflux.
- *Minor criteria*: Dyspnea on exertion, hepatomegaly, pleural effusion, bilateral ankle edema, nocturnal cough.

The presence of two major criteria, or one major + two minor criteria, indicates HF.

New York Heart Association Classification

The New York Heart Association (NYHA) classification of HF is as follows:

- *Class I*: Ordinary physical activity does not cause symptoms.
- *Class II*: Symptoms occur with ordinary exertion.
- *Class III*: Symptoms occur with less-than-ordinary exertion.
- *Class IV*: Symptoms occur at rest.

Staging of Heart Failure

The 2005 ACC/AHA update on the staging of HF is as follows:

- *Stage A*: Patients at high risk of HF but without structural heart disease or symptoms of HF.
- *Stage B*: Patients with structural heart disease but without symptoms of HF.
- *Stage C*: Patients with structural heart disease with previous or current symptoms of HF.
- *Stage D*: Patients with refractory HF requiring specialized interventions.

Anesthetic Management

The basic anesthetic principle of management is conditioned by the three basic principles of management of HF, that is, decrease preload, improve myocardial contractility, and decrease afterload.

Medications

- Digitalis and β-blockers are continued.
- Despite the well-known hypotensive effect of ACE inhibitors and angiotensin receptor blocker (ARB) antagonists, the 2014 ACC/AHA guidelines on perioperative cardiovascular evaluation and management of patients undergoing noncardiac surgery recommend continuing the therapy.
- Diuretics should be withheld on the day of surgery. As these patients are on diuretics and digitalis, checking preoperative electrolytes (especially potassium) is a must.

Choice of Anesthesia

CNBs are beneficial by a modest decrease in preload (venous return) and afterload (SVR). However, excessive hypotension should be avoided.

General Anesthesia

Induction: Etomidate is the induction agent of choice. Ketamine appears to be beneficial by its positive inotropic effect; however, tachycardia produced by ketamine may negate this effect by decreasing the diastolic filling time.

Maintenance: O_2 + N_2O and opioids. Inhalational agents can be used if the LV function is not significantly compromised.

Muscle relaxant: Vecuronium.

Inotropic support with dopamine or dobutamine may be required intraoperatively. The positive pressure ventilation is beneficial which decreases the preload as well as the afterload, consequently, decreased load on cardiac muscle.

Hypertension

Hypertension is considered as a leading risk factor of morbidity and mortality, accounting for 7% of disability-adjusted-life-years (DALYs) worldwide. Nearly one-third of adult surgical patients posted for noncardiac surgery and two-third of patients posted for coronary bypass had a preexisting history of hypertension. Hypertension can be staged as per **Table 14.3**.

As per 2014 JNC 8 guidelines, pharmacotherapy should be initiated when BP is ≥ 140/80 mm Hg in those < 60 years of age and ≥ 150/90 mm Hg in those ≥ 60 years of age.

Table 14.3 Classification of SBP in adults

Category	SBP (in mm Hg)	DBP (in mm Hg)
Normal	<120	<80
Prehypertension	120–139	80–89
Stage 1 hypertension	140–159	90–99
Stage 2 hypertension	≥160	≥100

Abbreviations: DBP, diastolic blood pressure; SBP, systemic blood pressure.

Hypertension can be classified into the following different:

- Resistant hypertension: Uncontrolled BP despite three or more antihypertensive drugs of different classes, including a nonpotassium-sparing diuretic, or the need for four or more drugs to achieve control.

- Refractory hypertension: Uncontrolled BP on five or more drugs.

- Hypertensive crisis is defined as BP > 180/120 mm Hg.

Anesthetic Considerations

Preoperative evaluation: All hypertensive patients should be considered as having IHD until proved otherwise. Other important considerations are as follows:

- Adequacy of BP control and the possibility of previously undiagnosed hypertension must be judged with the caveat of "white-coat" hypertension.

- Surgery must not be delayed until BP > 180/110 mm Hg or elevated BP with end-organ damage or the possibility of secondary hypertension in newly diagnosed hypertensives (e.g., children aged < 12 years, presence of renal bruit, flushing and sweating, presence of hypokalemia, etc.).

- The presence of postural hypotension should be checked, especially among the aged population.

- All antihypertensive drugs should be continued throughout the perioperative period with the possible exception of ARB antagonists and ACE inhibitors, which may be discontinued for 10 hours before surgery due to the risk of prolonged hypotension.

- Any elevated BP should not be decreased rapidly as cerebral autoregulation is set at a higher value.

- Premedication with a benzodiazepine helps alleviate anxiety.

Intraoperative Management

- Induction: Etomidate is the induction agent of choice. Propofol and thiopentone can be used, provided hypotension is avoided. Ketamine must not be used.

- Laryngoscopy response should be blunted by decreasing the duration, lignocaine, β-blockers and opioids.

- Induction can lead to profound hypotension due to volume depletion, especially in patients with chronic use of diuretics.

- Muscle relaxants: Vecuronium is most cardiostable. Rocuronium can be used for rapid sequence intubation. Atracurium is prone to histamine release specifically at induction dose. Cisatracurium is the choice in renal/hepatic compromised patients.

- Maintenance: These patients are more prone to hypotension. Prolonged use of ARB antagonists/ACE inhibitors and physiological factors (volume depletion, loss of vascular elasticity, baroreceptor desensitization) can lead to prolonged intraoperative hypotension. Any inhalational agent can be used, provided hypotension is avoided.

- Intraoperative hypertension is prevented by:

  ▶ Adequate depth of anesthesia.

  ▶ Avoid hypoxia, hypercarbia, and acidosis.

  ▶ Adequate analgesia and check for bladder distension.

  ▶ Pharmacotherapy—nitroglycerin (NTG), esmolol, labetalol, nicardipine, nitroprusside, clonidine, or dexmedetomidine.

  ▶ These patients are prone to increased risk of intraoperative blood loss. On the other hand, chronic hypertension can lead to a condition termed as HF with preserved ejection fraction (HFpEF); therefore, judicial fluid management is necessary.

Cardiomyopathy

As defined by the 2006 AHA expert consensus panel, "cardiomyopathies are a heterogeneous group of diseases of the myocardium associated with mechanical and/or electrical dysfunction that usually (but not invariably) exhibit inappropriate ventricular hypertrophy or dilation and are due to a variety of causes that frequently are genetic. Cardiomyopathies either are confined to the heart or are part of generalized systemic disorders, often leading to cardiovascular death or progressive HF-related disability."

Classification of Cardiomyopathies

- Primary cardiomyopathies are confined to cardiac myocytes only:

  ▶ *Genetic*: Hypertrophic cardiomyopathy (HCM), arrhythmogenic RV cardiomyopathy, glycogen storage disease, LV noncompaction, conduction system disease (Lenègre disease), ion channelopathies: long QT syndrome, short QT syndrome, Brugada syndrome.

  ▶ *Acquired*: Myocarditis (inflammatory cardiomyopathy) can be viral, bacterial, rickettsial, fungal, or parasitic (Chagas disease); stress cardiomyopathy; peripartum cardiomyopathy.

  ▶ *Mixed*: Dilated cardiomyopathy, primary restrictive non-HCM.

- Secondary cardiomyopathies: Systemic disease with pathophysiologic involvement of the heart:

  ▶ *Storage*: Hemochromatosis, glycogen storage disease, Niemann–Pick disease.

  ▶ *Infiltrative*: Amyloidosis, Gaucher disease, Hunter syndrome.

  ▶ *Inflammatory*: Sarcoidosis.

  ▶ *Endomyocardial*: Hypereosinophilic (Löffler) syndrome, endomyocardial fibrosis.

  ▶ *Toxic*: Drugs such as cocaine, alcohol; chemotherapy drugs like doxorubicin, daunorubicin, cyclophosphamide; heavy metals such as lead, mercury; and radiation therapy.

  ▶ *Autoimmune*: Lupus erythematosus, rheumatoid arthritis, scleroderma, dermatomyositis, polyarteritis nodosa.

  ▶ *Endocrine*: Diabetes mellitus, hyperthyroidism or hypothyroidism, pheochromocytoma, acromegaly.

  ▶ *Neuromuscular*: Duchenne–Becker dystrophy, neurofibromatosis, tuberous sclerosis.

Hypertrophic Cardiomyopathy

It is the most common genetic cardiovascular disease that is transmitted as an autosomal dominant trait with variable penetrance. The most common form of HCM presents as hypertrophy of the interventricular septum and anterolateral free wall.

Classification of HCM

- Obstructive: Peak pressure gradients > 30 mm Hg.
- Nonobstructive: With peak pressure gradients across the LVOT < 30 mm Hg (**Table 14.4**).
- Latent: Exercise-induced pressure gradients > 30 mm Hg.

Choice of Anesthesia

CNB (especially spinal) can increase LVOT by decreasing preload and afterload; therefore, it should be avoided.

General Anesthesia

Preanesthetic Evaluation

Most of the patients with HCM are young and maybe asymptomatic; therefore, family history of sudden death and 12-lead ECG is crucial. In previously diagnosed patients of HCM, calcium channel antagonists and β-blockers should be continued. In patients with implantable cardioverter defibrillator (ICD), the device should be disabled just before surgery and activated again in the recovery area.

Premedication

An anxiolytic (benzodiazepine) is important.

Induction

Etomidate is the induction agent of choice. A drug like ketamine, which stimulates the sympathetic system, is contraindicated. Sympathetic stimulation caused by intubation must be blunted by β-blockers or inhalational anesthetic agents. Preinduction volume loading may be helpful to counteract the hypotension following induction.

Maintenance

Opioids are preferred; however, inhalational agents at a moderate dose can be used if hypotension can be well controlled. Positive pressure ventilation with low-tidal volumes with a high respiratory rate should be applied. PEEP should be avoided.

Hypotension should be managed with volume infusion and pure α agonists like phenylephrine. However, hypervolemia may precipitate pulmonary edema. Ephedrine, dopamine, and dobutamine are contraindicated.

Table 14.4 Factors affecting outflow obstruction

Events that increase outflow obstruction	Events that decrease outflow obstruction

• Increased myocardial contractility
  ○ β-adrenergic stimulation (endogenous/exogenous catecholamines)
  ○ Digitalis
	• Decreased myocardial contractility
	  ○ β-adrenergic blockade
	  ○ Volatile anesthetics
	  ○ Calcium entry blockers

• Decreased preload
  ○ Hypovolemia
  ○ Vasodilators
  ○ Tachycardia
  ○ Positive pressure ventilation
	• Increased preload
	  ○ Hypervolemia
	  ○ Bradycardia

• Decreased afterload
  ○ Hypotension
  ○ Vasodilators
	• Increased afterload
	  ○ Hypertension
	  ○ α-adrenergic agonists

TOE is essential is these patient groups due to the unique pathology. Neither CVP nor PAC can accurately estimate the preload of LV in these patients. A cardioverter defibrillator should be present inside the OR all the time. It is vital to maintain the sinus rhythm as the atrial contraction is necessary to support adequate LV filling. Avoid anything that causes sympathetic activation like pain, hypoxia, hypercarbia, shivering, the lighter plane of anesthesia, acidosis, bowel/bladder distension, etc.

Muscle Relaxant

Vecuronium is the preferred muscle relaxant. Pancuronium is contraindicated due to its vagolytic action. Pulmonary edema in these patients cannot be treated by diuretics (decreases preload), nitrates (decreases afterload), and digitalis. β-blocker like esmolol is helpful in this situation.

Dilated Cardiomyopathy

Dilated cardiomyopathy is the most common type of cardiomyopathy, the third most common cause of HF, and the most common indication for cardiac transplantation.

Anesthetic Management

Since dilated cardiomyopathy is a cause of HF, the anesthetic management of these patients is the same as that described for other patients with HF. Regional anesthesia may be an alternative to GA in selected patients with dilated cardiomyopathy. However, anticoagulant therapy may limit this option.

Considerations in Patients on Cardiac Implanted Electronic Devices

The cardiac implanted electronic devices (CIEDs) include permanent pacemakers, ICDs, and cardiac resynchronization devices.

Anesthetic Considerations in a Patient with CIED

Preoperative Evaluation

- Focused history of comorbidity (hypertension, diabetes, MI, etc.), previous cardiac surgery, cardiomyopathy, peripheral vascular disease, valvular or CHD.

- Focused examination of previous cardiac disease, assessment of the device by pacemaker team (type, mode of pacing, programming, underlying rhythm, expected battery life, time since insertion, magnet response).

- Surgical details such as type, anatomic site, positioning during the surgery, electrocautery to be used, any other source of electromagnetic interference, anticipated blood loss.

- Investigations like 12-lead ECG with and without magnet, chest X-ray.

Preoperative Preparation

Disable all rate enhancement programming, consider increasing the lower limit to increase better oxygen delivery, reprogram to asynchronous mode at a rate higher than intrinsic HR, suspend antitachycardia pacing if present, CVP/PAC insertion may damage the pacemaker lead, and nerve stimulator use may interfere with pacing.

Choice of Anesthetic Technique

Vasodilation associated with CNB is poorly tolerated. GA is the technique of choice.

General Anesthesia

Induction: Ketamine and etomidate may cause myofasciculations, which may cause over sensing of the CIED. Volatile anesthetics increase the pacing threshold and atrioventricular (AV) nodal delay.

Maintenance: N$_2$O can accumulate in the pacemaker pocket with prolonged use. Maintain adequate hydration as hypovolemia is poorly tolerated. Monitor pacemaker spikes on the monitor. Cardiac arrhythmia may be difficult to detect; so, monitor pulse oximetry/arterial pressure waveform.

Considerations Regarding Electrosurgical Unit

- Prefer ultrasonic and bipolar over monopolar cautery.
- Pure "cut" electrocautery is preferred over "blend" or "coagulation."
- Positions return plate in such a way that the path of the current does not cross the generator or leads.
- Use the smallest burst of current for < 4 seconds separated by ≥ 2 seconds.
- Avoid electrocautery use within 6 inches of the generator/leads.

Causes of Pacemaker Failure Intraoperatively

- Generator failure: End of life, directly struck by cautery.

- Lead failure: Patient positioning, over or under sensing.
- Failure to capture: Change in the threshold (**Table 14.5**).

Pericardial Diseases (Constrictive Pericarditis/ Cardiac Tamponade)

Constrictive Pericarditis

Diagnostic features are as follows:

- Clinical examination: Jugular venous distension (JVD) with Kussmaul's sign (increase in JVD with inspiration) and Friedreich's sign (a rapid decrease in JVD in early diastole), pulsatile hepatomegaly.
- Auscultation: "Pericardial knock," which is a high-pitched sound in early diastole.
- CT/MRI: Thickened pericardium > 2 mm.
- Cardiac catheterization: Right atrial (RA) pressure leads to "M"/"W" waveform with prominent y-descent; ventricular pressure tracing leads to "dip and plateau" sign or "square root sign."
- Echocardiography: Ventricular septal "bounce."

Table 14.5 Factors affecting the threshold of pacemaker

Factors increasing the threshold	Factors decreasing the threshold
• Increased K$^+$ • Hypoxemia • Hypoglycemia • Alteration in pH • Decreased body temperature • Antidysrhythmic medication (e.g., quinidine, procainamide, lidocaine, propafenone) • Local anesthetics (lidocaine) • Myocardial ischemia • MI (scar tissue) • Acute inflammation around lead tip during the first month after implantation	• Decreased K$^+$ • Increased catecholamine levels • Hyperthyroidism • Hypermetabolic states • Sympathomimetic drugs • Anticholinergics • Glucocorticoids • Stress or anxiety

Abbreviation: MI, myocardial infarction.

Cardiac Tamponade

Diagnostic features are as follows:

- Beck's triad: Muffled heart sound, JVD, and hypotension.

- Pulsus paradoxus, ECG: Electrical alternans, chest X-ray—right costophrenic (CP) angle < 90°.

- Echocardiography: Minimal (50–100 mL) < 5 mm; small (100–250 mL) is 5 to 10 mm; moderate (250–500 mL) is 11 to 20 mm; and large (>500 mL) > 20 mm.

Patients with pericardial diseases are in low cardiac output state; therefore, CNBs are contraindicated. Pericardiocentesis should be done under local anesthesia before proceeding to GA.

General Anesthesia

Induction: Ketamine, by stimulating the sympathetic system, will increase the cardiac output.

Maintenance: Combinations of opioids and benzodiazepines with or without low doses of volatile anesthetics are appropriate for the maintenance of anesthesia.

Muscle relaxant: Drugs with minimal hemodynamic consequences are the best choices, although the modest increase in HR observed with pancuronium is also acceptable.

Conclusion

The patients with cardiac abnormalities pose great challenges to anesthetists during the perioperative period. The anomalies can involve any structure of the heart with complex pathophysiology, and their management often gets complicated by the cardiovascular effects of anesthetic agents. The patients may require invasive monitoring (invasive BP monitoring, central venous catheter), based on the type and complexity of the surgery. Choosing appropriate drugs in the appropriate dosage and maintaining the cardiac grid for the given cardiac condition are crucial for the optimal outcome of such a group of patients.

CHAPTER 15

Anesthesia for Respiratory Diseases

Heena Garg and Puneet Khanna

Introduction

Respiratory illnesses often complicate anesthetic management of patients in elective as well as emergency surgeries. Patients with respiratory diseases are at risk of desaturation, laryngospasm, and bronchospasm during the perioperative period. Anesthetists need to be acquainted with commonly encountered respiratory illnesses and acquire appropriate airway skills to provide optimal patient care. This chapter will discuss the following respiratory illnesses in detail, including anesthetic considerations:

- Asthma.
- Chronic obstructive pulmonary disease (COPD).
- Restrictive lung disease.
- Tuberculosis.
- Respiratory tract infection (RTI).
- Thoracotomy and pneumonectomy.

Asthma

Asthma is characterized by episodes of recurrent wheezing, dyspnea, and dry cough caused by airway obstruction, airway inflammation, and airway hyperresponsiveness.

Preoperative Assessment

Preoperative evaluation should focus on:

- Duration and frequency of symptoms.
- Sputum amount and its characteristics.
- Current medications.
- Asthma precipitating triggers, for example, dust, smoke, exercise, drugs, or any RTI.
- Activity level.
- History of airway complications in prior anesthesia exposure.
- History of hospital admission for asthma exacerbations.

Physical Examination

It should focus on the assessment of wheeze, the presence of prolonged expiratory wheeze, and signs of respiratory distress. Cyanosis and drowsiness should be noted and documented. Oxygenation status should be confirmed using pulse oximeter and blood gas analysis (if required).

Investigations

- Pulmonary function tests (PFT).
- Forced expired volume in the first second (FEV1)/peak expiratory flow rate (PEFR) ratio.
- PEFR variability.

Preparation for Surgery

Patients should take all asthma medications on the morning of surgery.

Anesthetic Management

The goal of anesthetic management is to avoid airway manipulations to the minimum, ensure adequate depth of anesthesia as well as analgesia during airway handling, and use anesthetic drugs with maximal bronchodilation properties. Induction of general anesthesia (GA), airway manipulation, and emergence from anesthesia represent the most critical times for potential airway complications during a general anesthetic.

The effects of various anesthetic agents and airway devices on the airway are as follows:

- Fentanyl is preferred over morphine due to the histamine-releasing property of the latter.

- All volatile anesthetics have direct bronchodilation properties except desflurane. Halothane followed by sevoflurane is the most effective bronchodilator.

- Desflurane is an airway irritant and is avoided in asthmatics.

- Propofol is superior to etomidate and thiopental in terms of lowering airway resistance but has inferior bronchodilator properties compared to volatile anesthetics.

- Ketamine has a direct bronchodilation activity and blunts airway reflex; bronchoconstriction, although coming at the cost of increased secretions, can complicate airway management.

- Neuromuscular blocking drugs (NMBDs) improve intubating conditions in adults. Preferred ones are rocuronium and vecuronium. Atracurium has histamine-releasing properties.

- The use of noninvasive such as supraglottic airway (SGA) carries a lower risk of postoperative hypoxemia and coughing compared to the endotracheal tube (ETT) in adults.

- In patients with airflow obstruction, prolongation of the expiratory phase of ventilation occurs. Increase the inspiratory:expiratory (I:E) ratio to allow ample time for expiration, in order to avoid dynamic hyperinflation (autopositive end-expiratory pressure [PEEP] or breath stacking).

- Extubation in a deep plane of anesthesia should theoretically decrease the risk of bronchospasm caused by the stimulus of the ETT.

Chronic Obstructive Pulmonary Disease

COPD is a chronic progressive, an irreversible inflammatory condition resulting in expiratory airflow limitation. It includes:

- Emphysema.

- Chronic bronchitis.

- Small airway disease.

Risk factors for COPD include:

- Cigarette smoking.

- Increased airway responsiveness to various exogenous stimuli.

- Respiratory infections.

- Occupational exposures (coal mining, gold mining, and cotton textile dust).

- Ambient air pollution.

- Genetic: Severe antitrypsin (α1 AT) deficiency.

Preoperative Evaluation

- History should focus on exercise tolerance, change in trend of symptoms, addition of new medication or escalation of previous medications, number of hospitalizations related to exacerbations, need of mechanical ventilation, and presence of any comorbid illness.

- Physical examination:

  ▶ Nutritional status: Body mass index (BMI), outside the normal range, increases the risk of pulmonary complications.

  ▶ Auscultation: The presence of diminished breath sounds, prolonged expiration, wheeze, and rhonchi are predictors of postoperative pulmonary complications.

  ▶ Fever, purulent sputum, worsening cough, and dyspnea also add to the risk of complications.

- Investigations:
  - ▸ Routine preoperative blood tests.
  - ▸ Electrocardiogram: To rule out right-sided heart disease or concomitant ischemic heart disease.
  - ▸ Chest X-ray: For hyperinflated lung fields.
  - ▸ Spirometry: For COPD diagnosis and assessment of severity.
  - ▸ Formal exercise testing: The functional status of patients.
  - ▸ A baseline arterial blood gas (ABG).

Preoperative Preparation

Preoperative preparation should target on smoking cessation. Smoking cessation anytime before surgery has been found to reduce complications (e.g., pneumonia, length of intensive care stay, and need for mechanical ventilation), but maximum benefit is seen with at least 8 weeks of abstinence before surgery. Chest physiotherapy is warranted in patients with a large volume of sputum to optimize patient outcomes.

Anesthetic Management

GA with tracheal intubation is associated with laryngospasm, bronchospasm, cardiovascular instability, barotraumas, and hypoxemia, resulting in increased rates of postoperative pulmonary complications. Therefore, regional anesthesia (RA) is preferred.

General Anesthesia

- **Preinduction**

  Preoxygenation should be used in any patient who is hypoxic on-air before induction. The use of continuous positive airway pressure (CPAP) during induction may be used to improve the efficacy of preoxygenation and reduce the development of atelectasis in patients with severe hypoxia. Ventilatory management is an essential consideration in a patient of COPD, and the following points are noteworthy:

  - ▸ Avoid auto-PEEP: It can be achieved by reducing the frequency of breaths or I:E ratio. Exhalation time should be more to prevent breath stacking.
  - ▸ Application of PEEP: Extrinsic PEEP (usually 80% of intrinsic PEEP) helps to decrease the work of breathing.
  - ▸ Treatment of bronchospasm: It can be treated with any of the following:
    - ○ Use of inhaled bronchodilators.
    - ○ Deepening the plane of anesthesia with either propofol or increasing concentration of inhaled anesthetic.

At the end of the surgery, extubation should be done cautiously and preferably in the presence of an experienced anesthetist. Before extubation, oxygenation and reversal of the neuromuscular blockade must be ensured. Switching from tracheal intubation to noninvasive ventilation (NIV) may lessen the work of breathing and air trapping in select high-risk patients.

Postoperative Care

- Close monitoring of patients with severe COPD is required to prevent respiratory failure.
- Opioids should be avoided for pain management because of the risk of respiratory depression.
- Appropriate analgesia techniques and drugs in proper concentration should be used for pain control.
- Mucus plugging and consequent ventilatory failure should be prevented by physiotherapy, saline nebulization, and suctioning.

Restrictive Lung Disease

Restrictive respiratory diseases are characterized by a reduction in all lung volumes (restriction) and decreased compliance on pulmonary function testing; however, there is preservation of expiratory flow. Patients with restrictive respiratory disorders are at high risk of perioperative morbidity and mortality. Conditions that may cause such restriction include:

- Intrinsic disorders: Interstitial lung diseases.

- Extrinsic disorders: Abnormalities of the chest wall (pectus excavatum, kyphoscoliosis), pleura (effusion, trapped lung), or abdomen (ascites, obesity, masses) that mechanically compress the lungs or limit their expansion.

- Neuromuscular diseases affecting chest wall nerves and muscles, resulting in chronically reduced lung volumes and restrictive physiology.

Anesthetic Considerations

- Potential difficult bag and mask ventilation (BMV) and rapid desaturation (decreased functional residual capacity [FRC]).

- Altered respiratory physiology, for example:

  ▶ Hypoxemia (V/Q mismatch).

  ▶ Decreased compliance and risk of barotrauma and pneumothorax.

  ▶ Pulmonary hypertension and cor pulmonale.

- Increased risk of perioperative respiratory complications:

  ▶ Pneumonia, pneumothorax, respiratory depression (sensitive to opioids), and respiratory failure.

▶ Higher risk if vital capacity (VC) < 15 mL/kg, forced vital capacity (FVC) < 50% or 500 mL, or pCO_2 > 45 cm H_2O.

▶ Cancel elective procedures if there is an acute and reversible process.

- Management may include the use of a high-performance ventilator, using small tidal volumes with rapid rates, and may require postoperative ventilation and ICU care.

- Medications:

  ▶ Steroids, immunosuppressive, oxygen, pulmonary hypertension treatment.

  ▶ History of bleomycin, amiodarone use.

- **Goals**

  ▶ Preoperative optimization, if possible.

  ▶ Minimally invasive (local anesthetic or regional) or maximum support (slow wean).

  ▶ Lung protective ventilation: Low-tidal volume, fast respiratory rate, inverse ratio, pressure control, PEEP.

  ▶ Minimize exposure to oxygen if history of previous bleomycin use.

  ▶ Avoid precipitants of pulmonary hypertension (hypercarbia, hypoxia, acidosis, pain).

  ▶ Excellent pain management to minimize the risk of postoperative respiratory failure.

Tuberculosis

Tuberculosis, a common pulmonary disease in developing countries, can present with the involvement of any organ, but lungs being the most common. The usual presentation is with a chronic productive cough and hemoptysis. Patients can also present with fever, night sweats, loss of weight, or failure to thrive.

Preoperative Considerations

It is important to evaluate the condition under the following headings:

- Patient assessment:
  - ▶ A complete history and examination of the patient is necessary.
  - ▶ Investigations: Chest X-ray, laboratory test results, liver function tests, pulmonary function tests, ABG, ventilation, and perfusion scans.
- The impact of the disease on organ function.
- The current medications.
- Potential for drug interactions.

  Antitubercular drugs and anesthetic agents interact at pharmacokinetic levels due to induction or inhibition of cytochrome enzymes by antitubercular drugs.
  - ▶ Rifampicin is an enzyme inducer, while isoniazid is an enzyme inhibitor. Both of them can alter the plasma level of drugs metabolized by particular hepatic enzymes, resulting in either subtherapeutic level or toxicity, for example, patients on protease inhibitors.
  - ▶ Induction agents: Increased metabolism can cause awareness during total IV anesthesia.
  - ▶ LA: Reduced risk of local anesthetic toxicity as a result of fastened metabolism.
  - ▶ Risk of halothane hepatitis with antituberculosis treatment (ATT). Newer inhalational agents have minimal metabolism and are not affected by ATT.
  - ▶ NMBDs: The effect of succinylcholine remains unchanged until a significant decrease in pseudocholinesterase level as sequelae of liver dysfunction. Streptomycin may potentiate the effects of nondepolarizing agents. Therefore, the dose of nondepolarizing agents should be titrated and supported by neuromuscular monitoring.
  - ▶ Pretreatment with rifampicin decreases the analgesic effect of morphine. Duration of action of other opioids like fentanyl and alfentanil is shortened because of extensive metabolism by hepatic cytochrome enzymes.
  - ▶ Nonsteroidal anti-inflammatory drugs (NSAIDs): The effect of diclofenac is decreased with rifampicin, while that of ibuprofen is unchanged, making it a safer option.
- The risk of transmission of tuberculosis to staff and other patients: ATT is continued on the day of surgery. The patient should wear a mask when leaving the room. If possible, the patient should wear the mask until the induction of anesthesia. Procedures should be performed in a negative air-pressure room, if possible, to avoid exposing other patients and personnel.

Intraoperative Care

The exposure to OT personnel should be minimized by scheduling such cases at the end of the day. Disposable anesthetic equipment should be used wherever possible, and every measure should be taken to not contaminate the nondisposable anesthesia equipment and machines.

- Patients with tuberculosis who must undergo surgery are at particular risk of hyperthermia as well as hypothermia. Temperature monitoring to maintain the core body temperature is a must.
- The patient's reduced ability to clear secretions can cause pneumonia and lung abscess as sequelae of bronchial plugging by mucus.

Respiratory Tract Infection

An acute upper respiratory tract infection (URTI) is the most common illness in the general population, primarily the pediatric age group. It is not uncommon for patients with active or recent URTI to present for elective or emergency surgery. An acute viral URTI may result in a variety of signs and symptoms, including sneezing, rhinorrhea, sore throat, cough, low-grade fever, headache, malaise, as well as sinusitis or uncomplicated bronchitis. Implications for patients undergoing GA, depending on the anatomical involvement of the infection, patient comorbidities, and the planned surgical procedure or intervention, are as follows:

- Children undergoing GA with a current or recent URTI are at increased risk of perioperative respiratory adverse events mostly related to airway hyperreactivity. These include laryngospasm, broncho-spasm, atelectasis, coughing, airway obstruction, hypoxia, stridor, and breathe holding.

- Although most of the adverse events can be easily managed, perioperative cardiac arrests can occur in children due to respiratory cause, most commonly with laryngospasm.

Mechanisms of Airway Hyperreactivity

- Chemical mediators and neurologic reflexes.

- Bronchoconstriction: Due to the release of inflammatory mediators like bradykinin, prostaglandin, histamine, and interleukin.

- Viral neuraminidases inhibit M2 receptors and increase the release of acetylcholine, leading to bronchoconstriction.

- Viral infections may inhibit the activity of neutral endopeptidase, resulting in

an increased smooth muscle constrictor response to tachykinins.

The risk of perioperative complications is increased for up to 6 to 8 weeks following a URTI attack and is maximal with ongoing RTI. The induction of anesthesia with propofol is associated with lesser complications compared to inhaled anesthetics. Complications are highest with thiopentone and in case of inadequate neuromuscular blockade recovery. The rate of complications goes down in the presence of an experienced anesthetist.

Preoperative Assessment

- Elder children with mild URTI can be safely anesthetized without significant morbidity. In contrast, in children < 1 year of age, respiratory complications are much higher, and there should be a low threshold to cancel surgery in children in this age group.

- Elective surgeries should be postponed for at least 4 weeks in children with severe symptoms.

- Laboratory tests: Chest X-ray should be done to rule out lower respiratory infection (if history and clinical examination suggest so).

Anesthetic Management

The goals of anesthetic management are to minimize secretions and avoid or limit the stimulation of a potentially irritable airway. The airway should only be suctioned under deep anesthesia. The patient should be well-hydrated, and a humidifier may be helpful to clear secretions and prevent bronchial mucus plugging. The other important considerations are:

- Preoperative bronchodilators given 10 to 30 minutes before surgery have been found to reduce perioperative respiratory events.

- A combination of beta-2 agonists such as salbutamol and inhaled corticosteroids are more effective than inhaled beta-2 agonist alone in minimizing intubation-related bronchoconstriction.

- A laryngeal mask airway (LMA) or facemask is preferred, and tracheal intubation should be avoided if possible, particularly in children less than 5 years.

- Lubricating the LMA with lignocaine gel reduces the incidence of airway complications in children with URTI.

- The incidence of adverse respiratory events is less when propofol is used as the induction agent compared with sevoflurane.

Thoracotomy and Pneumonectomy

Open pulmonary resection is most commonly performed to treat a known intrathoracic malignancy such as lung cancer or to diagnose pathology of a suspicious nodule or mass. Other indications for pulmonary resection include the management of thoracic trauma, pulmonary infection, and bronchopleural fistula. Surgical procedures for these indications include sublobar resection (segmentectomy, wedge resection), lobectomy, or removal of more than one lobe (bilobectomy, lobectomy plus segmentectomy). The patients are usually elderly, with a long history of smoking and consequent comorbid pathology; evaluation of cardiorespiratory requires more attention.

Preoperative Assessment

Routine investigations required are:

- Complete blood count (CBC).

- Chest X-ray.

- ABG: A $PaCO_2$ of > 50 mm Hg and a PaO_2 of < 60 mm Hg correlates with an elevated risk of postoperative pulmonary complications.

- Spirometry: Spirometry helps to identify the presence and severity of obstructive and restrictive lung disease and should be performed in all cases. The following parameters correlate with pulmonary complications following pneumonectomy:

  ▶ FVC < 50% of predicted or < 1.75 to 2 L.

  ▶ Forced expiratory volume (FEV1) > 2 L, mortality = 10%, < 2 L, mortality = 20 to 45%.

Perfusion lung scanning with radioactive isotopes can estimate the relative blood flow to each lung, and predicted postoperative FEV1 > 800 mL identifies a patient safe for pneumonectomy.

The single most important preoperative clinical indicator before pneumonectomy is the patient's exercise tolerance.

Preoperative Preparation

Preoperative respiratory preparation is centered around smoking cessation, treating respiratory infections, education, training of breathing exercises, as well as incentive spirometry. An adequate amount of blood products should be arranged and kept ready in the blood bank to deal with blood loss during surgery.

Anesthetic Management

- A large-bore cannula.

- Standard monitoring: ECG, noninvasive blood pressure (NIBP, SpO_2, $ETCO_2$, minimum alveolar concentration (MAC).

- Invasive blood pressure: For repeated ABG.

- Central venous pressure (CVP): For postoperative fluid management, particularly following pneumonectomy.

- A volatile agent or a volatile agent with or without nitrous oxide, an opiate, and a short- to intermediate-acting muscle relaxant is a safe anesthesia technique.

- One-lung ventilation (OLV) is an integral component of anesthetic care during lung resection surgeries and may be required in the following conditions:

  ▶ To prevent cross-contamination of a noninvolved lung from blood or pus.

- To control the distribution of ventilation in cases where there is a major air leak, such as bronchopleural fistula, tracheobronchial trauma, or in major airway surgery.

- To perform bronchopulmonary lavage.

- Thoracic aneurysm repair, pneumonectomy, and upper lobectomy.

- Middle and lower lobectomy, esophagostomy, and thoracoscopic and thoracic spinal procedures may require double-lumen tube (DLT).

Left-sided DLTs are commonly used because of increased safety of margin. 39 or 41 Fr DLT is preferred for males, while 37 or 35 Fr is optimal for females. With OLV, maintaining adequate oxygenation is of paramount importance and can be achieved with the help of the following:

- Maintain constant minute ventilation during OLV.

- Peak inspired pressure should be < 35 cm H_2O.

- Plateau pressure of < 25 cm H_2O.

- The FiO_2 may be increased to 1.0, if necessary, to preserve oxygenation.

- 2 to 5 cm H_2O of CPAP with 100% oxygen to the operative lung (following lung re-expansion).

Postoperative Complications

- Atelectasis.
- Pneumothorax.
- Cardiac herniation.
- Hemorrhage.

- Arrhythmias.
- Right heart failure.

Fluid Management

The judicious use of fluids is warranted in the postoperative period to avoid the risk of pulmonary edema. The use of colloids can add to pulmonary edema, so they should be avoided.

Postoperative Analgesia

Thoracotomy is one of the most painful operative procedures. Excellent analgesia is essential to prevent hypoventilation, due to pain, which may increase the risk of postoperative pulmonary complications. Analgesia can be achieved through one of the following:

- Systemic opioids: Patient-controlled analgesia (PCA).

- NSAIDs: Opioid-sparing benefits.

- Epidural analgesia.

- Intercostal nerve blocks.

- Interpleural analgesia.

Conclusion

Respiratory diseases are commonly encountered during anesthesia practice. They are unique and challenging due to decreased pulmonary reserve and pose patients at risk of hypoxia during the perioperative course. Preoperative identification and optimization minimize the risk of respiratory complications. Patients with tuberculosis are contagious to OT personnel, and appropriate precautions must be practiced to avoid transmission of tubercular bacilli.

CHAPTER 16

Anesthesia for Central Nervous Diseases

Heena Garg and Nishant Patel

Introduction

Patients with diseases of the central nervous system (CNS) may require diagnostic, therapeutic as well as a surgical intervention under anesthesia. The pharmacodynamic effects of anesthetic agents are mediated through their action on various proteins in the CNS. These agents may cause long-term neurological sequelae in patients with underlying pathology of CNS. The patients with CNS disorders may have cognitive, sensory, motor, and autonomic deficit that make preoperative assessment difficult and in addition make intraoperative and postoperative care challenging. This chapter highlights salient anesthetic considerations of common CNS disorders.

Parkinson's Disease

Parkinson's disease (PD) is characterized by the loss of dopaminergic neurons in the substantia nigra. The common clinical manifestations include:

- Resting tremors—characteristic pill-rolling tremor in hands.
- Bradykinesia.
- Limb rigidity.
- Gait and balance problems.

Drugs such as phenothiazines, butyrophenones, and metoclopramide can inhibit dopaminergic receptors and result in Parkinsonism.

Anesthetic Considerations

- Interruption of anti-Parkinson's drug therapy should be as brief as possible and should be continued on the day of surgery with a sip of water.

- Avoid dopaminergic drugs like metoclopramide as premedication. Prokinetic agents such as cisapride or domperidone do not interact with dopaminergic receptors and are an acceptable alternative to metoclopramide.

- The autonomic function should be evaluated preoperatively, as these patients are at the risk of orthostatic hypotension and altered response to vasopressors.

- Regional anesthesia is preferred over general anesthesia because general anesthetics and muscle relaxants can mask tremors.

- The patients taking levodopa are at increased risk of tachyarrhythmias, especially with halothane and ketamine.

- Propofol has the potential to produce dyskinesias and ablation of resting tremor, suggesting that it may have both excitatory and inhibitory effects in this patient population.

- Opioids like alfentanil and fentanyl can cause exacerbation of muscle rigidity, while morphine has a dose-related effect on dyskinesia (dyskinesia decreases at low dose and increases at a higher dose).

- Nondepolarizing muscle relaxants do not affect the symptoms of PD. However, suxamethonium has been reported to cause hyperkalemia in PD.

- The glycopyrrolate bromide is the anticholinergic agent of choice, as it does not cross the blood–brain barrier (BBB).

- Adequacy of ventilation and return of airway reflexes should be ensured prior to extubation.

The patient's anti-Parkinson's drugs should be resumed as soon as possible in the postoperative period to avoid exacerbation of symptoms.

Alzheimer's Disease

Alzheimer's disease (AD) is the most common neurodegenerative disorder among the elderly. It is characterized by profound memory disturbances and irreversible impairment of cognitive function.

Anesthetic Considerations

- Loss of memory and cognitive dysfunction makes the patient disoriented, uncooperative, confused, and at times violent. Besides, the clinical history and examination may remain incomplete, and obtaining consent is difficult.

- Perioperative sedation may aggravate mental confusion, and hence attention should be paid before prescribing them. Benzodiazepines often result in worsening of acute confusion and delirium.

- Regional anesthesia is potentially challenging because of poor cooperation and disorientation.

- Fragile skin, weak bones, bradykinesia, and stiff joints with limited range of motion demand careful and gentle intraoperative positioning and adequate padding.

- Prolonged immobilization increases the incidence of deep venous thrombosis (DVT) and pulmonary embolism (PE).

- The recovery of mental status to the preoperative level is delayed due to slow metabolism and excretion of drugs.

- Glycopyrrolate is preferred over atropine or scopolamine as antisialagogue because it is impermeable to the BBB.

- The dose of intravenous (IV) anesthetics and minimum alveolar concentration (MAC) of inhaled anesthetics should be kept low and titrated to achieve an adequate balance between the anesthetic effect and the harmful effects.

- Postoperative cognitive dysfunction (POCD) and delirium are possible consequences of anesthetic agents interacting with acetylcholine receptors (AChRs) to produce inhibition of central cholinergic transmission already impaired by age-related changes.

Epilepsy

The burden of epilepsy in the general population ranges from 0.5 to 1.0%. Epilepsy is the paroxysmal, abnormal cerebral electrical discharge associated with a clinical change. It can be either generalized or focal.

Anesthetic Considerations

- The preoperative assessment should focus on duration, frequency, and control of seizure symptoms with medications.

- All the current medications and their dosage should be reviewed.

- Patients should continue their medications on the day of the surgery.

- The potent anticonvulsant action of thiopentone makes it the drug of choice for refractory status epilepticus.

- Propofol decreases cortical activity during both anesthesia and status epilepticus. However, it has been reported to cause excitation of the CNS in a 10% population.

- Ketamine produces a state of dissociative anesthesia. It should normally be avoided in epileptics.

- The myoclonus due to etomidate should not be misdiagnosed as an epileptiform activity.

- Inhalational anesthetics cause burst suppression on the electroencephalogram (EEG) and are safe for use in epileptics, except enflurane, which causes epileptiform activity.

- All of the commonly used anticonvulsants cause enzyme induction in the liver. This can lead to markedly reduced duration of activity of the aminosteroidal muscle relaxants, particularly those which are excreted via the liver (vecuronium and pancuronium).

- The extrapyramidal effects and dystonic reactions due to dopamine antagonists may be confused with epileptic activity and should be avoided.

- Metabolic disturbances due to prolonged fasting should be avoided as they may precipitate seizures.

- Hypocarbia and hypoventilation should be avoided.

- The shivering and confusion in the post-operative period should not be confused with seizure activity.

Stroke

Acute stroke is the second leading cause of death worldwide and the leading cause of long-term disability, of which ischemic stroke accounts for 87% of cases.

Anesthetic Considerations

- The preoperative assessment should focus on the level of consciousness, fasting status, allergies, airway assessment, comorbidities, and hemodynamic stability.

- The neurological deficit should be evaluated and documented during the preoperative evaluation. The risk of perioperative stroke and exacerbation of neurological deficit should be explained to patients, and consent for the same must be obtained.

- General anesthesia is advantageous over local anesthesia or sedation in terms of better immobility, pain control, and airway protection but at the cost of hemodynamic changes with intubation.

- On the other hand, local anesthesia or sedation provides smooth hemodynamics and allows intraprocedural clinical neurological evaluation. However, it has disadvantages like lack of airway protection, continued patient movement, uncontrolled pain and agitation, and prolonged procedure time.

- Patients can also present for other surgeries poststroke, and they may be in different stages of recovery.

- Patients with a recent history of stroke < 3 months should be taken up only for emergency surgeries. The anesthetic concerns for such patients include:

  ▸ Perioperative recurrence of stroke.

  ▸ Re-emergence of neurological deficits postoperatively.

- Perioperative stroke increases risk of mortality by eightfold compared with patients without stroke.

- Exacerbation of prior unrecognized or unreported neurological deficits can occur following both neuraxial and general anesthesia due to compromised cerebral perfusion.

- Antihypertensive medications and statins should be continued preoperatively, and adequate hydration should be ensured.

- Sedative premedication should be avoided or used in minimal dosages.

- Apart from standard American Society of Anesthesiologists (ASA) monitoring, invasive arterial blood pressure, central venous pressure, urine output, and neuromuscular monitoring on the unaffected side may be required.

- Cerebral electrophysiological monitoring and transcranial Doppler (TCD) are restricted to patients at high-risk repeat stroke. Cerebral oximetry is useful to detect ischemia during high-risk cardiac or major vascular surgery and surgeries in the beach chair position.

- IV anesthetic agents offer cerebral protection by decreasing cerebral metabolism. Inhalational agents are vasodilators and, therefore, may be beneficial.

- Addition of intermediate- or short-acting opioids reduce the dose of induction agents, thereby reducing hemodynamic instability during induction.

- Succinylcholine can cause life-threatening hyperkalemia in patients of stroke with loss of significant muscle function.

- Avoid hypotension as it can reduce the focal cerebral blood flow and predispose the patient to postoperative stroke. Intraoperative blood pressure should be maintained at baseline or slightly elevated levels.

- Avoid hypoxia, hypercarbia and hypocarbia, and acidosis.

- Avoid hypoglycemia and hyperglycemia. Tight glucose control is beneficial in stroke patients.

- Ascertain protective airway reflexes prior to tracheal extubation. The neurological function should be assessed at the earliest after recovery from anesthesia.

- High-dependency unit care is required for patients with major neurological deficits.

Multiple Sclerosis

Multiple sclerosis (MS) is an autoimmune inflammatory disease, leading to demyelination and axonal damage to the CNS.

Anesthetic Considerations

- A thorough baseline neurologic history and examination should be performed and documented during the preoperative assessment.

- Patients should continue to take corticosteroid therapy and may require stress dosing.

- Strict temperature monitoring is required. Even slight increase in body temperature may precipitate a decline in neurologic function postoperatively.

- The use of succinylcholine should be avoided as it may increase the risk of hyperkalemia.

- Patients with MS may have altered sensitivity to nondepolarizing muscle relaxants. Therefore, cautious use of these drugs is advised along with neuromuscular monitoring.

- The limited neurologic and respiratory reserve increases the risk of postoperative residual paralysis in such a group of patients. Patients with baseline weakness or pharyngeal dysfunction will require comprehensive monitoring and care postoperatively.

- Patients with MS may be expected to have some MAC reduction and delayed emergence proportionate to the severity of their disease.

- Demyelination of the spinal cord makes patients of MS more susceptible to the neurotoxic effects of local anesthetics.

Syringomyelia

Syringomyelia is a rare, slowly progressive neurological condition characterized by the presence of a syrinx within the spinal cord. Syringomyelia is a chronic progressive disorder of the nervous system characterized by a cystic cavity (syrinx) in the spinal cord which fills with cerebrospinal fluid (CSF). It is commonly associated with Arnold–Chiari malformation.

Anesthetic Considerations

- The anesthetic management plan for a patient with syringomyelia should include strategies to avoid any increase in intracranial pressure (ICP).
- Any rise in ICP may result in herniation of the cerebellum/brainstem or further extension of the syrinx.
- Patients with syringomyelia may also be sensitive to nondepolarizing neuromuscular blockade due to muscle wasting, atrophy, and hyperkalemic responses to succinylcholine administration.
- These patients usually present with a difficult airway.
- Neuraxial anesthesia has been performed in such patients successfully without any complications, especially in pregnancy.

Amyotrophic Lateral Sclerosis

Amyotrophic lateral sclerosis (ALS) is a rare but rapidly progressive neuromuscular degenerative disorder. Clinical manifestations include muscular weakness, atrophy, fasciculations, spasticity, and hyperreflexia.

Anesthetic Considerations

- Preoperative evaluation should identify inherent muscle weakness and associated respiratory insufficiency.

- Short-acting anesthetic drugs with rapid recovery form the goal of anesthetic management in these cases.
- Regional anesthesia may cause exacerbation of pre-existing neurologic damage. Epidural anesthesia may be beneficial over spinal as the concentration of local anesthetic in the CSF is smaller as compared to that of spinal anesthesia in a patient with neurological disease.

Guillain–Barré Syndrome

Guillain–Barré syndrome (GBS) is an immune-mediated polyneuropathy characterized by progressively ascending symmetric paralysis that often follows a viral or bacterial illness within the preceding 4 weeks. Some patients may have respiratory compromise requiring prolonged ventilatory support and bulbar dysfunction.

Anesthetic Considerations

- Vital capacity, maximal inspiratory, and expiratory pressures provide information about the power of respective groups of respiratory muscles.
- Tracheostomy is required if prolonged respiratory support is likely to be needed.
- Suxamethonium must not be used in GBS patients.
- Monitoring of the electrocardiogram (ECG), blood pressure, and fluid balance is advisable because of autonomic dysfunction in 70% cases. Invasive blood pressure is advisable, keeping autonomic instability in mind.
- Patients with autonomic dysfunction may be susceptible to the development of paralytic ileus. This may be treated with prokinetic agents such as metoclopramide or erythromycin.

- Compression nerve palsies, pressure sores, and contractures can occur due to limb position and pressure. Careful position and padding should be done to prevent such complications.
- There may be increased sensitivity to nondepolarizing neuromuscular blocking agents.
- Epidural anesthesia may be useful to avoid postoperative opioid use.

Autonomic Dysfunction

The incidence of severe autonomic failure is about 1 in 1,000 persons. Autonomic failure may be secondary to diseases like diabetes mellitus, amyloidosis, or bronchogenic carcinoma or be due to a primary autonomic disorder such as multiple system atrophy (MSA; Shy–Drager syndrome) or pure autonomic failure. The clinical features are:

- Orthostatic hypotension.
- Postprandial hypotension.
- Urinary bladder dysfunction with urinary retention.
- Decreased gastrointestinal motility and erectile dysfunction.
- Supine hypertension.

Anesthetic Considerations

- Preoperative evaluation should focus on detailed clinical history and examination, measurement of blood pressure and heart rate while supine, and again after 1 and 3 minutes of standing.
- Tests for autonomic dysfunction are:
  - ▸ Orthostatic and tilt-table testing.
  - ▸ The Valsalva maneuver.
  - ▸ The cold pressor test.
  - ▸ Deep breathing.
  - ▸ Hyperventilation.
  - ▸ Thermoregulatory sweat test.

  - ▸ Quantitative sudomotor axon reflex test.
- Ensure adequate hemodynamic stability with fluids and pharmacologic means.
- Alpha-1 adrenoreceptor agonist (phenylephrine) is preferred for hypotension under anesthesia.

Spinal Cord Transection

Spinal cord transection is common in trauma patients. The patients are in spinal shock during the first 1 to 3 weeks due to sympathetic cutoff; therefore, they are vulnerable to hypotension and bradycardia. In the case of old spinal cord injuries (especially transection above T6), the patients develop autonomic hyperreflexia characterized by severe hypertension and reflex bradycardia.

Anesthetic Considerations

- Care should be taken to immobilize the trauma victims during interhospital as well as intrahospital transport.
- The urgent nature of airway interventions usually requires direct or indirect laryngoscopy with manual in-line stabilization (MILS).
- Prevention of secondary injury through adequate oxygenation, blood pressure support through volume replacement, and immobilization is necessary.
- Multimodality neuromonitoring is adequately sensitive and specific for detecting intraoperative neurologic injury during spine surgery, and the choice of anesthetic has an impact on its quality.
- Corticosteroids may be used only after careful consideration of associated risks and benefits.
- For autonomic hyperreflexia, both regional anesthesia and general anesthesia, are equally good. Succinylcholine should not be used due to extrajunctional receptors.

Psychiatric Disorders

The patients with mental disorders and substance abuse are not uncommon. The potential interaction of psychotropic medications with anesthetic agents make anesthetic care challenging and tricky in such a group of patients. The common psychiatric disorders and their anesthetic implications are described below:

a. Depression: It is a common psychiatric disorder affecting 6 to 7% of the population. The females are affected more often than males. The abnormalities of amine neurotransmitter pathways are considered the most likely etiologic factors; however, the true pathway is still not known.

Anesthetic Considerations

- The potential to commit suicide should be evaluated in all patients.
- The patients taking monoamine oxidase inhibitors (MAOIs) can be safely taken for elective surgeries (earlier recommendation was to discontinue MAOIs 14 days prior to elective surgeries).
- Benzodiazepines are safe for preoperative anxiety.
- Sympathetic stimulants like ketamine should be avoided.
- The general anesthesia with volatile anesthetic is acceptable. However, the requirement of anesthetic is more due to increased epinephrine levels in the CNS.
- Spinal and epidural anesthesia are acceptable, but they may be associated with a higher risk of hypotension and, consequently, an increased need for vasopressors.
- A lighter plane of anesthesia and directly acting vasopressors should be avoided to decrease the incidence of systemic hypertension.
- Multimodal analgesia with nonsteroidal anti-inflammatory drugs (NSAIDs) and opioids is safe. However, meperidine should not be used in patients who are on MAOIs.

b. Bipolar disorder: It is characterized by mood swings, ranging from depressive episodes to manic or hypomanic episodes, with normal behavior in between.

Anesthetic Considerations

- Preoperative evaluation should review the most recent serum lithium concentration.
- ECG monitoring is mandatory to detect lithium-induced conduction defects or dysrhythmias.
- Neuromuscular monitoring is required because lithium can prolong the duration of action of both depolarizing as well as nondepolarizing muscle relaxants.

c. Schizophrenia: It is a psychotic mental disorder with features of abnormal reality testing or thought processes. The dopamine hypothesis suggests the disease symptoms occur due to the dysfunction of the neurotransmitter dopamine.

Anesthetic Considerations

- Antipsychotic medications have the potential to cause postural hypotension, QT prolongation, seizures, and elevation of liver enzymes.
- Drug-induced sedation decreases the requirement of anesthetic drugs.
- The poor cooperation from patients makes general anesthesia as the preferred choice of anesthesia.

d. Substance abuse: It may be defined as drug use by self-administration which deviates from accepted medical or social use; if sustained, it can lead to physical and psychological dependence.

Anesthetic Considerations

- Preoperative psychiatric evaluation is essential in patients with substance abuse.
- Patients must not be posted for elective surgeries if in acute withdrawal.
- Patients with cocaine abuse are at risk of myocardial ischemia and dysrhythmias; therefore, any drug or event with potential to cause sympathetic stimulation must be avoided.
- Thrombocytopenia associated with cocaine abuse may influence selection of regional anesthesia.
- Unexpected agitation in the postoperative period may suggest cocaine ingestion.
- The patients addicted to opioids should be maintained on opioids or methadone during the perioperative period.
- Opioid agonist–antagonist should be avoided in opioid addicts because of risk of withdrawal reactions.

- Opioid addicts experience exaggerated pain in the postoperative period (for unknown reasons).
- Alcoholics must be evaluated for associated medical illnesses like dilated cardiomyopathy, cirrhosis, pancreatitis, metabolic disorder (hypoglycemia), and nutritional disorder (Wernicke–Korsakoff syndrome).

Conclusion

Patients with neurological disorders are challenging in nature during the entire perioperative course. The preoperative assessment may be difficult due to altered mental status, complicating assessment of neurological status, and perception of pain during the postoperative period. Anesthesia and surgery alter the hemodynamic and electrolyte balance, leading to neuronal insult and precipitation of seizures, respectively. The effects of anesthetic agents on cerebral physiology should be understood and applied carefully to avoid neurologically adverse events.

CHAPTER 17

Anesthesia for Liver Diseases

Ushkiran Kaur, Neel Prakash, and Sandeep Sahu

Preoperative Evaluation of Liver Function

Evaluation should be directed at establishing the etiologic diagnosis, then grading or estimating how severe the disease is, and finally staging the disease. The severity or activity of the disease is assessed and graded accordingly as mild, moderate, or severe. Estimation of the point in the course of the natural history of the disease, early or late, precirrhotic, cirrhotic, or end-stage, is referred to as the stage of the disease.

History

The relevant history, including symptoms and signs, is summarized in **Table 17.1**.

Investigations

Biochemical tests or liver function tests include the following:

- Serum bilirubin: Normal value of 0.3 to 1.5 mg/dL for total bilirubin and 0.3 mg/dL for conjugated bilirubin. It forms the basis of grading the severity of the liver injury and is a critical component of scores like *Child–Turcotte–Pugh (CTP) score or Child Criteria* and model for end-stage liver disease or MELD score (**Table 17.2**).

- Serum enzymes: *The aminotransferases (transaminases) are sensitive indicators of liver cell injury.* Aspartate aminotransferase (AST) is found in the liver, cardiac muscle,

Table 17.1 Symptoms and signs of liver disease

Symptoms	Signs
• Fatigue, weakness, nausea, poor appetite, malaise	• Icterus
• Jaundice	• Pallor due to anemia
• Light or clay-colored stools with high colored urine (suggestive of obstructive jaundice)	• Tenderness in the abdomen: *Murphy's sign*—seen in cholecystitis cholangitis
• Itching	• Xanthoma due to hypercholesteremia
• Abdominal pain	• Ecchymosis due to vitamin K deficiency
• History of fever: Fever with arthralgia at the onset of jaundice is indicative of viral hepatitis, fever with rigors could be due to cholangitis, low-grade fever over several days can be seen in neoplasm	• Hepatosplenomegaly
	• Pedal edema due to hypoproteinemia
	• Ascites
• Bloating and dyspepsia	• Distended and palpable gall bladder (*Courvoisier's sign*) seen in malignant obstruction of common bile duct
• History of multiple blood transfusion, vaccinations	
• Drug intake: The history of ingestion of hepatotoxic drugs, e.g., antitubercular drugs	• Encephalopathy
• Family history of diseases such as Wilson's disease, alpha-antitrypsin deficiency, etc.	
• History of substance abuse especially alcohol	
• History of any previous surgery	

Table 17.2 CTP score and MELD scores

Parameter	1 point	2 points	3 points
Encephalopathy	Absent	Mild to moderate (grade 1–2)	Severe (grade 3–4)
Serum bilirubin (mg/dL)	<2.0	2.0–3.0	>3.0
Serum albumin (g/dL)	>3.5	3.5–2.8	<2.8
Prothrombin time (prolongation [s])	1–4	4–6	>6
Prolongation of INR	<1.7	1.7–2.3	>2.3
Ascites	Absent	Mild-to-moderate (responsive to diuretics)	Severe (refractory to diuretics)

Abbreviations: CTP, Child–Turcotte–Pugh; MELD, model for end-stage liver disease.
Notes: The CTP score is a system to assess the strength of treatment and the necessity of liver transplant of chronic liver disease, primarily cirrhosis. The scores are added, and then the patients are divided into the following categories:

- Class A: 5–6 points,
- Class B: 7–9 points,
- Class C: >10 points,

with the 1-year survival being 100% for class A, 80% for class B, and 45% for class C.
MELD score is used for assessing the severity of the chronic liver disease (CLD), and it uses the patient's values for serum bilirubin, serum creatinine, and the international normalized ratio (INR) for prothrombin time to predict survival.

skeletal muscle, kidneys, brain, pancreas, lungs, leukocytes, and erythrocytes. Alanine transferase (ALT) is found mainly in the liver. *The normal range is 10 to 40 IU/L.* Modest elevations up to 300 IU/L are nonspecific, while elevations more than 1,000 IU/L are seen in viral hepatitis, ischemic liver injury (prolonged hypotension or acute heart failure), or toxin/drug-induced liver injury. AST:ALT ratio is typically < 1 in patients with chronic viral hepatitis and nonalcoholic fatty liver disease (NAFLD). As cirrhosis develops, ratio rises to > 1. AST:ALT ratio > 2:1 is suggestive, and > 3:1 is highly suggestive of alcoholic liver diseases. Alkaline phosphatase, 5′–nucleotidase, and gamma-glutamyl transpeptidase (GGT) are elevated in cholestatic jaundice.

- **Tests for biosynthetic functions:**
  - Serum albumin: Half-life of 18 to 20 days, with 4% degrade per day. Minimal changes are seen in acute events, but their levels are decreased (<3 g/dL) in chronic liver disease (CLD). In ascites, the level could be low due to an increased volume of distribution even with normal production.
  - Serum globulins: A group of gamma globulins produced by B lymphocytes and primarily produced by hepatocytes. Diffuse polyclonal increase in IgG is seen in autoimmune hepatitis, while elevations in IgM levels are seen in primary biliary cirrhosis, and IgA levels are higher in alcoholic liver disease.
  - Coagulation factors: Liver synthesizes all clotting factors *except Factor VIII* (it is synthesized by vascular endothelium). *Vitamin k is required for posttranslational modification of factors II, VII, IX, and X.* Their serum half-lives are much smaller than albumin, and hence the measurement of the clotting factors is not only the single best *acute measure of synthetic hepatic function* but also helpful in diagnosing and assessing the parenchymal function of the liver.

▶ Other tests: Other tests that may be needed in the specific patient are serum ammonia level, abdominal ultrasound, endoscopic retrograde cholangiopancreatography (ERCP), etc.

Anesthetic Considerations in Patients with Liver Diseases

Preoperative

- Postpone elective surgery in acute liver disease.
- Optimize patients in terms of coagulopathy, encephalopathy, ascites, metabolic derangements (electrolytes and blood sugar), and anemia before the surgery.
- Avoid benzodiazepines for premedications, as these patients are highly sensitive to sedatives.

Intraoperative

- Practice universal precautions (if the patient is seropositive for hepatitis B and C).
  Splanchnic vasodilation (especially in patients of CLD) leads to a decrease in effective circulatory volume. Therefore, such patients are susceptible to develop hypotension under anesthesia.
- Avoid neuraxial anesthesia because of the existence of low-circulatory volume and coagulopathy.
- The dose of intravenous (IV) anesthetics is increased due to increased volume of distribution; on the other hand, a decrease in the metabolism of the drug leads to prolonged action.
- Propofol is the induction agent of choice (short-acting and extrahepatic metabolism).
- Sevoflurane is the inhalational agent of choice (preserve hepatic blood flow, no trifluoroacetic acid on metabolism).

Isoflurane and desflurane are acceptable alternatives

- Avoid nitrous oxide (as it can increase pulmonary pressure in patients with portopulmonary hypertension).
- Cisatracurium and atracurium are muscle relaxants of choice (because of organ independent Hoffman elimination).
- Succinylcholine can have prolonged action (if the level of pseudocholinesterase decreases to 25% or less).
- Remifentanil is the opioid of choice (organ independent metabolism).
- Care should be taken to avoid:
  ▶ *Hypotension* (risk of hepatic injury).
  ▶ *Hypoglycemia* (patients are already prone to hypoglycemia).
  ▶ *Alkalosis* (increased conversion of ammonium to ammonia and precipitation of hepatic encephalopathy).
  ▶ *Sepsis* (precipitation of encephalopathy).

Blood product should be arranged after cross-matching like packed red blood cells (PRBC), frozen fresh plasma (FFP), cryoprecipitate, and platelets, as per the need.

Static variables of preload such as central venous pressure (CVP) and pulmonary capillary wedge pressure (PCWP), although being used traditionally, have been shown to be poor predictors of fluid responsiveness. *Dynamic variables like stroke volume variation (SVV) obtained by FloTrac/Vigileo system and the pulse pressure variation (PPV) have the ability to predict fluid responsiveness and should be used if the facility is available.*

Postoperative

- Oxygen supplementation to prevent hypoxia.
- Aseptic care of the wound and surgical sites to prevent infection.

- Adequate volume replacement and monitoring of urine output.

Anesthesia for Obstructive Jaundice

This is discussed under the following headings:

- Pathophysiology of obstructive jaundice.
- Preoperative assessment and preparation.
- Selection of anesthesia.
- Postoperative management.

Pathophysiology of Obstructive Jaundice on Patient Physiology

Jaundice affects the functions of the following organs which are important to know before giving anesthesia and optimization, if possible:

- Hepatic: Can cause severe liver injury, including hepatocellular necrosis and apoptosis, which leads to fibrosis.
- Renal: These patients are at high risk of renal failure due to the presence of enteric endotoxins, which can cause vasoconstriction of the renal vasculature. Severe disturbance of body fluid compartment due to fluid shift and blood loss can also play a role in renal complications. Thus correction of volume deficits and optimum intraoperative fluid management can reduce the risk of renal complications in the perioperative period.
- Cardiovascular: Jaundiced heart or hepatic cardiomyopathy is commonly seen in these patients and is ascribed to altered beta-adrenergic signaling, alteration in membrane fluidity, and downregulation of beta receptors.
- *Bile acids* can cause negative ionotropic effects; hence, preoperative bradycardia can affect the management of hypotensive crises during the perioperative period.

- Gastrointestinal system: Malnutrition is a common finding in these patients. Impaired enterohepatic circulation can cause decreased availability of fat-soluble vitamins, leading to their deficiency. Intestinal mucosal damage and increased permeability can lead to an escape of pathogens in systemic circulation and cause sepsis, leading to multiorgan failure.
- Hematological: Anemia and deranged coagulation profile are common, which can be attributed to malnutrition and compromised synthetic function of the liver, respectively.

Preoperative Assessment, Preparation, and Optimization

- The *decrease in preoperative hematocrit (<30%), increased indirect bilirubin, and malignancy* are three independent risk factors determining the prognosis of patients with obstructive jaundice.
- Vitamin K therapy, maintenance of serum protein values to close to the normal, rational use of antibiotics and active fluid therapy, and maintenance of hydration are the cornerstones in preparation of the patients for surgery.
- Oral bile salts and H2 receptor antagonist should be used.
- Improvement of the nutritional status of the patient should be given a priority with high-protein, high-carbohydrate, and a low-fat diet. Parenteral nutrition can be initiated in patients with severe malnutrition 5 to 7 days before the surgery and continued after.
- A written informed consent detailing all the implications of surgery and anesthesia should be clearly explained to the patient and must be documented.

Conduct of Anesthesia and Selection of Agents

Combined general and epidural anesthesia is a preferred choice as it can maintain more stable hemodynamics and provide a balanced anesthetic effect. It also reduces the requirement of general anesthetic and hence can help in the early awakening and extubating of the patient.

Anesthetic Goal

The goal is to maintain hepatic blood flow and renal function and thus factors that could lead to its reduction should be avoided such as:

- Sympathetic stimulation, hypotension, hypocapnia, and hypoxemia.
- Pressure effects due to surgical retraction and tumors.
- A position like head low, and intermittent positive pressure ventilation (IPPV) with positive end-expiratory pressure (PEEP),

can lead to hepatic venous congestion and hence should be looked after.

- The use of a low dose of dopamine can be considered to maintain the pressure head for renal vasculature.

The principles of intraoperative and postoperative management of patients with biliary obstruction are the same as highlighted above.

Conclusion

The liver is the principal organ that not only plays an important role in synthesis, metabolism, and detoxification but is also an important immune system component. Derangement of liver function has multisystem manifestation, with significant alteration in the metabolism and excretion of anesthetic agents. Preoperative identification, optimization, selection of appropriate anesthetic agents, and avoiding further damage to the liver during the perioperative period are crucial to managing such patients.

CHAPTER 18

Anesthesia for Renal Diseases

Ushkiran Kaur, Neel Prakash, and Sandeep Sahu

Anesthesia for Chronic Kidney Disease

Chronic kidney disease (CKD) is the progressive, irreversible deterioration of renal function that results from a wide variety of diseases. Patients having a *glomerular filtration rate (GFR) less than 60 mL/min/1.73 m² for more than 3 months* are defined as having CKD. This disease, however, affects not only kidneys per se but has widespread pathophysiological manifestations affecting multiple organ systems, which play an important role in the anesthetic management when such a patient is posted for surgery (**Table 18.1**).

Special Anesthetic Considerations in the Perioperative Period

- Maintain renal perfusion by maintaining adequate blood pressure.
- Administer intravenous (IV) fluid judiciously; maintain adequate perfusion but avoid fluid overload.
- Avoid any nephrotoxic drugs and insults.

The various pathophysiological abnormalities and their anesthetic implications are as follows:

1. **Fluid and electrolytes:**
   - **Hyperkalemia:** This is caused by the inability of kidneys to excrete potassium, the majority of which is dependent on renal excretion. It may be aggravated by factors such as drugs (beta-blockers, K⁺ sparing diuretics, angiotensin-converting enzyme [ACE] inhibitors) and extracellular acidosis.

     Anesthetic implication: All patients should undergo preoperative estimation of serum potassium levels, and if elevated, then ECG should be done. *Succinylcholine should be avoided if serum potassium is > 5.5 mEq/L.*

   - **Hypokalemia:** Hypokalemia poses a patient at risk of arrhythmias. Mild hypokalemia (>3 mEq/L) do not require treatment in most of the cases.

     Anesthetic implication: Vigilant ECG monitoring (as patients are at risk of arrhythmias), avoid factors which can aggravate hypokalemia (e.g., hyperglycemia, hyperventilation).

   - **Chronic metabolic acidosis:** This occurs due to loss of ability to secrete protons and buffers in exchange for bicarbonate. Initially, it is of normal anion gap variety but progresses to high-anion gap variety in advanced renal failure.

     Anesthetic implication: Acidosis can be precipitated in the perioperative period and should be watched for and avoided.

   - **Sodium and water retention:** This is usually mild in nature. It is the cause of hypertension, fluid overload, and pulmonary edema.

     Anesthetic implications: Perioperative IV fluid administration should be judicious to avoid precipitation of overload and pulmonary edema. Usual

Table 18.1 Summary of the multisystemic manifestations of CKD and their anesthetic implications

Effect on various organ systems	Anesthetic implication
Fluid and electrolytes	
• Hyperkalemia	• Monitor potassium level
	• Avoid succinylcholine
• Chronic metabolic acidosis	• Monitor blood gases
• Sodium and water retention	• Avoid fluid overload
• Hypocalcemia	• Increased tendency to fractures during positioning
• Hypermagnesemia	• Potentiation of neuromuscular blockade
Cardiovascular system	
• Hypertension and LVH	• Increased risk of cardiovascular morbidity and mortality
• Accelerated atherosclerosis and IHD	• Detailed evaluation and optimization required
• Metastatic calcific VHD	
Hematological system	
• Anemia	• Consider transfusion if Hb < 7 g/dL
• Coagulopathy	• Prepare for increased risk of bleeding
Pulmonary system	
• Pulmonary congestion and edema	• Avoid fluid overload
• Atelectasis	• Appropriate ventilator strategies required
Gastrointestinal system	
• Delayed gastric emptying	• Aspiration prophylaxis and rapid sequence induction
• Gastrointestinal bleeding	required
• Nausea and vomiting	• Antiemetics and prokinetics are given
Immune system	
• Uremic immune dysfunction	• Adhere to strict aseptic precautions
Neurological system	
• Uremic encephalopathy	• Antiseizure prophylaxis may be required
• Peripheral neuropathy	• Pre-existing sensory or motor losses should be documented
• Autonomic neuropathy	• Autonomic hemodynamic responses may be blunted
Endocrine system	
• Altered temperature regulation	• Intraoperative hypothermia common

Abbreviations: CKD, chronic kidney disease; IHD, ischemic heart disease; LVH, left ventricular hypertrophy; VHD, valvular heart disease.

fluid intake and urine output should be recorded.

- **Hypocalcemia:** Its causes are as follows:

    a. Decreased production of vitamin D by kidneys, leading to reduced intestinal absorption of calcium.

    b. Hyperphosphatemia, resulting from impaired renal excretion of phosphates, causes deposition of calcium phosphate in the skin and soft tissues while also inhibiting the renal synthesis of vitamin D.

Hypocalcemia and hyperphosphatemia lead to *secondary hyperparathyroidism*, which results in increased osteoclastic and osteoblastic activity, causing ostetitis fibrosa cystica.

Anesthetic implications: Hypocalcemia can cause laryngospasm and hypotension. Therefore, symptomatic hypocalcemia must be treated before surgery. Avoid hyperventilation and alkalosis during the perioperative course, which can aggravate hypocalcemia.

- **Hypercalcemia:** Hypercalcemia manifests as tetany, circumoral numbness, and carpopedal spasm.

  Anesthetic implications: Maintain hydration and adequate urine output to precipitate hypercalcemia. Anticipate need for higher doses of nondepolarizing muscle relaxants.

- **Hypermagnesemia:** This results from reduced renal excretion of magnesium.

  Anesthetic implications: It may lead to muscle weakness and potentiation of the action of nondepolarizing muscle relaxants. Acidosis and dehydration can add to hypermagnesemia and must be avoided.

- **Hypomagnesemia:** The causes of hypomagnesemia in chronic renal failure are increased urinary loss and decreased dietary intake.

  Anesthetic implication: It can cause ventricular arrhythmias and may be associated with refractory hypokalemia as well as hypocalcemia.

2. **Cardiovascular manifestations:**

- **Hypertension:** This is caused by sodium and water retention along with hyperreninemia. It leads to left ventricular hypertrophy.

- **Accelerated atherosclerosis and ischaemic heart disease:** This is the result of decreased plasma triglyceride clearance, hypertension, and fluid overload, causing left ventricular hypertrophy and failure.

- **Metastatic calcific valvular heart disease:** This may be a manifestation of hypocalcemia and hyperphosphatemia.

  Anesthetic implications: Cardiovascular disease (CVD) is a major cause of perioperative morbidity and mortality in CKD patients, necessitating the need for detailed cardiovascular evaluation and optimization preoperatively. *Thrombosis of central veins may make cannulation difficult.*

3. **Hematological abnormalities:**

- **Anemia:** It is a normochromic normocytic in character. It is caused by the following:

  a. Insufficient erythropoietin production.

  b. Iron deficiency.

  c. Blood retention in the dialyzer.

  d. Gastrointestinal (GI) bleeding.

  e. Reduced red blood cells (RBC) life due to uremia.

  Anesthetic implication: A transfusion trigger of Hb < 7 g/dL is generally acceptable.

- **Prolongation of bleeding time:** It is caused by the following:

  a. Decreased activity of platelet factor.

  b. Abnormal platelet aggregation and adhesiveness.

  c. Impaired prothrombin consumption.

  Anesthetic implications: CKD patients should undergo platelet count, standard coagulation tests, and further qualitative analysis, if required, especially if regional anesthesia is planned. There may be increased bleeding tendency intraoperatively, and it is managed with transfusion of cryoprecipitate, platelets, or desmopressin. *Heparin should be avoided during preoperative dialysis to lessen intraoperative bleeding.*

4. **Pulmonary abnormalities:**

   - **Pulmonary congestion and edema:** It occurs primarily due to fluid overload but can occur even in the absence of the latter.

   - Increased predisposition to atelectasis and infections.

5. **Gastrointestinal abnormalities:**

   - Anorexia, nausea, and vomiting are common.

   - GI bleeding can be caused by uremia.

   - Delayed gastric emptying, decreased residual volume, and decreased pH lead to increased risk of peptic ulcer disease and aspiration.

     Anesthetic implication: Increased risk of aspiration should be managed with aspiration prophylaxis and rapid sequence induction and intubation.

6. **Immune system dysfunction:**

   - **Uremic immune dysfunction:** It is caused by inhibition of cell-mediated immunity and humoral defense mechanisms.

     Anesthetic implication: Catheter and fistula site infections are common.

7. **Neurological manifestations:**

   - Uremic encephalopathy.

   - Peripheral neuropathy: Distal glove-and-stocking sensory loss, progressing to motor loss.

   - Autonomic neuropathy.

   - Dialysis dementia: It is caused by aluminum toxicity from the dialysate.

   - Dialysis disequilibrium syndrome: It is caused by a reverse urea effect at the start of dialysis.

     Anesthetic implication: Caution with regional anesthesia in case of documented peripheral neuropathy.

8. **Endocrine disturbances:**

   - Temperature regulation is altered.

     Anesthetic implication: Patients are prone to hypothermia intraoperatively.

Changes in Drug Pharmacokinetics

Broadly, the pharmacokinetic effects may be classified on the basis of lipid solubility:

- **Lipid soluble drugs:** Termination of action of these drugs is dependent on redistribution and metabolism, rather than renal excretion. The metabolites are usually inactive and harmless even when retained. *This class includes most anesthetic drugs such as narcotics, benzodiazepines, barbiturates, phenothiazines, butyrophenones, local anesthetics, and ketamine.*

- **Lipid insoluble drugs:** They are excreted unchanged in the urine, and kidney dysfunction can cause their duration of action to be prolonged. *This class includes muscle relaxants and cholinesterase inhibitors.*

The effect of renal dysfunction on individual anesthetic drugs is as follows (**Table 18.2**):

- **Induction agents:**

   a. **Propofol**: Its pharmacokinetics is not affected by renal dysfunction, nor does it adversely affect renal function.

   b. **Thiopentone**: The free fraction of thiopentone is increased, owing to hypoalbuminemia and the presence of acidosis, necessitating dose reduction.

Table 18.2 Summary of the effects on drug handling in CKD for commonly used anesthetic drugs

Drug	Effect	Anesthetic implication
Propofol	No significant effect	No dose alteration required
Thiopentone	Increased free fraction	Dose reduction required
Morphine	Accumulation of nephrotoxic metabolites	Dose and frequency reduction required
Fentanyl	No significant effect	No dose alteration required
Succinylcholine	Increases serum K^+	Avoided in hyperkalemia
Vecuronium Rocuronium Pancuronium	Reduced clearance Prolonged elimination half-life Prolonged duration of action	Dose and frequency reduction required
Atracurium	No significant effect	No dose alteration required
Cholinesterase inhibitors	Delayed excretion	No dose alteration required
Local anesthetics	Shortened duration of action	Dose reduction required
Sevoflurane	No evidence of nephrotoxicity by Compound A in humans	No dose alteration required
Desflurane Enflurane Isoflurane	Safe	No dose alteration required

Abbreviation: CKD, chronic kidney disease.

- **Opioids:**
  a. **Morphine:** Its glucuronide conjugate can accumulate in renal failure and lead to life-threatening respiratory depression. Thus, its dose and frequency should be reduced.

  b. **Fentanyl:** Its clearance is not altered by renal failure.

  c. **Remifentanil:** It is the opioid of choice, as it is rapidly metabolized by plasma esterases.

- **Neuromuscular blocking drugs:**
  a. **Succinylcholine:** It is to be avoided in patients with serum potassium > 5.5 mEq/L. It is otherwise safe in renal dysfunction.

  b. **Vecuronium, rocuronium, and pancuronium:** Their clearance is reduced in kidney dysfunction, leading to prolonged elimination half-life and duration of action.

  c. **Atracurium:** Its metabolism and elimination are not dependent on kidneys, and therefore the elimination half-life and duration of action remain unchanged in CKD.

Muscle relaxants of choice are cis-atracurium and atracurium (because of renal independent Hoffman elimination).

- **Cholinesterase inhibitors:** Excretion of all cholinesterase inhibitors is delayed in patients with renal dysfunction to the same extent as muscle relaxants.

- **Local anesthetics:** Their duration of action is shortened, owing to altered protein binding, and requires dose reduction.

- **Inhalation anesthetics:**
  a. **Sevoflurane:** Compound A, formed on reaction with soda lime, had nephrotoxic potential in rats, but no evidence of renal dysfunction has been found in humans.

b. **Desflurane, enflurane, and isoflurane:** They have been reported to be safe in renal failure.

- **Regional anesthesia:** Presence of uremic coagulopathy and peripheral neuropathy mandates *avoiding central neuraxial blocks as well as peripheral nerve blocks in CKD patients.*

- **Fluids:** Traditionally, normal saline used to be preferred over Ringer lactate because of the absence of potassium in normal saline. However, the recent literature suggests a higher risk of hyperchloremic metabolic acidosis-induced hyperkalemia with normal saline. Therefore, Ringer lactate and other balanced salt solutions (plasmalyte) are preferred now. Avoid colloids (hydroxyethyl starch) as it can cause renal injury.

Anesthesia for Transurethral Resection of Prostate

Transurethral resection of the prostate (TURP) is the surgical procedure by which a resectoscope inserted through the urethra is used to resect prostatic tissue using an electrically powered metal loop, which may be monopolar or bipolar. The bladder is continuously irrigated with an irrigating solution, which allows direct vision and washes away debris and blood. The importance of TURP to the anesthetist lies chiefly because of its potential complications, especially TURP syndrome.

Irrigation Solutions

An ideal irrigation solution, having the qualities of being isotonic, electrically inert, nontoxic, transparent, easy to sterilize, and inexpensive, does not exist. The available irrigation solutions are highlighted in **Table 18.3**:

- *Glycine 1.2 and 1.5%:* It is the most commonly used irrigation solution. However, it has the potential to cause water intoxication as well as visual disturbances (due to glycine toxicity).

- *Normal saline:* It can be used with bipolar and laser TURP, but not with monopolar TURP, because it is highly ionized and

Table 18.3 Characteristics of various irrigation solutions

Irrigation solution	Osmolality (mOsm/kg)	Advantages	Disadvantages
Distilled water	0	• Improved visibility	• Hemolysis • Hemoglobinuria • Hemoglobinemia • Hyponatremia
Normal saline	308	• Isosmolar	• Highly ionized
Glycine 1.5%	220	• Less likelihood of TURP syndrome	• Transient postoperative visual loss • Hyperammonemia • Hyperoxaluria
Sorbitol 3.3%	165	• Same as glycine	• Hyperglycemia • Lactic acidosis • Osmotic diuresis
Mannitol 5%	275	• Isosmolar • Not metabolized	• Osmotic diuresis • Possibility of acute intravascular volume expansion

Abbreviation: TURP, transurethral resection of the prostate.

disperses the high-frequency current from a monopolar resectoscope.

- *Distilled water:* Its extreme hypotonicity and the consequent risk of hemolysis makes it unfit for use.
- *Glucose 2.5 to 4%.*
- *Sorbitol 3.5%.*
- *Mannitol 3 to 5%.*
- *Cytal (a mixture of sorbitol and mannitol).*
- *Urea 1%.*

Choice of Anesthetic Techniques

Spinal anesthesia is the anesthetic technique of choice for TURP, owing to its following advantages over general anesthesia:

- It allows for continuous monitoring of the patient's mental status, which may alter if TURP syndrome sets in.
- It allows early recognition of capsular tears and bladder perforation in which the conscious patient complains of abdominal and shoulder pain, apart from hemodynamic disturbances and restlessness. *However, the level of the sensory blockade should not go above T9 for this pain to be apparent.*
- It provides good postoperative analgesia.
- It reduces the hypercoagulable tendency, thus reducing the incidence of deep vein thrombosis.
- It reduces operative blood loss.
- It is useful for patients with significant respiratory disease.

TURP Syndrome

Excessive absorption of irrigating solutions from the large prostatic venous sinuses leads to a constellation of signs and symptoms, due to water intoxication, hyponatremia and hypo-osmolality, collectively termed the TURP syndrome (**Fig. 18.1**). The amount of irrigation solution absorbed depends upon the following:

- Height of the container of irrigation solution from the surgical table, which determines the hydrostatic pressure.
- The time of resection.

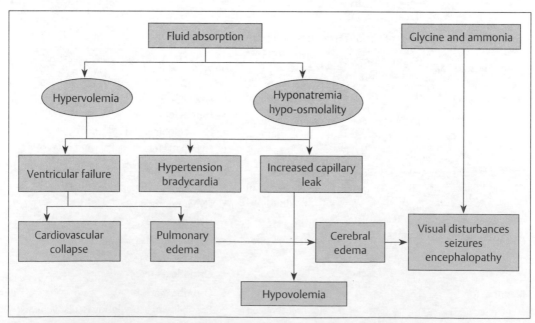

Fig. 18.1 Features of the transurethral resection of the prostate (TURP) syndrome.

Rule of Sixty

Based on the above factors, the rule of sixty should be followed to prevent TURP syndrome: *Resection time limited to less than 60 minutes and height of container not more than 60 cm from the surgical table.*

The features of this syndrome are as follows:

- **Central nervous system (CNS) effects:** Agitation, confusion, nausea, disorientation, seizures, coma, and visual disturbances
- **Cardiovascular effects:** Hypotension, bradycardia, tachycardia, congestive heart failure, pulmonary edema, myocardial infarction, hypertension, and ECG changes.

Treatment of TURP Syndrome

The following should be the approach to treat TURP syndrome:

- Surgery should be stopped.
- IV fluids must be stopped.
- Support airway and breathing by intubation and ventilation.
- Support circulation with vasopressors.
- Anticonvulsants for seizures (benzodiazepines and magnesium).
- Diuretics for fluid overload—furosemide or mannitol.

- 3% hypertonic saline if severe hyponatremia is present.

Complications of TURP

The complications of this procedure include the following:

- TURP syndrome.
- Glycine toxicity.
- Ammonia toxicity.
- Bladder perforation.
- Bleeding and coagulopathy.
- Transient bacteremia and septicemia.
- Hypothermia.
- Clot retention.
- Postoperative cognitive dysfunctions.

Conclusion

The kidney is the most important organ for the excretion of anesthetic agents. Kidney dysfunction results in poor handling of water and electrolytes, leading to fluid overload and electrolyte disturbance under anesthesia and after the surgery. Choosing an anesthetic agent with minimal effect on kidney function is important to avoid further renal damage. TURP requires vigilant monitoring to identify TURP syndrome early and manage the same.

CHAPTER 19

Anesthesia for Endocrine Disorders

Neha Garg

Introduction

Endocrine disorders are not uncommon in clinical practice. The abnormalities can range from subclinical hypothyroidism to overt pheochromocytoma. An uncontrolled and poorly optimized state can lead to intraoperative as well as postoperative complications. Therefore, it is mandatory to do a proper clinical evaluation in order to identify and diagnose the abnormal functioning of the pancreas, thyroid, and adrenal glands. This chapter highlights the important perioperative considerations of common endocrine disorders.

Diabetes Mellitus

It is one of the most common endocrine disorders encountered in clinical practice. It is the hyperglycemic state caused either due to a decrease in insulin level or due to decreased peripheral utilization of glucose. It is a multisystem disease that requires optimization before elective surgery. The important considerations are mentioned below.

Preoperative

- Sugar control: Fasting less than 140 mg/dL and postprandial less than 180 mg/dL can be accepted for surgery.
- Assess complications of diabetes.
  - ▶ Microvascular complications include:
    - ○ Retinopathy.
    - ○ Nephropathy leading to renal failure.
    - ○ Peripheral neuropathy with risk of foot ulcers, amputations, and Charcot's joints.

  - ○ Autonomic neuropathy: Fluctuations in BP, delayed gastric emptying.
  - ▶ The macrovascular complications are:
    - ○ Ischemic heart disease.
    - ○ Stroke.
    - ○ Cerebrovascular disease.
    - ○ Peripheral arterial disease.
- Omit oral hypoglycemic agents and insulin on the morning of surgery.
- On the morning of surgery, measure fasting blood glucose and urine ketones for all patients, and serum potassium if the patient is on insulin.
- If autonomic neuropathy is suspected, then give tablet ranitidine and metoclopramide on the night before surgery to prevent any residual food in the stomach.

Intraoperative

- May encounter difficult intubation due to stiff joint syndrome (atlantoaxial joint, thyromental joint, and interarytenoid joints).
- Avoid dehydration, hypotension, nephrotoxic drugs; judicious use of contrast; hourly urine output monitoring in major cases to prevent acute kidney injury in those already compromised with nephropathy.
- Target intraoperative serum glucose between 120 and 200 mg/dL. Blood sugars beyond 200 will lead to glycosuria and dehydration.
- Avoid hypoglycemia, as its detection may be delayed due to the effect of sedatives, anesthetics, beta blockers, and sympatholytics.

- Autonomic neuropathy may lead to labile blood pressure.
- Avoid the use of drugs causing sympathetic stimulation and resulting in hyperglycemia such as ketamine, atropine, pancuronium, and desflurane > 6%.

Postoperative

- Fine sugar control.
- Pain control to prevent sympathetic stimulation leading to hyperglycemia; infection control as diabetics are more prone to infection.
- ECG monitoring for perioperative silent myocardial infarction (MI).

Thyroid Disorder

Hypothyroidism

Hypothyroidism, also known as myxedema, is known to affect 0.5 to 0.8% of the population. The slow and progressive nature of hypothyroidism leads to a gradual slowing of mental and physical activities in the long term. It can have a myriad of end-organ effects that need to be identified and optimized wherever possible.

Preoperative

- If the patient is clinically hypothyroid or thyroid-stimulating hormone (TSH) value increased (however, a slight increase may be taken for surgery), surgery to be deferred. Any change in dose of thyroxin, wait up to 3 weeks for repeat TSH.
- These patients are sensitive to the depressive effects of sedatives; so alprazolam premedication is generally not indicated.
- Gastric emptying may be delayed; tablet metoclopramide and ranitidine is indicated one night before surgery.

- Associations such as hyponatremia, bradycardia, anemia, mental slowing, hypoglycemia, etc., must be noted and corrected wherever possible.
- Continue thyroxine dose on the morning of surgery.

Intraoperative

- Most patients may be obese and have neck mass (look for signs of retrosternal extension); so keep difficult intubation cart ready.
- These patients are sensitive to opioids and muscle relaxants; so use judiciously.
- Maintain body temperature, as they are prone to hypothermia.

Postoperative

- Patients may have airway obstruction due to hematoma, recurrent laryngeal nerve palsy, and hypocalcemia on account of hypoparathyroidism or tracheomalacia.
- The residual effect of opioids and neuromuscular blockade may be present.

Hyperthyroidism

It refers to the hyperfunctioning of the thyroid gland, with the resultant secretion of thyroid hormones in excess. Grave's disease, multinodular goiter, and a toxic adenoma are common etiologies for hyperthyroidism. The perioperative considerations are as follows:

Preoperative

- Look for signs of hyperthyroidism—arrhythmias, tachycardia, cardiac failure, hyperdynamic circulation, and MI.
- Rule out upper airway compromise due to the presence of goiter.
- The euthyroid state must be ensured before elective surgery.

- Continue antithyroid on the day of surgery.
- Give anxiolytics on the day of surgery.

Intraoperative

- Thiopentone is preferred as it decreases peripheral conversion of T4 to T3.
- Ketamine is avoided due to sympatho-mimetic action.
- Pancuronium is best avoided due to its vagolytic effect.
- During induction, keep patients deep by giving a good dose of opioids to avoid thyroid storm.
- A difficult intubation cart should be kept ready in case of the thyroid mass. Phenylephrine, a directly acting alpha-adrenergic receptor agonist, is the drug of choice for hypotension.
- Avoid adrenaline-containing solutions and indirectly acting vasopressors like ephedrine and mephentermine.
- Avoid epinephrine-containing local anesthetics in regional anesthesia.

Postoperative

- Patients may have airway obstruction due to hematoma, recurrent laryngeal nerve palsy, hypoparathyroidism, or tracheomalacia.

Adrenal Disorder

Pheochromocytoma

These are catecholamine-secreting tumors that arise from chromaffin cells of the sympatho-adrenal system. These are potentially lethal and can be truly cured with antihypertensives. The majority of them are isolated, while 10% are familial in nature. The noteworthy perioperative considerations are described below.

Preoperative

- Correct hypertension by giving alpha blockers (phenoxybenzamine, prazocin, terazocin, doxazocine) and beta blockers.
- Beta blockers are never used before alpha blockers, as it may lead to life-threatening hypertension due to unopposed alpha action.
- Preoperative alpha blockers also correct the contracted intravascular volume.
- Preoperative hematocrit must be in the normal range.
- Cardiac evaluation by preoperative 12 lead ECG and echocardiography to diagnose left ventricular hypertrophy (LVH), bundle branch block, diastolic dysfunction, and dilated cardiomyopathy.
- Benzodiazepines are administered 1 day before surgery to alleviate anxiety.
- Continue both alpha and beta blockers on the day of surgery. Still, long-acting alpha blockers must be replaced with short-acting alpha blockers to avoid the postoperative residual effect of these drugs.
- Electrolytes on the morning of surgery for possible hyponatremia.

Intraoperative

- Blunt any sympathetic stimulation by the use of opioids, beta blockers, propofol, diltiazem, nitroglycerin (NTG) at the time of intubation or during tumor handling.
- Use of large-bore IV access and central line for fluid resuscitation and vasopressor infusion, respectively.
- An arterial line for the beat-to-beat monitoring of blood pressure.
- Avoid factors that can cause catecholamine release, for example, fear, stress, pain, shivering, hypoxia, and hypercarbia.

- Theoretically, morphine and atracurium should be avoided because of their potential to cause sympathetic stimulation through histamine release.
- Atropine, pancuronium, and succinylcholine can cause sympathetic stimulation, so they should be avoided.
- Ensure optimal volume status before tumor vein ligation because of risk of precipitous fall in blood pressure due to decreased catecholamines in the systemic circulation.

Postoperative

- More than half of the patients remain hypertensive after surgery. Therefore, frequent monitoring of and treatment of blood pressure is required.
- Treat hypoglycemia if hypoadrenalism is present.
- Treat hypotension by fluids and vasopressor infusion, if required.

Cushing's Disease

It occurs due to long-term exposure to an excess of glucocorticoids. The perioperative considerations are described below.

Preoperative

- Due to glucocorticoid excess, patients have hyperglycemia, hypertension, hypokalemia, and volume overload.
- Osteoporosis and the consequent risk of fracture should be anticipated.
- Difficult airway due to obesity may be present.

Intraoperative

- Careful shifting from trolley to OR table due to the risk of osteoporosis-related fracture.

- Judicious use of muscle relaxants in case of significant muscle weakness.
- Be watchful for pneumothorax, as adrenalectomy is a significant risk factor for it.

Postoperative

- Steroid supplementation with fludrocortisone if bilateral adrenalectomy is performed.
- Delayed wound healing and increased risk of infections due to glucocorticoids excess.

Glucocorticoid Deficiency

Exogenous glucocorticoid leads to hypothalamic-pituitary-adrenal (HPA) suppression. Thus, patients who have taken steroids in the past 1 year (prednisolone more than 5 mg/day for more than 3 weeks or equivalent by any route) must be supplemented with the intraoperative steroid of 100-mg hydrocortisone thrice daily on the day of surgery, which may be continued up to 48 hours postoperatively. Etomidate should be avoided as it can cause adrenal suppression.

Pituitary Dysfunction

Acromegaly

It is characterized by excessive secretion of growth hormone, most commonly by a pituitary adenoma. The multiorgan effects of growth hormone necessitate a thorough evaluation of each organ system and optimization. The peculiar perioperative considerations are:

Preoperative

- Almost always a difficult airway is observed due to:
  ▶ Prognathism.
  ▶ Macroglossia.

- ▸ Narrowing of vocal cords due to over-growth (use a smaller size tracheal tube).
- ▸ Overgrowth of epiglottis, making visualization of vocal cords difficult.
- Cardiovascular: Hypertension, LVH, diastolic dysfunction, arrhythmias, coronary artery disease, or cardiomyopathy may be present.
- Respiratory: Obstructive sleep apnea, pulmonary hypertension must be noted.
- Peripheral neuropathies must be recorded preoperatively and may be a contraindication for regional anesthesia.
- Vision: Document visual acuity and visual field defects, if any.
- Correct hyperglycemia.
- May have difficult landmarks for regional anesthesia.

Intraoperative

- Keep difficult airway cart ready.
- Cautious cannulation of the radial artery, because of the possibility of inadequate collateral circulation.
- Monitoring of blood glucose levels in case of diabetes mellitus.
- Peripheral nerve stimulation should be used to guide the dosing of muscle relaxants if skeletal muscle weakness is present.

- A titrated dose of sedative and anesthetics should be used to avoid respiratory depression in the postoperative period.

Postoperative

- Monitor patient for cerebrospinal fluid (CSF) leak after transsphenoidal surgery.
- Monitor fluid status and sodium level, as there is a chance of diabetes insipidus.
- Look for bleeding at the operative site.
- Use opioids judiciously for pain management due to the risk of respiratory depression.

Conclusion

Endocrine disorders are becoming increasingly common with time. Patients with diabetes, thyroid, adrenal, and pituitary disorders can be identified, based on history and examination during the preoperative period. Such disorders may only be observed for the first time during preoperative evaluation. A thyroid storm can occur in poorly controlled hyperthyroidism. Similarly, a patient with diabetes can become ketotic if sugars are not controlled. Identifying them and optimizing such patients help in avoiding complications under anesthesia and in the postoperative period.

CHAPTER 20

Anesthesia for Patients with Neuromuscular Diseases

Neha Garg

Introduction

Neuromuscular disorders are not a familiar entity to anesthetists. Although rare, patients with neuromuscular disorders require judicious use of muscle relaxants, vigilant neuromuscular monitoring to minimize the risk of pulmonary aspiration, and ventilatory failure in the postoperative period. This chapter highlights the anesthetic considerations of major neuromuscular disorders.

Myasthenia Gravis

Myasthenia gravis (MG) is an autoimmune disorder characterized by IgG-mediated destruction or inactivation of postsynaptic acetylcholine receptors at the neuromuscular junction, leading to reduced numbers of receptors and degradation of their function. Clinical manifestations include easy fatigability and muscle weakness with ocular paresis being the most common. Patients may also present with myasthenia crisis and need mechanical ventilation for respiratory support. Patients afflicted with MG receive acetylcholinesterase inhibitors as a part of their medical management. Corticosteroids and other immunosuppressive agents may be used to suppress the exaggerated autoimmune response of the body in such a group of patients.

Anesthetic Concerns

Use of acetylcholinesterase inhibitors (physostigmine, pyridostigmine) *also inhibit plasma pseudocholinesterase and can lead to prolongation of duration of succinylcholine and local anesthetics (ester-type).*

The salient anesthetic concerns are as follows:

- Use regional anesthesia wherever possible.
- These patients are *resistant to depolarizing muscle relaxants but sensitive to nondepolarizing muscle relaxants;* therefore, neuromuscular monitoring is a must to prevent postoperative respiratory complications.
- Train of four (TOF) > 0.9 must be ensured before extubation.
- A combination of rocuronium and sugammadex is an attractive alternative with the due concern of inhibition of plasma pseudocholinesterase by acetylcholinesterase inhibitors.
- Certain drugs can prolong the duration of neuromuscular blockade and potentiate weakness. The commonly implicated drugs are the following:
  - ▶ Antibiotics like macrolide (azithromycin, clarithromycin), aminoglycosides (gentamicin, neomycin, streptomycin, tobramycin), and fluoroquinolones (ciprofloxacin).
  - ▶ Lithium, phenytoin, and chlorpromazine.
  - ▶ Antiarrhythmics (quinidine, procainamide), beta-blockers, and verapamil.
  - ▶ Magnesium, lidocaine, corticosteroids, and nondepolarizing muscle relaxants.

Lambert-Eaton Syndrome

It is an autoimmune disease caused by IgG antibodies against voltage-gated calcium channels at the presynaptic membrane. A decrease in voltage-gated calcium channels results in a lower level of acetylcholine in synapse and clinically resembles MG in terms of weakness. It has been historically linked with the paraneoplastic syndrome, but it can also occur in patients without cancer. The use of the drug 3,4-diamino-pyridine (3,4-DAP) does improves muscle strength, but *anticholinesterases are not effective at all.*

Anesthetic Concerns

- Increased sensitivity to both depolarizing and nondepolarizing muscle relaxants.
- Avoid general anesthesia (GA) whenever possible and use regional anesthesia.
- Use neuromuscular monitoring and target a TOF > 0.9 before extubation.

Dermatomyositis and Polymyositis

Dermatomyositis and polymyositis are immune-mediated multisystem diseases which manifest as muscle weakness (flexors of the neck, muscles of shoulder and hip) along with cutaneous changes (periorbital edema, discoloration of the upper eyelid, and malar rash). The weakness of pharyngeal and respiratory muscles can lead to dysphagia and ventilatory insufficiency, respectively.

Anesthetic Concerns

- Consider the possibility of aspiration in patients with polymyositis.
- In the past, there had been concerns of abnormal response to muscle relaxants, but recent evidence suggests a normal response to both depolarizing and nondepolarizing muscle relaxants.

Periodic Paralysis

It is clinically characterized by an intermittent acute attack of skeletal muscle paresis or paralysis caused by a mutation in voltage-gated calcium channels or inward rectifier potassium channels. It may be associated with both hypokalemia as well as hyperkalemia, with the latter form being rarer. *Acetazolamide is the standard of care for periodic paralysis.*

Anesthetic Concerns

- Nondepolarizing muscle relaxants are safe.
- Avoid factors which can precipitate muscle weakness (e.g., hypothermia, hypocalcemia, use of steroids, etc.).

Muscular Dystrophies

Muscular dystrophies are inherited disorders caused by the breakdown of the dystrophin-glycoprotein complex, leading to painless degeneration of muscle fibers. There is a progressive weakness of skeletal muscle with preserved skeletal muscle innervation. There is no sensory loss, and reflexes are preserved. The common muscular dystrophies include the following:

- Duchenne muscular dystrophy.
- Becker muscular dystrophy.
- Limb-girdle muscular dystrophy.

Anesthetic Concerns

- Keep the possibility of pulmonary aspiration in mind (because of decreased gastrointestinal [GI] motility and associated weak laryngeal reflexes).
- Succinylcholine is contraindicated (threat of hyperkalemia and consequent cardiac arrest).
- Ensure availability of dantrolene in OT complex, as there is heightened risk of malignant hyperthermia.
- Anticipate postoperative pulmonary dysfunction which can be delayed by up to 36 hours.

Malignant Hyperthermia

Malignant hyperthermia (MH) is a progressive, life-threatening hyperthermic reaction occurring during GA, with an incidence of 1 in 14,000 administrations of anesthesia, and the incidence rise *to 1 in 2,500 patients undergoing squint repair. The mutations in the* RYR1 *gene, which codes for the ryanodine receptor (RyR), is the most common defect.*

A variety of anesthetic agents can trigger malignant hyperthermia as listed below:

- *Neuromuscular blocking agent*: Succinylcholine.
- *Volatile anesthetics*: Halothane, isoflurane, sevoflurane, enflurane, desflurane, ether, and methoxyflurane.

Presentation

A persistent *rise in end-tidal CO_2 (EtCO_2) despite increasing minute ventilation is the cardinal feature of MH.* An unexplained tachypnea, rise in core body temperature, and muscle rigidity despite muscle relaxants are other signs which hint toward MH. Also, there can be rhabdomyolysis, leading to hyperkalemia and acute kidney injury due to tubular plugging by free hemoglobin molecules.

Confirmation of Diagnosis

In vitro contracture testing (IVCT) using freshly *excised muscle biopsy* specimens remains the only definitive means of demonstrating that an individual is not susceptible to MH.

The muscle specimens are exposed to increasing concentrations of *halothane or caffeine. The interpretation of this testing is beyond the scope of this book, and readers can refer to this testing in detail for better understanding.*

Clinical Management

- Stop administration of the volatile anesthetic agent.
- Cancel or conclude surgery as soon as possible.
- Hyperventilate with >10 L/min of 100% oxygen to increase the elimination of triggering agents and CO_2.
- Administer dantrolene (2.5 mg/kg) IV over 5 minutes and repeat if required.
- Switch off active warming devices and initiate active cooling measures (cold fluids, cold sponging).
- Use 1 to 2 meq/kg of sodium bicarbonate to correct metabolic acidosis.
- Treat hyperkalemia with calcium chloride (10 mg/kg) or insulin (0.2 U/kg) in 50% dextrose (1 mL/kg).
- Follow advanced cardiac life support protocol in case of dysrhythmias or cardiac arrest.
- Insert arterial and central venous catheters.
- Maintain urine output of 2 mL/kg/h with additional mannitol and furosemide if needed.
- Repeat venous blood gas analyses and electrolytes every 15 minutes until these and the vitals stabilize.

A patient who has been successfully treated for MH inside the operation theater needs intensive care to continue treatment and monitor late manifestations of the disorder. Late events range from mild pain to multiorgan failure.

Conclusion

Myasthenia gravis is associated with increased pulmonary complications like intubation failure (due to large thymus) and extubation failure due to neuromuscular weakness. The use of muscle relaxants without neuromuscular monitoring can delay the recovery from neuromuscular blockade. Such patients are resistant to depolarizing muscle relaxants and sensitive to nondepolarizing muscle relaxants. Malignant hyperthermia is associated with grave complications and identifying patients at risk of this complication is crucial (an unexpected demise of the first-degree relative under anesthesia suggests the possibility of malignant hyperthermia).

CHAPTER 21

Anesthesia for Immune-Mediated and Infectious Diseases

Ruchi Kapoor

Introduction

The immune system plays a pivotal role in protecting an individual from many infectious agents and leading a healthy life. The abnormal response can result in life-threatening anaphylaxis, and a weak or absence of response poses risks to individuals to acquire infection. The immune system's exaggerated response can cause diseases involving multiple organ systems and may complicate anesthetic management. This chapter is an overview of common immune-mediated and infectious disorders.

Anaphylaxis

Anaphylaxis is a life-threatening manifestation of immersive antigen-antibody in which prior antigen detection has evoked antigen-specific IgE antibodies. Vasoactive mediators generated by mast cells and basophils are responsible for anaphylaxis's clinical symptoms. During anesthesia, anaphylaxis occurs 1 in 5,000 to 20,000 cases. The estimated mortality is 3 to 6%. Risk factors include:

- Asthma history.
- Female sex preponderance.
- Multiple previous procedures.
- Systemic mastocytosis.

Diagnosis

The clinical symptoms of anaphylaxis may resemble pulmonary embolism, acute myocardial infarction, aspiration or vasovagal reaction. Hypotension and cardiovascular arrest can be the only manifestations of anaphylaxis in general anesthesia patients. The plasma tryptase concentration is elevated within 1 to 2 hours of the alleged reaction, while the plasma histamine returns to baseline 30 to 60 minutes after the anaphylactic reaction. A positive intradermal test result (wheal and flare response) may be obtained, indicating the existence of unique IgE antibodies. The primary and secondary treatment of anaphylaxis is highlighted in **Box 21.1**.

Drug Allergy

Drug allergy causes 3.4 to 4.3% of deaths due to anesthesia. Regardless of the cause responsible for life-threatening allergic drug reactions, the manifestations and treatment are identical to those of anaphylaxis.

Allergic drug reactions have been observed for most medications that could be administered during anesthesia except ketamine and benzodiazepines. *Muscle relaxants are responsible for about 60% of perioperative allergic reactions.* The cardiovascular arrest can be the primary manifestation of a life-threatening allergic reaction in an anesthetized patient. Bronchospasm occurs in fewer patients. Latex allergy may also cause these reactions. Onset usually reaches 30 minutes after exposure. Skin tests can enhance latex hypersensitivity. Questions regarding scratching, conjunctivitis, rhinitis, rash, or wheezing after inflating toy balloons, wearing latex gloves, or dental or gynecological examinations involving latex gloves may help recognize these patients. *Operating room staff and spina bifida patients had increased chances of latex sensitivity.* Other sources of these allergic reactions are antibiotics, blood,

Box 21.1 Management of anaphylactic reaction under anesthesia

Primary Treatment

General measures

- Inform the surgeon.
- Call for help.
- Stop administration of all drugs, colloids, and blood products.
- Maintain airway and provide 100% oxygen.
- Elevate legs if feasible.

Epinephrine administration

- Titrate dose according to symptom severity and clinical response.
- Adults: 10 µg to 1 mg by bolus, repeat every 1–2 min(s) as needed intravenous (IV).
- Infusion: 0.05–1 µg/kg/min.
- Children: 1–10 µg/kg bolus, repeat every 1–2 min(s) as needed.

Fluid therapy

- Crystalloid: Normal saline 10–25 mL/kg over 20 min and more as needed.
- Colloid: 10 mL/kg over 20 mins.

Anaphylaxis resistant to epinephrine

- Glucagon: 1–5 mg bolus followed by 1–2.5 mg/h IV infusion.
- Norepinephrine: 0.05–0.1 µg/kg/min IV infusion.
- Vasopressin: 2–10 unit IV bolus followed by 0.01–0.1 unit/min IV infusion.

Secondary Treatment

Bronchodilators

- β_2-Agonist for symptomatic treatment of bronchospasm.

Antihistamines

- Histamine 1 antagonist: Diphenhydramine 0.5–1 mg/kg IV.
- Histamine 2 antagonist: Ranitidine 50 mg IV.

Corticosteroids

- Adults: Hydrocortisone 250 mg IV or methylprednisolone 80 mg IV.
- Children: Hydrocortisone 50–100 mg IV or methylprednisolone 2 mg/kg IV.

plasma volume expanders (dextran, colloids), protamine, radiocontrast media, etc.

Local anesthetic-induced allergic reactions are uncommon. Ester-type local anesthetics are metabolized to strongly antigenic para-aminobenzoic acid and are more likely to evoke an allergic response than amide-type local anesthetics not metabolized to this compound. Anaphylaxis can also be caused by inducing antibody production by the preservative and not by the local anesthetic. This is why it is appropriate to treat patients with an allergy background with amide-based local anesthetics.

Rheumatoid Arthritis

Rheumatoid arthritis is a multisystem auto-immune disease with female preponderance.

Preoperative Evaluation

- Focus on airway involvement (cervical spine, temporomandibular joint, and cricoarytenoid joints). Atlantoaxial sub-luxation may be present.

- Rule out vertebral artery involvement by asking the patient for any discomfort or symptoms during various head position (flexion, extension, and side rotation).
- Rule out other system involvement (cardiac, pulmonary, and hematological).
- Consider the effect of nonsteroidal anti-inflammatory drugs (NSAIDs) on platelet functions.
- Collect detailed drug history (corticoster-oids and other antirheumatoid drugs).

Anesthetic Management

- Regional anesthesia (spinal/epidural) can be safely performed as the lumbar spine's involvement is unusual in rheumatoid arthritis.
- General anesthesia is challenging because of:
  - ▶ Airway involvement (awake intubation is preferred with minimal neck move-ment as an excess of movement in atl-antoaxial subluxation can cause spinal cord damage and quadriplegia).
  - ▶ Difficult arterial cannulation due to calcified arteries.
  - ▶ Central venous cannulation may be difficult due to limited neck movement.
  - ▶ Postextubation laryngeal obstruction can happen if there is the involvement of cricoarytenoid joints.

Systemic Lupus Erythematosus

It is characterized by antinuclear antibody production with a multisystem chronic inflam-matory process.

Preoperative Evaluation

- Assessment should focus on multiorgan involvement (central nervous system [CNS], heart, liver, kidneys, and skin).
- Detailed drug history and their side effects should be considered (steroids, NSAIDs, and quinine).
- Cricoarytenoid arthritis and recurrent laryngeal nerve palsy can be there.

Anesthetic Management

- Spinal and epidural can be performed without much concern.
- Drug selection and dose adjustment should be titrated to organ dysfunction.
- Postoperative respiratory distress can occur in a patient with poor pulmonary reserve.
- Patients may require perioperative steroids to prevent acute adrenal insufficiency.

Ankylosing Spondylitis

It is a chronic inflammatory disease that involves articulations of the spine and the adjacent soft tissues. The disease involvement can vary from isolated sacral involvement to the fusion of entire vertebral bodies.

Preoperative Evaluation

- Focus on the involvement of the spine and associated pulmonary (restrictive lung disease) and cardiac dysfunction (aortic regurgitation) deserve special attention.
- Assessment of neck movement is important if endotracheal intubation is planned.

Anesthetic Management

- Spinal/epidural is challenging through the midline approach. However, paramedian approach can be used with much ease in such patients.

- Endotracheal intubation may require assistance with video laryngoscope or fiberoptic in case of limited neck flexion and extension.
- Neurologic monitoring is needed in patients undergoing corrective spinal surgeries.
- A sudden increase in systemic vascular resistance should be avoided in patients with significant aortic regurgitation.

Scleroderma

Scleroderma is characterized by:
- Inflammation and autoimmunity.
- Vascular injury with eventual vascular obliteration.
- Fibrosis and accumulation of excess matrix in many organs.

Preoperative Evaluation

- Preoperative assessment should focus on organ involvement (cardiac, lung, kidneys, and gastrointestinal [GI] tract).
- Pulmonary hypertension, interstitial fibrosis, renal artery stenosis, and gut hypomotility should be ruled out.
- Patients may have coagulation abnormalities due to malabsorption of vitamin K.
- Tight facial skin and nonpitting skin may cause difficult mouth opening and poor IV access, respectively.

Anesthetic Management

- Decreased mandibular motion and narrow oral aperture due to taut skin should be kept in mind before induction of anesthesia.
- Oral and nasal telangiectasias may bleed profusely if endotracheal intubation is a traumatic one.

- Intra-arterial catheterization may lead to Raynaud's phenomenon.
- Induction of anesthesia can cause significant hypotension because of underlying vasomotor instability.
- Hypotonia of the lower esophageal sphincter puts the patient at risk of regurgitation and aspiration.
- Poor pulmonary compliance may require high airway pressure to achieve adequate ventilation.
- The dose of drugs should be adjusted to renal dysfunction.
- Regional anesthesia may be complicated by joint and soft-tissue involvement.
- Eyes should be protected to prevent corneal abrasions.
- Peripheral vasoconstriction should be minimized by ensuring optimum OT temperature (>21°C).

Acquired Immunodeficiency Syndrome

Acquired Immunodeficiency Syndrome (AIDS) is an acquired form of immunodeficiency with multisystem involvement.

Preoperative Evaluation

- Highly active antiretroviral therapy (HAART) used to treat AIDS can impact several organ systems. Therefore, complete blood count (CBC), metabolic panel, renal function, liver function tests, and coagulation factors assay should be ordered.
- Focal neurological lesions in these patients can increase intracerebral pressure, precluding neuraxial anesthesia.

Anesthetic Management

- Any patient must be considered potentially infectious, and all personnel must take universal precautions during surgery.

- Following an event involving a high-risk body fluid, such as (hollow) needlestick injury, postexposure prophylaxis should begin as soon as possible after the incident, preferably within 1 to 2 hours and maybe considered up to 1 to 2 weeks after the injury.

- Neurological involvement can render the usage of succinylcholine hazardous.

- Unexplainable hypotension should be treated with steroid supplementation.

Conclusion

Anaphylaxis is a rare event that anesthetists encounter in their practice. However, once it occurs, identification of triggering agents and timely management are vital. Antibiotics and neuromuscular blockers are the most common agents implicated in allergy and anaphylaxis. Patients with autoimmune disorders have multisystem involvement and often have a difficult airway due to limited mouth opening and movements at the cervical spine.

CHAPTER 22

Anesthesia for Disorders of Blood

Neha Garg

Introduction

Blood is the carrier of oxygen because of hemoglobin in the red blood cells (RBCs). It also plays an important role in the cessation of bleeding by virtue of its components, that is, platelets, coagulation factors, and fibrinogen. Deficiency and/or loss of functional capability of these components can cause life-threatening bleeding during the perioperative period. Thorough knowledge of blood disorders makes the anesthesia provider confident and efficient in managing such a group of patients.

Anemia

Anemia is defined as a decrease in the oxygen-carrying capacity of blood due to a decrease in red cell mass. It is often encountered in surgical populations preoperatively and can result from iron deficiency, deficiency of vitamin B12, chronic disease states (e.g., tuberculosis, malignancy, etc.), and hemoglobinopathies. It is not simply a laboratory diagnosis but an important predictor of negative clinical outcomes. Preoperative evaluation for the cause of anemia and optimization of the same improves patient's outcome drastically. WHO defines anemia as follows:

- Hemoglobin < 13 g/dL in men.
- Hemoglobin < 12 g/dL in nonpregnant females.
- Hemoglobin < 11 g/dL in pregnant females.

Anesthetic Concerns in Anemia

Preoperative

- Rule out hyperdynamic circulation and consequent heart failure in preoperative evaluation.
- The optimal cutoff of hemoglobin to post a patient for elective surgery is not known. *However, hemoglobin of ≥ 8 g/dL for the normal healthy patient and ≥ 10 g/dL for patients with cardiac morbidities, stroke, and epilepsy is usually considered safe.*
- Rule out neurological deficit due to vitamin B12 deficiency.

Intraoperative

- Minimize blood loss with controlled hypotension.
- Estimate blood loss with a visual inspection of the surgical field, drainage container, and number of blood-soaked pads and their weight.
- Use restrictive approach to replace blood lost during surgery to avoid complications of allogeneic blood transfusion.
- Avoid triggers of increased oxygen demand (e.g., pain, shivering).
- Avoid regional anesthesia in patients with documented neurological deficit.
- Avoid nitrous oxide in vitamin B12 deficiency because nitrous oxide can cause megaloblastic anemia.

- Cautious use of intravenous and inhaled anesthetics in patients with hyperdynamic circulation (*vasodilatory effects of anesthetic agents can cause precipitous fall in blood pressure*).

Postoperative

- Avoid shivering as it increases oxygen demand and can cause myocardial ischemia in susceptible patients.

- Provide adequate analgesia as hyperventilation due to pain will shift the oxygen dissociation curve to left and hence decrease the tissue oxygen delivery.

Sickle Cell Disease

Sickle cell hemoglobinopathy occurs due to mutation in the β-globin subunit, leading to the abnormal assembly of beta proteins of hemoglobin A and consequent sickling of red cells when exposed to triggers (e.g., dehydration, pain, hypoxia, static blood flow, etc.).

Anesthetic Concerns

Preoperative

- Rule out vasoocclusive end-organ damage:
  - ► Central nervous system (CNS): Stroke, proliferative retinopathy, peripheral neuropathy.
  - ► Pulmonary: Acute chest syndrome, restrictive lung disease.
  - ► Gastrointestinal tract (GIT): Liver disease, cholelithiasis.
  - ► Hematological: Hemolytic anemia.
  - ► Orthopedic: Osteomyelitis, dactylitis.
  - ► Vascular: Leg ulcers.
- Cancel or postpone the surgery if the patient is in acute sickle cell crisis.
- Avoid preoperative dehydration to prevent sickling. Also, address anxiety and stress with benzodiazepines.

- Target hemoglobin of 10 g/dL (hematocrit [HCT] of 30%) with HbS < 30% and prophylactic transfusion in moderate-to-high risk cases.

- HbS level < 5% is considered optimal for the patient undergoing cardiac bypass surgery.

Intraoperative

- All techniques of regional block appear to be safe in sickle cell disease. Bier's block is no more an absolute contraindication in patients afflicted with sickle cell disease.

- Avoid hypoxia, hypothermia, dehydration, and acidosis in the intraoperative period to prevent sickling.

- The use of tourniquets is not absolutely prohibited in sickle cell patients; however, their use is definitely associated with increased risk of complications.

Postoperative

- Ensure early mobilization.

- Oxygen supplementation, bronchodilator, and pulmonary toileting tailored to patient's need to minimize the risk of acute chest syndrome.

- Pain assessment with pain scoring systems and effective analgesia with opioids as well as regional anesthesia should be done to prevent pain crisis.

Thalassemia

The pathophysiology of thalassemia includes a decrease in the synthesis of either alpha or beta chain of hemoglobin with consequent precipitation of unpaired hemoglobin chains, leading to premature destruction of RBC. Chromosome 16 contains two copies of alpha-globin chains. The variants of thalassemia are highlighted in **Table 22.1**.

Thalassemia minor is not of much concern, while patients with thalassemia major are at

Table 22.1 Variants of alpha thalassemia

Condition Genotype		Phenotype
Salient carrier	αα/α -	Asymptomatic
Minor (alpha thalassemia trait)	α -/α -; αα/- -	Asymptomatic
Hb H	α-/- -	Moderate-to-severe hemolytic anemia
Alpha thalassemia major (Hb Bart's)	- -/- -	Causes nonimmune hydrops fetalis

heightened risk of perioperative morbidity and mortality.

Anesthetic Concerns

- Chronic hemolytic anemia with a compensatory rise in cardiac output and plasma volume. Therefore, rule out features of heart failure during preoperative assessment.

- Patients can present with cardiomyopathy, features of pulmonary hypertension, diabetes, and hepatic fibrosis as sequelae of iron overload (because of multiple transfusion).

- May have potential difficult airway due to maxillary overgrowth (from bone marrow stimulation).

- Regional anesthesia may be difficult because of cortical thinning and vertebral destruction.

Polycythemia

It is characterized by an increase in blood viscosity accompanied by raised HCT. The tissue oxygen delivery gets saturated at the HCT of 33 to 36%, and further rise beyond this HCT causes deterioration of microcirculation and threatens tissue perfusion. Patients can present with headache and easy fatigability in milder forms and with thrombosis in severe forms.

Anesthetic Concerns

- Heightened risk of perioperative thromboses.

- Target preoperative HCT of 45 and 42% in males and females, respectively, to minimize the risk of thromboses.

- Cytoreduction with hydroxyurea can be considered in patients > 60 years and previous history of thrombosis.

G-6-PD Deficiency

It is an X-linked recessive genetic disease with impaired capacity to handle oxidative stress by red cells. Patients can present with hemolytic anemia, intermittent hemolysis, and hemolysis only with stressors.

Anesthetic Concerns

- Assess the severity and acuity of anemia.

- Avoid exposure to oxidative drugs:[a]

  ► Isoflurane.

  ► Sevoflurane.

  ► Metoclopramide.

  ► Penicillin.

  [a] *Codeine, ketamine, benzodiazepines (except diazepam), propofol, and fentanyl are safe.*

- Avoid drugs that can cause methemoglobinemia (e.g., prilocaine, lidocaine, benzocaine, and silver nitrates), as methemoglobinemia increases the risk of hemolysis in G-6-PD.

- Address acidosis, hypothermia, hyperglycemia, and infections aggressively, as they can precipitate hemolysis.

Porphyria

These disorders are characterized by enzymatic defects (aminolevulinic acid) of heme synthesis which can be either inherited or acquired.

Anesthetic Concerns

Preoperative

- Suspect acute attack of porphyria in patients who present with pain abdomen, changes in mental status, dark-colored urine, and positive family history of porphyria.

Intraoperative

- No absolute contraindication to regional anesthesia but detailed evaluation and proper documentation of established neuropathy is a must.
- Avoid regional anesthesia in the settings of acute crisis, as there is a rapid onset of neuropathy, compounded by poor cooperation due to altered mental status.
- Avoid drugs with the potential to induce enzyme aminolevulinic acid synthetase (e.g., benzodiazepines, etomidate, and halothane).
- Propofol, nitrous oxide, opioids, muscle relaxants isoflurane, and enflurane are safe.
- Ketamine is usually considered safe.
- Prolonged fasting, dehydration, and infection can trigger an acute crisis.
- Barbiturates are absolutely contraindicated in acute intermittent porphyria.

Postoperative

- Continue monitoring for porphyric crisis up to 5 days because of delayed presentation.
- Frequent neurologic assessment is warranted.
- Avoid metoclopramide as antiemetic therapy.

Disorders of Hemostasis

Platelet Disorders

Platelets are the important soldiers to stop blood loss by forming the primary hemostatic plug at the site of bleeding. Both acquired and inherited platelet conditions cause skin and mucosal bleeding. Platelet dysfunction can be quantitative (i.e., decrease in platelet counts with normal function) as well as qualitative (platelet counts are normal with the decreased functional capability). Platelet dysfunction can cause life-threatening bleeding during the surgical procedure, and that mandates proper evaluation of platelet disorders preoperatively by the anesthetists.

Anesthetic Concerns

Ensure procedure-specific cutoff for platelet count:[a]

- Surgery on brain/posterior eye: At least 1 lakh/mm^3.
- Regional anesthesia: 80,000/mm^3.
- Major non-neuraxial surgery/liver, renal biopsy: 50,000/mm^3.
- Central line/diagnostic enteroscopy/bronchoscopy with lavage: 20,000/mm^3.

[a] *Symptomatic patients (spontaneous bleeding) require platelet transfusion irrespective of platelet counts.*

Hemophilia and Related Clotting Disorders

Hemophilias are X-linked genetic disorders. Hemophilia A and B are due to deficiency of factor VIII and IX, respectively. The sex-linked origin of some of these disorders means that hemophilia occurs almost exclusively in the male children of female carriers; men do not transmit the disease to their male children. The acquired deficiency of clotting factors can occur due to vitamin K deficiency. Factors' deficiencies lead to bleeding in deep tissues such as muscles and inside the joints and cause severe blood loss during the perioperative period. Therefore, preoperative evaluation of coagulation disorder is vital to the anesthesia provider's practice.

Anesthetic Concerns

- In elective surgery, levels of the deficient coagulation factor should be assayed 48 hours preoperatively and the level restored to 40% of normal before the surgical procedure.

- Careful temperature control during surgery (hypothermia decreases factor activity and increases the risk of bleeding).

- Avoid trauma to patients during anesthesia care (during patient transfer to OT/transfer from trolley to OT table).

- Caution with regional anesthesia.

- Use of local anesthetics with vasoconstrictors can decrease blood loss.

- Ensure availability of the adequate amount of required clotting factors for a major surgery.

Hypercoagulable States

The excess of prothrombin proteins or decrease in antithrombotic proteins poses a patient at risk of hypercoagulability. The defect can be either congenital (congenital ATIII deficiency and factor V mutation) or acquired (malignancy, nephrotic syndrome, pregnancy, and use of oral contraceptives). These patients often require long-term anticoagulation with heparin, warfarin, and other anticoagulants.

Anesthetic Concerns

- Assess the risk of thrombosis and the risk of bleeding during and after the surgery.

- Consider bridging therapy with unfractionated heparin or low-molecular weight heparin in patients at moderate-to-high risk of thrombosis.

- The central neuraxial block is preferred as it decreases the risk of thromboembolism.

- Target antithrombin level > 80% for at least 5 days in the postoperative period in patients with antithrombin deficiency.

- Correct protein C and protein S deficiency in the preoperative period with fresh frozen plasma.

Conclusion

The disorders of blood compromise oxygen-carrying capacity (due to anemia) and may lead to poor hemostasis at the surgical site (because of thrombocytopenia and coagulopathy). The decreased oxygen-carrying capacity and excessive blood from the surgical site amplifies the risk of myocardial infarction and delayed wound healing. Identifying such disorders, ensuring the availability of adequate blood products, and minimizing blood loss during surgery is paramount. Avoiding dehydration is essential to avoid thrombotic complications in hypercoagulable states.

Section V
Subspecialty Management

CHAPTER 23

Neurosurgical Anesthesia

Ranjitha Nethaji and Puneet Khanna

Introduction

Patients with diseases involving the central nervous system (CNS) may require surgery to treat the underlying cause. The patient's positioning, need for vigilant monitoring during surgery, and risk of acute and long-term neurologic sequelae make neurosurgical procedures unique. The knowledge of cerebral physiology and the effect of anesthetic drugs on cerebral homeostasis are a must to ensure optimal patient care with improved outcomes. This chapter will overview the important neurosurgical conditions along with the anesthetic considerations.

Cerebral Physiology and Pharmacology

Almost two-third of total oxygen consumption by the brain is used for adenosine triphosphate (ATP) production to support neuronal electrical activity. Interruption of cerebral perfusion for 10 seconds or more results in complete unconsciousness. Failure of restoration of blood flow within 3 to 8 minutes results in irreversible cellular injury. Important cerebral physiological parameters are discussed below.

Cerebral Blood Flow

Cerebral blood flow (CBF) depends on cerebral metabolic activity, cerebral perfusion pressure, arterial carbon dioxide, and oxygen tension. CBF averages 50 mL/100 g/min at a $PaCO_2$ of 40 mm Hg in an awake healthy individual with intact autoregulation. The flow in gray matter is around 80 mL/100 g/min and white matter is 20 mL/100 g/min. The total flow in adults averages is

750 mL/min (15 to 20% of cardiac output). CBF can be measured by various methods like CT perfusion scans directly, but bedside monitoring of CBF is not possible by these methods. Indirect measures to estimate the adequacy of CBF and brain tissue oxygen delivery are transcranial Doppler (TCD), infrared spectroscopy, and brain tissue oximetry. The CBF is autoregulated and depends on multiple factors, as discussed below:

1. Cerebral perfusion pressure (CPP): It is the difference between mean arterial pressure (MAP) and intracranial pressure (ICP) or central venous pressure (CVP) if greater than ICP:

$$CPP = MAP - ICP \ (or \ CVP).$$

CPP is 80 to 100 mm Hg. Moreover, ICP is normally less than 10 mm Hg. *Hence, CPP is proportional to MAP.* CPP values less than 50 mm Hg often show slowing on the EEG, whereas those with a CPP between 25 and 40 mm Hg show flat EEG; less than 25 mm Hg can lead to irreversible brain damage.

Cerebral vasculature rapidly adapts to change in CPP. A decrease in CPP results in cerebral vasodilation, whereas elevations induce vasoconstriction. It remains constant between MAP of 60 and 160 mm Hg; outside these limits, blood flow will become pressure dependent.

2. Extrinsic factors:

- **Arterial tension of carbon dioxide:** CBF changes approximately 1 to 2 mL/100 g/min per mm Hg change in $PaCO_2$. Marked hyperventilation ($PaCO_2$ < 20 mm Hg causes cerebral vasoconstriction with consequent fall in CBF).

- **Temperature:** CBF changes 5 to 7% per 1°C change in temperature.

- **Viscosity:** A decrease in hematocrit decreases viscosity and can improve CBF and vice versa with elevated viscosity.

3. Autonomic factors: The sympathetic and parasympathetic systems innervate intracranial vessels. Sympathetic stimulation induces vaso-constriction and limits CBF.

Cerebrospinal Fluid

It is a clear fluid present in the subarachnoid space. It is produced at 450 to 500 mL per day by the choroid plexus located in the lateral, third, and fourth ventricles. It is reabsorbed into the bloodstream through the arachnoid villi.

Effect of Anesthetic Agents on Cerebral Physiology

The anesthetic agents can affect the various aspects of cerebral physiology, as shown in **Table 23.1**.

It is important to understand the concept of flow-coupling metabolism to realize the effect of anesthetic agents on cerebral physiology.

According to the flow-coupling metabolism theory, the CBF correlates with cerebral metabolism. The inhaled anesthetic decreases the cerebral metabolic rate, leading to a decrease in CBF. However, these agents are intrinsic vasodilators, causing a rise in CBF. Therefore, metabolism suppression-related decline in CBF is compensated by increased blood flow due to intrinsic vasodilation and matches at 1 MAC. All the inhaled anesthetics do not increase CBF and ICP and are safe even in patients with raised ICP.

General Anesthetic Considerations

The important anesthetic considerations for patients undergoing neurosurgical procedures are:

- Provision of optimal operating conditions.

- Use of physical/pharmacological means to maintain a stable ICP.

- Maintenance of stable hemodynamics, oxygenation, and ventilation.

- Maintaining appropriate CPP and oxygenation.

- Early detection and prompt management of intraoperative complications:

Table 23.1 Effect of anesthetic agents on cerebral physiology

Agent	CMR	CBF	CSF production rate	CSF absorption	CBV	ICP
Isoflurane	Decreases	Increases	Same	Increases	Increases	Increases
Desflurane	Decreases	Increases	Increases	Decreases	Increases	Increases
Sevoflurane	Decreases	Increases	Unknown	Unknown	Increases	Increases
Nitrous oxide	Decreases	Increases	Same	Same	Same	Increases
Propofol	Decreases	Decreases	Unknown	Unknown	Decreases	Decreases
Benzodiazepines	Decreases	Decreases	Same	Increases	Decreases	Decreases
Opioids	Same	Same	Same	Increases	Same	Same

Abbreviations: CBF, cerebral blood flow; CBV, cerebral blood volume; CMR, cerebral metabolic rate; CSF, cerebrospinal fluid; ICP, intracranial pressure.

- ▶ Venous air embolism (VAE) in posterior fossa surgery.
- ▶ Intracranial bleeding during cerebral aneurysm rupture.
- Controlled but rapid emergence from anesthesia to enable early assessment and monitoring of neurological status.

Anesthesia for Craniotomy

A craniotomy is one of the commonly performed procedures in neurosurgical patients. The anesthetic implications and their management is being discussed here.

Preoperative Assessment

Preoperative evaluation should focus on:

- Detailed past medical and surgical history.
- Documentation of level of consciousness, presence, and extent of neurological deficit.
- Observe breathing pattern (tachypnea, labored, or Cheyne–Stokes pattern).
- Rule out bulbar involvement by assessing cough and gag reflex.
- Rule out features of raised ICP (vomiting, headache, focal neurological signs, and papilledema).
- Assess the volume status and possible electrolyte imbalance in patient who has been vomiting, fluid restricted/receiving diuretic therapy.
- Assess glycemic control in diabetic patients being treated with dexamethasone.
- Rule out endocrine dysfunction in patients with pituitary malignancies.
- Based on an overall assessment, identify patients who would require postoperative ventilation in ICU–Glasgow coma scale (GCS) ≤ 6, evidence of raised ICP, large or deep-seated tumor.

Premedication

- Opioid premedication often avoided as it causes hypercarbia, leading to increased CBF and ICP.
- Short-acting benzodiazepines in titrated form can be given intravenously (IV) in OT before induction.

Induction

- Confirm availability of ICU or high-dependency unit (HDU).
  - ▶ Establish venous access with large bore cannula (cannulation of the saphenous vein is preferred, as the anesthetist is at the foot end, and it avoids the need for extension tubings).
  - ▶ Monitoring for temperature, neuro-muscular blockade, invasive arterial and CVP monitoring in addition to standard American Society for Anesthesiologists (ASA) monitoring.
  - ▶ Preoxygenation with 100% oxygen for 3–5 minutes.
  - ▶ Lignocaine (1–1.5 mg/kg) or esmolol (0.5–1 mg/kg) can be used to blunt sympathetic reflex during airway manipulation.
  - ▶ Suxamethonium transiently increases ICP; hence, best avoided in elective cases (except in difficult intubation) but should not be withheld in emergency cases.
  - ▶ Ensure adequate paralysis before attempting laryngoscopy and intubation.
  - ▶ Protect the pressure points using pads if the patient in a prone position.
  - ▶ Maintain head-up tilt of 15 to 20 degrees, avoid extreme neck flexion or rotation, and recheck endotracheal tube (ETT) placement after positioning.

- Head is often secured using Mayfield 3-point fixator; hence, an additional dose of fentanyl before the pins is useful.
- Use mannitol 0.5–1 g/kg and/or frusemide 0.5 mg/kg to lower raised ICP. Mannitol infusion is best started at the time of skin incision, so that the peak effect is seen during the dural opening.
- Target PaO_2 > 100 mm Hg and $PaCO_2$ between 30 and 35 mm Hg.

Maintenance of Anesthesia

- Total intravenous anesthesia (TIVA) with propofol, neuromuscular blockers (NMB) drug, opioid, and intermittent positive pressure ventilation with O_2-air mixture is the preferred choice OR.
- Inhalation technique with a volatile agent (sevoflurane is preferred because of smooth induction, rapid onset, and offset) can also be used.
- Paralysis is achieved through intermittent or continuous infusion of neuromuscular blocking agents.
- Nitrous oxide increases CBV and ICP. Besides, the chances of pneumoencephalocele are high. Hence, it should be avoided.

Fluid Management

The goal of IV fluid administration is to maintain euvolemia and hemodynamic stability. Dextrose containing fluids, being hypoosmolar, can cause transcellular fluid shift and lead to cerebral edema. Besides, hyperglycemia can cause impaired neurological recovery. Ringer's lactate is also hypoosmolar and can cause hyperglycemia through the metabolism of lactate and increases ICP. Hence, 0.9% saline is the preferred crystalloid but may cause hyperchloremic acidosis when large doses are transfused. Blood loss may be torrential; adequate blood should be reserved.

Temperature Control

Normothermia should be achieved before the patient awakens to avoid shivering, which may increase O_2 demand.

Thromboembolic Prophylaxis

Neurosurgical patients are at risk for deep vein thrombosis (DVT) and pulmonary embolism. Heparin should not be used because of the risk of bleeding in a confined cavity. Instead, graduated compression stockings and intermittent pneumatic leg compression are used.

Management of Emergence

- Emergence after the surgical procedure should be complete and smooth to do neurological assessment in a timely fashion.
- Coughing can increase ICP and, therefore, should be avoided during extubation.
- The volatile and/or IV anesthetic agent should be switched off in time, so that patient is fully awake and has no residual paralysis at the time of extubation.

Postoperative Management

- Regular neurologic monitoring to catch any neurological deterioration (should raise suspicion of intracranial bleeding [ICB]/edema).
- Hemodynamics should be closely monitored to maintain adequate cerebral perfusion pressure.

Anesthesia for Posterior Fossa Surgery

Posterior fossa surgeries are peculiar because of the vital structures it contains, the patient's positioning during surgery, and the risk of fatal VAE.

Preoperative Assessment

- Document the level of consciousness and focal neurological deficit.
- Rule out bulbar involvement and insert a nasogastric tube in case of inadequate gag reflex.
- Assess the need for postoperative mechanical ventilation (based on GCS, size of the tumor, and chances of damage to cranial nerves IX and X).
- Anticipate blood loss based on the size of the tumor and its vascularity.

Premedication

Premedication should be avoided wherever possible (especially in patients with raised ICP).

Position

Surgery can be performed in prone, lateral, or semiprone (park-bench) position. Sitting is rarely adopted because of the very high risk of VAE. Extreme care must be taken while turning the patient. Avoid extreme flexion of the neck, which may cause venous and lymphatic obstruction (can cause raised ICP and upper airway edema, respectively). It can also cause cord hypoperfusion leading to quadriparesis.

Induction and Maintenance of Anesthesia

The principles of induction and maintenance of anesthesia are the same as those for craniotomy.

Special Intraoperative Consideration

Since surgery in the posterior fossa can damage the vital respiratory and cardiovascular centre, monitoring is crucial.

- Look for any arrhythmia or hypertension and notify the surgeon at the earliest.
- A precipitous decrease in heart rate (HR) often signifies brainstem ischemia, and surgical retraction must be removed immediately.

The discussion of posterior fossa surgery would be incomplete without a word on VAE.

Venous Air Embolism

It is characterized by the ingress of air into the vascular system. Arterial air embolism can occur during:

- Paradoxical air embolism via heart defect.
- Direct arterial cannulation during cardiac surgery or angioplasty.

It is classically seen in sitting craniotomy. Besides, it has also been reported in laparoscopic, pelvic, and orthopedic procedures.

Prerequisites

- Direct communication between the source of air and vasculature.
- Pressure gradient favoring passage of air into the circulation (**Flowchart 23.1**).

Factors that favor entrainment of air are:

- Subatmospheric venous pressure.
- The surgical field above the level of the heart.
- Central venous cannulation during spontaneous respiration.
- Infusion of air or other gas under pressure into the venous system.
- Insufflation of CO_2 in laparoscopic surgery.
- Venturi jet ventilation.
- Pressurized IV infusion set.

Clinical Manifestations

- Sudden fall in end-tidal CO_2 due to a reduction in pulmonary blood flow.
- Hypotension.
- Tachy/bradyarrhythmia.
- *Millwheel murmur* via esophageal/precordial stethoscope.
- Arterial hypoxemia due to reduced pulmonary blood flow and ventilation perfusion (V/Q) mismatch.

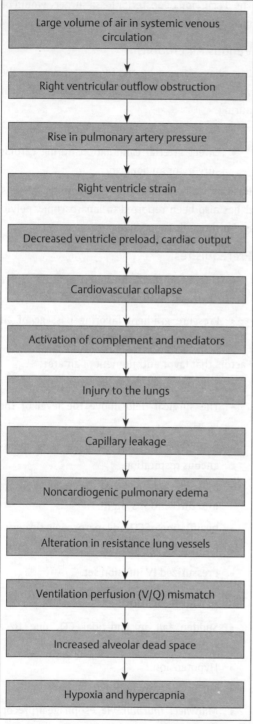

| Large volume of air in systemic venous circulation |
| ↓ |
| Right ventricular outflow obstruction |
| ↓ |
| Rise in pulmonary artery pressure |
| ↓ |
| Right ventricle strain |
| ↓ |
| Decreased ventricle preload, cardiac output |
| ↓ |
| Cardiovascular collapse |
| ↓ |
| Activation of complement and mediators |
| ↓ |
| Injury to the lungs |
| ↓ |
| Capillary leakage |
| ↓ |
| Noncardiogenic pulmonary edema |
| ↓ |
| Alteration in resistance lung vessels |
| ↓ |
| Ventilation perfusion (V/Q) mismatch |
| ↓ |
| Increased alveolar dead space |
| ↓ |
| Hypoxia and hypercapnia |

Flowchart 23.1 Pathophysiology of venous air embolism.

- Peaked P waves, suggestive of right heart strain.
- ST segment elevation or depression, nonspecific T wave.
- Sudden increase in CVP with reduced cardiac output and increased pulmonary vasculature resistance.

Neurological signs: Occur secondary to paradoxical air embolism across a patent foramen ovale and characterized by:

- Delayed emergence.
- Cerebral irritation.
- Convulsions.
- Localized neurological signs.

Management of Venous Air Embolism

- Notify the surgeon and start sprinkling saline over the surgical field.
- Increase inspired oxygen concentration to 100%.
- Durant position (make patient left lateral and head low, so that entrained air lies near the apex of the right ventricle and does not enter the pulmonary circulation).
- Resuscitate with rapid fluid bolus administration.
- Start vasopressor/inotrope in case of inadequate response to the fluid bolus.

Anesthesia for Cerebrovascular Surgery

Subarachnoid hemorrhage (SAH) is the leading cause of rising morbidity and mortality in neurosurgical patients. Patients present with sudden onset of unusually severe headache, followed by a period of unconsciousness. It may cause compression of adjacent neural structures, headache, and cranial nerve palsies. The optimal timing of surgery for SAH is controversial.

- Early surgery within 48 hours provides suboptimal surgical conditions but may reduce the incidence of rebleeding and vasospasm.

- Surgeries performed between days 7 and 10 is associated with a high risk of angiographic and clinical vasospasm.

- Delayed surgery provides time for edema to subside.

Anesthetic Considerations

- Problems common to neurosurgical procedures.

- Problems associated with ruptured intracranial aneurysm.

- Control of intracranial hypertension.

- Prevention and treatment of cerebral vasospasm.

- Problems during intraoperative management.

- Stringent control of intraoperative blood pressure (BP) within narrow limits.

- The intraoperative rupture of the aneurysm may cause rapid and massive blood loss.

Preoperative Assessment

- Assess and document neurological status.

- Assess volume status and electrolyte imbalance (secondary to syndrome of inappropriate antidiuretic hormone [SIADH] secretion).

- Look for hypertension and optimize it before surgery.

- Patients may have ECG changes that may mimic myocardial injury.

- Basal atelectasis in patients with prolonged bed rest.

- Aspiration pneumonia in comatose patients.

- Neurologic pulmonary edema.

Goals of Management of SAH

- To maintain normal CPP.

- Avoidance of extreme hypertension.

- Maintenance of normal fluid balance.

- Triple-H therapy (hypertension, hypervolemia, hemodilution) in an attempt to improve CPP and prevent ischemic neurological deficit caused by vasospasm.

Anesthetic Management

- Well-formulated and planned discussions about surgical conditions and hemodynamic parameters are essential.

- Invasive BP monitoring and CVP monitoring before the commencement of anesthesia.

- Prevent wide fluctuation in BP:

  ▶ Ensure smooth induction (prevent hypertension during intubation and hypotension after induction).

  ▶ Intraoperative BP should be maintained within 10 to 20% of baseline BP.

  ▶ A rise in BP risks aneurysm rupture, while hypotension risks cerebral ischemia.

  ▶ Rapid transfusion device should be primed and ready for volume resuscitation.

Induced Hypotension in Excision of Arteriovenous Malformation

- Systolic BP 60 to 80 mm Hg should be adequately achieved by:

  ▶ Volatile anesthetic.

  ▶ Beta-blockers and/or

  ▶ Sodium nitroprusside.

- When arteriovenous malformation (AVM) is excised, reperfusion of surrounding tissue may cause cerebral edema and raise ICP.

Neuroprotective Measures in Difficult Aneurysm Surgery/Intraoperative Aneurysm Rupture

- Hypothermia to 32°C.
- Thiopentone infusion to reduce cerebral metabolic oxygen consumption.
- Intensive neurologic and hemodynamic monitoring for all the patients.
- Prolonged surgery or intraoperative complications may necessitate sedation and ventilation postoperatively.
- Neurological status should be assessed as soon as feasible and regular assessment should be made after that.
- The decrease in GCS or development of new neurological deficit indicate:

▸ Vasospasm.

▸ ICB.

▸ Hydrocephalus.

Urgent CT may be needed for definitive diagnosis and further management plan.

Conclusion

The anesthetic agents have their unique effect on cerebral metabolism, cerebral metabolism, and cerebral autoregulation. Anesthetic goals during the neurosurgical procedure include maintaining optimal cerebral perfusion pressure, avoiding a rise in intracranial pressure, and ensuring smooth emergence from anesthesia. Venous air embolism, a dreaded complication during surgery on the posterior fossa, must be identified and managed immediately to prevent cardiovascular collapse.

CHAPTER 24

Anesthesia for Obstetrics

Anju Gupta and Bhavya Krishna

Introduction

Pregnancy is unique to all clinicians because of the responsibilities of two lives. Physiological changes occur in pregnancy due to hormones secreted by corpus luteum and placenta, like progesterone, and the mechanical effects by the gravid uterus. Interaction between mother and fetus both at physiological as well as pharmacokinetic level make anesthetic management challenging in such a group of patients. Following is the detailed discussion about physiological changes in pregnancy:

1. Cardiovascular system

Changes occur to provide the growing needs of the fetus, to maintain adequate fetal oxygenation, as well as to compensate for reduced venous return in the mother. These changes in the cardiovascular system are illustrated in **Table 24.1**.

Note: Remember diastolic murmur in pregnancy is always pathological.

Supine hypotension syndrome: In this phenomenon, circulatory collapse occurs due to diminished venous return and because of gravid uterus compressing over inferior vena cava (IVC) in the supine position in parturients by 13 to 15 weeks. This causes hypotension and decreased cardiac output. Turning the patient to lateral position (left) restores venous return and corrects hypotension. The gravid uterus also compresses over the aorta, which occurs by 28 to 30 weeks, compromising uteroplacental flow which, in turn, leads to reduced fetal perfusion in the supine position. This aortocaval compression is a preventable because of fetal distress; *hence, left uterine displacement should be done with a wedge (Crawford wedge) of >15° under the right hip as a precaution in the OT.*

2. Hematological system

Maternal hematological changes begin to occur early in pregnancy as mentioned in **Table 24.2**.

3. Respiratory System

Changes in the respiratory system during pregnancy are summarized in **Table 24.3**.

4. Gastrointestinal system

Changes in the gastrointestinal (GI) system are tabulated in **Table 24.4**.

Mendelson's syndrome: It is the most common cause of death during general anesthesia (GA) in obstetrics. It is caused by pulmonary aspiration of gastric contents. It can be prevented by:

- Empty stomach: Fasting for solids > 6 hours, clear liquids > 2 hours, before any anesthesia induction.

- Reduction in gastric acid secretion by administering H2 blockers like ranitidine.

- Neutralization of any acid produced in the stomach by giving 30 mL of 3M non-particulate antacid, like sodium citrate, 30 minutes before the induction of anesthesia.

- Increasing lower esophageal sphincter tone and increasing gastric emptying by prokinetic drugs like metoclopramide.

- Sellick maneuver (backward pressure on cricoid cartilage).

5. Renal system

Renal system changes in pregnancy are as mentioned in **Table 24.5**.

6. Central nervous system

Pregnancy-related central nervous system (CNS) changes are summarized in **Table 24.6**.

Table 24.1 Cardiovascular changes in pregnancy

Cardiovascular parameter	Change	Anesthetic implication
Heart rate	+20–30%	Due to hyperdynamic circulation—more prone to CHF
Stroke volume	+20–50%	
Cardiac output	+30–50% • Increases from 5th week onwards • Reaches maximum by 32 weeks during pregnancy • Highest is in the immediate postpartum period (increase by up to 75%)	
Uterine perfusion	Increased to 10% of cardiac output	Uterine perfusion not autoregulated
Supine hypotension syndrome	• IVC compression by 13–16 weeks • Aortic compression by 28–30 weeks	Supine hypotensive syndrome requires left lateral tilt by wedge placement of 15–20°, exacerbates hypotension caused due to GA and RA
Central venous pressure	Unchanged	
Pulmonary capillary wedge pressure	Unchanged	
Systemic vascular resistance	–20%	Hypotension common under RA and GA
Blood pressure	A slight decrease in the second trimester by 10–15 mm Hg. Both systolic as well as diastolic pressure fall	
Pulmonary vascular resistance	–30%	
Pulmonary artery pressure	–30%	
Wide, loud, and split S1, S3 and soft ejection systolic murmur on auscultation		
ECG: Left axis deviation—due to upward displacement of heart by the uterus		
Arrhythmias: Sinus tachycardia, ventricular ectopics, paroxysmal supraventricular tachycardia, paroxysmal atrial complexes, ventricular arrhythmias		

Abbreviations: CHF, congestive heart failure; GA, general anesthesia; IVC, inferior vena cava; RA, regional anesthesia.

Placental Transfer of Anesthetic Drugs

The drugs given to pregnant women may cross the placenta and have adverse effects on the fetus.

- The processes by which this transfer can happen are:
  - *Simple diffusion*: Transfer occurs along concentration gradient following Fick's principle, for example, paracetamol and midazolam.
  - *Facilitated transport*: Simple diffusion requiring carrier molecule, for example, glucocorticoids.
  - *Active transport*: Transfer occurs against concentration and requires carrier and energy, for example, dopamine and norepinephrine.

Table 24.2 Hematological changes in pregnancy

Parameter	Change	Anesthetic implication
Blood volume	+45%	Dilutional/physiological anemia of pregnancy
Plasma volume	+55%	
Red blood cell volume	+30%	

Coagulation factor		Change/effect
Factor II		Unchanged
Factor VII		Increased
Factors VIII, IX, X, XII		Increased
Factor XI		Reduced
Fibrinogen		Increased
Platelets		Dilutional thrombocytopenia
↑ Coagulation factors		Thromboembolic complications (DVT prophylaxis)
↓ Albumin and colloid osmotic pressure		Edema, decreased protein binding of drugs

Abbreviation: DVT, deep vein thrombosis.

Table 24.3 Changes in the respiratory system during pregnancy

Parameter	Change	Cause	Anesthetic implication
1. Respiratory mechanics			
Pulmonary resistance	Decreases by 50%	Due to bronchiolar dilatation by progesterone	
FEV1, FEV1/FVC	No change		
Type of breathing	Diaphragmatic type	Limited thoracic cage movement and pressure of gravid uterus and upward displacement of the diaphragm	The potential risk of hypoxemia in the supine and Trendelenburg positions
Mucosal edema and increased friability			• Difficult laryngoscopy and intubation; bleeding during attempts • Smaller endotracheal tube preferred (size 6–7 mm OD) • Increased work of breathing
2. Respiratory physiology at term gestation[a]			
Tidal volume, minute and alveolar ventilation *Respiratory rate unchanged*	+45%	Increased oxygen demand and increased requirement for CO_2 elimination	Faster inhalation induction
FRC	−20%		*Shorter apnea time during intubation; hence, parturients desaturate faster*
Closing capacity	Unchanged		
Total lung capacity, expiratory reserve volume, residual volume	Reduced		Preoxygenation for 5 mins reduces the rate of desaturation

(*Continued*)

Table 24.3 (*Continued*)

3. Blood gas parameter[b]	Nonpregnant	First trimester	Second trimester	Third trimester	Comments
PaCO$_2$ mm Hg	40	30	30	30	
PaO$_2$ mm Hg	100	107	105	103	*Increase is due to increase in minute ventilation*
pH	7.40	7.44	7.44	7.44	Respiratory alkalosis of pregnancy
Bicarbonate	24	21	20	20	

Abbreviations: FEV, forced expiratory volume; FRC, functional residual capacity; FVC, forced vital capacity; OD, outer diameter.
Notes: [a]Progesterone sensitizes the respiratory center to CO$_2$ and is responsible for the increase in ventilation.
[b]The rightward shift of the oxygen dissociation curve occurs during pregnancy.

Table 24.4 Gastrointestinal changes in pregnancy

Gastrointestinal parameter	Cause	Anesthetic implication
↑ Intragastric pressure ↓ Barrier pressure	• Progesterone and gastrin relaxes smooth muscles and impairs gastric and intestinal motility • Reduced motilin • Gravid uterus causes upward displacement of stomach and diaphragm	• ↑ Aspiration risk • Antacid prophylaxis • RSI with cricoid pressure • After 12 weeks gestation, parturients should be considered full stomach • ETI preferred over LMA insertion—for airway protection • RA preferred over GA
Residual volume of the stomach ↑	Increased gastrin secretion	
Increased cortisol and human placental lactogen	Reduced glucose tolerance	Hyperglycemia and ketosis can be encountered

Abbreviations: ETI, endotracheal intubation; GA, general anesthesia; LMA, laryngeal mask airway; RA, regional anesthesia; RSI, rapid-sequence intubation.

Table 24.5 Renal changes in pregnancy

Renal parameter change	Cause	Anesthetic implication
↑ Renal plasma flow ↑ GFR by 50%	• Increased cardiac output during pregnancy • Elevated creatinine and uric acid clearance	Normal urea and creatinine may mask impaired renal function
↓ Reabsorptive capacity		• Glycosuria up to 1–10 g/day • Proteinuria up to 300 mg/day
Dilatation of calyces, pelvis, ureters		Leads to urinary stasis—frequent UTI

Abbreviations: GFR, glomerular filtration rate; UTI, urinary tract infection.

Table 24.6 CNS changes in pregnancy

CNS change	Cause	Anesthetic implication
1. RA		
↑ Epidural vein engorgement	Due to the compression of IVC by gravid uterus—swelling of epidural veins and increased CSF pressure due to raised intraabdominal pressure	Bloody tap more common
↓ Epidural and subarachnoid space volume		More extensive local anesthetic spread in subarachnoid space leading to an *increased chance of high spinal*
↑ Sensitivity to LA		Dose requirement of LA reduced by 30%
↑ Lumbar lordosis		More cephalad spread of LA
2. GA		
↑ Sensitivity to opioids and sedatives	Production of endogenous opioids and production of progesterone	The lesser requirement of those drugs
Reduced MAC of volatile anesthetics by 25–40%		
Altered pain threshold		

Abbreviations: CNS, central nervous system; CSF, cerebrospinal fluid; GA, general anesthesia; IVC, inferior vena cava; LA, local anesthesia; MAC, minimum alveolar concentration; RA, regional anesthesia.

- ▶ *Pinocytosis*: Molecule gets engulfed by placental membrane.
- The extent of transfer depends on:
  - ▶ Molecular weight: <500 D cross placenta, for example, bupivacaine and succinylcholine.
  - ▶ Degree of lipid solubility: Lipid-soluble drugs easily cross the placenta, for example, thiopentone, benzodiazepines, and local anesthetics (LAs).
  - ▶ Protein binding: Highly protein-bound molecules do not cross the placenta, for example, bupivacaine and succinylcholine.
  - ▶ Degree of ionization and pKa: Ionized drugs are not able to cross the placenta, for example, glycopyrrolate, succinylcholine, neostigmine, and nondepolarizing muscle relaxants.
  - ▶ Other factors: Route of administration, maternal metabolism, maternal pH, placental blood flow, fetal pH, and fetal circulation.

Once a drug crosses the placenta, the fetal pH and protein binding affect drug disposition. The fetal liver gets exposed first. Hepatic drug uptake by a fetus may protect it from the harmful effects of certain drugs. Hence, to avoid the placental transfer of drugs, regional anesthesia (RA) is preferred over GA.

There is no anesthetic agent known to cause any teratogenicity in humans directly.

Table 24.7 enlists drugs with the differential capability to cross the placenta.

Table 24.8 summarizes the maternal and fetal effects of various anesthetic agents.

Table 24.7 Uteroplacental transfer of drugs

Anesthetic drugs that undergo transplacental transfer	Anesthetic drugs that do not undergo transplacental transfer
• Atropine • Benzodiazepines (diazepam, midazolam) • Intravenous Induction agents (propofol, thiopentone, ketamine, etomidate) • LA (except chloroprocaine) • Opioids (morphine > fentanyl) • Alpha 2 agonists (clonidine, dexmedetomidine) • Antihypertensive drugs (beta-blockers, NTG) • Ephedrine	• Glycopyrrolate • Heparin • Depolarizing and nondepolarizing neuromuscular blocking agents • Phenylephrine • Neostigmine • Insulin • Volatile anesthetics

Abbreviations: LA, local anesthetic; NTG, nitroglycerin.

Table 24.8 Maternal and fetal effects of anesthetic drugs

Anesthetic drug	Properties	Placental transfer	Effects on fetus/neonate	Maternal effects
1. Induction agents				
Thiopentone	Highly lipid-soluble, weak acid	+++	Quickly cleared by neonate after delivery	Narcosis
Propofol	Lipid soluble	+++	Transient depression of Apgar score and neurobehavioral effects in the neonate	
Ketamine	Weak base	++++		
2. Inhalational agents				
Volatile anesthetics	Highly lipid-soluble, low-molecular weight	+++	Greater sedative effect if dose-delivery time increased	*Decreased MAC, reduced uterine tone, hypotension*
Nitrous oxide		++	Possible diffusion hypoxia in the neonate, Prolonged exposure may inhibit DNA synthesis; avoid in the first trimester	
3. Opioids				
Morphine	Less lipid-soluble, low-protein binding	++	Neonatal respiratory depression. May require naloxone 0.01 mg/kg dose for reversal through the umbilical vein	Increased maternal sensitivity
Fentanyl	Lipid soiuble	+++		
Pethidine	50% plasma protein-bound	++	Prolonged depression due to active metabolites	
Remifentanil		+	Rapidly metabolized by fetus	

(Continued)

Table 24.8 (*Continued*)

Anesthetic drug	Properties	Placental transfer	Effects on fetus/neonate	Maternal effects
NSAIDs		-	Premature ductus arteriosus closure, avoid after 28 weeks; *ketorolac contraindicated*	
Benzodiazepine	Highly lipid-soluble	++ Diazepam > midazolam	Neonatal depression	
4. Muscle relaxants				
Nondepolarizing neuromuscular blockers	Large molecules, poorly lipid-soluble, highly ionized	-	No significant clinical effect	
Succinylcholine				Possible prolonged action
5. Anticholinergics				
Atropine	Lipid soluble	++	Fetal tachycardia	
Glycopyrrolate	Fully ionized	-		
Neostigmine	Small molecule	+++	May cause fetal bradycardia	
6. LA				
Lignocaine	Less lipid-soluble, low protein binding	++	Can accumulate in fetus causing *fetal acidosis* (known as ion trapping)	Use lower intrathecal doses in late pregnancy
Bupivacaine, Ropivacaine	Highly lipid-soluble, high protein binding	++		
7. Anticoagulants				
Warfarin	Crosses the placenta		Teratogenic	
Heparin	Does not cross the placenta			
8. Anticonvulsants				
Phenytoin, carbamazepine, sodium valproate			Congenital malformations (NTD)	
Magnesium sulfate				*Muscle weakness, interaction with neuromuscular blocking agents*
Thiazides			Neonatal thrombocytopenia	

Abbreviations: LA, local anesthetic; MAC, minimum alveolar concentration; NSAID, nonsteroidal anti-inflammatory drug; NTD, neural tube defect.

Anesthesia for Cesarean Section

Options of anesthesia are: GA and RA (spinal, epidural, combined spinal-epidural [CSE]).

Choice of anesthesia: Choice of anesthesia is RA unless contraindicated.

Regional Anesthesia

For RA in parturients, we have to consider several factors as mentioned in the physiological changes section such as:

- Enhances sensitivity to LA: Hormonal factors, engorgement of epidural venous plexus, decreased epidural space and cerebrospinal fluid (CSF) volume, the more cephalic spread of LA during spinal and epidural.
- Lower doses of LA used: Due to altered pharmacokinetics and pharmacodynamics.
- Lignocaine: Less protein-bound, can cross the placenta, and cause fetal acidosis.

Advantages of RA over GA:

- Better newborn Apgar score.
- Lower risk of maternal aspiration.
- Postoperative pain control better.

Contraindications of epidural/spinal:

- Maternal coagulopathy.
- Spinal deformity.
- Patient refusal.
- Skin infection at the injection site.

Complications of RA:

- Hypotension.
- Total spinal.
- Dural puncture.
- Postdural puncture headache (PDPH).
- Infection.
- Failed epidural/spinal.

1. **Spinal anesthesia:** The merits and demerits of spinal anesthesia are enlisted in **Table 24.9**.

   Choice of the drug: Hyperbaric bupivacaine 0.5% (2–2.5 mL) is the most commonly used drug for the subarachnoid block, and the block effect lasts for 1.5 to 2 hours.

   The level of block required is T4 to S1 for the lower segment cesarean section (LSCS). Because of sympathetic blockade leading to hypotension, coloading with intravenous (IV) bolus of crystalloid or colloid is often given. *Phenylephrine or ephedrine are vasopressors of choice in case of hypotension (phenylephrine is superior to ephedrine as per the recent literature).*

2. **Epidural anesthesia: Table 24.10** summarizes the advantages and disadvantages of epidural anesthesia.

   For obstetric cases, the epidural catheter is placed at L2–3/L3–4 space, and boluses/infusion of LA is given through the catheter. To confirm the placement of the catheter in the epidural space, intravascular and intrathecal placement need to be ruled out. The catheter must be aspirated before use, and test dose given as described below:

Table 24.9 Advantages and disadvantages of spinal anesthesia

Advantages	Disadvantages
• Quick onset within minutes	• Profound hypotension
• Avoids risks of GA	• Not suitable for postoperative analgesia
• Complete pain relief	• The short duration of anesthesia (2–3 h)
• Dense sensory and motor block	• Higher incidence of PDPH
• A minimal amount of LA required	

Abbreviations: GA, general anesthesia; LA, local anesthetic; PDPH, postdural puncture headache.

Table 24.10 Advantages and disadvantages of epidural anesthesia

Advantages	Disadvantages
• Avoidance of GA • Maintains uteroplacental flow if no undue hypotension • Improves intervillous blood flow • Complete and prolonged pain relief • Postoperative analgesia • The reduced stress response to surgery • Stable cardiac output	• Risk of hypotension • Hematoma • *Slow onset of action 20–30 mins, hence not suitable for emergency* • Time-consuming procedure • Variable effect • Technically difficult • A large dose of LA required • Chance of intravascular/intrathecal injection high

Abbreviations: GA, general anesthesia; LA, local anesthetic.

Table 24.11 Epidural test dose regimens

Test dose components	Positive intravascular test dose	Positive intrathecal test dose
Combined intrathecal and IV test dose		
Lignocaine 2% with epinephrine 5 µg/mL (1:200000)– 3 mL	Heart rate + 20 BPM within 1 min	Motor blockade at 3–5 mins
Bupivacaine 0.25% with epinephrine 5 µg/mL		
IV test dose		
Lignocaine 100 mg/bupivacaine 25 mg/fentanyl 100 µg	Tinnitus, circumoral numbness, dizziness	
Intrathecal test dose		
Lignocaine 40–60 mg/ bupivacaine 7.5 mg		Motor blockade at 3–5 mins

Abbreviations: BPM, beats per minute; IV, intravenous.

Epidural test dose regimens: Table 24.11 summarizes various epidural test dose regimens.

LA must be administered in fractionated dose after ruling out intrathecal and intravascular placement. For surgical anesthesia, about 8 to 10 mL of 0.25% bupivacaine can be given.

This technique is usually not the sole mode used for surgical anesthesia and is combined with a subarachnoid block. This is called combined spinal-epidural (CSE). It has the advantage of providing rapid onset of dense surgical anesthesia, while also being able to prolong analgesia postoperatively through the epidural catheter.

3. General anesthesia: GA carries 16 times more mortality in obstetric anesthesia than RA. Currently, indications of GA for cesarean delivery are limited in emergencies like:

- Maternal bleeding.
- Coagulopathy.
- Patient refusal for regional technique.
- Life-threatening fetal compromise (nonreassuring fetal condition).
- Decompensated heart disease, hemodynamically unstable status.

Table 24.12 gives a summary of the merits and demerits of GA.

Conduct of GA:

- *Aspiration prophylaxis:* As mentioned before, before the induction of anesthesia, prophylaxis should be given (metoclopramide, antacid, H2 blocker) to avoid Mendelson's syndrome.

- *Patient preparation and position:* Routine monitors should be connected and left uterine displacement should be done by placing a wedge under right hip.

- *Preoxygenation:* Judicious preoxygenation should be done for 5 minutes with 100% oxygen, or four vital capacity breaths should be taken.

- *Induction:* Rapid sequence induction and intubation with cricoid pressure (Sellick's maneuver) should be done. Thiopentone and succinylcholine are commonly used. Endotracheal intubation is recommended (avoid placement of laryngeal mask airway [LMA]).

- *Maintenance:* Oxygen/nitrous oxide with the volatile anesthetic. An opioid is given for analgesia after baby's delivery, and the cord is cut. All fluorinated inhalational agents relax the uterus and increase the chance of postpartum hemorrhage (PPH) in a dose-related fashion. *Halothane is the best uterine relaxant.* Drugs to facilitate uterine contraction are usually given after baby delivery like oxytocin (5–20 IU oxytocin IV).

- Extubation once the patient is fully awake.

Labor Analgesia

Pain Pathway during Labor

- During the first stage of labor: Pain impulses arise from the uterus. Uterine contractions cause myometrial ischemia, leading to bradykinin, histamine, and serotonin release. There is also stretching and distension of the lower uterine segment and cervix, which causes dull and poorly localized pain in the distribution of T10, T11, T12, and L1 spinal segments.

- In the second stage of labor: Pain is due to the stretching of the perineum and is localized in the distribution area of S2, S3, and S4 levels.

Level of the block to be achieved:

- First-stage labor: T10–L1.
- Second-stage labor: S1, S2, S3.
- LSCS: T4.

Labor pain can be alleviated with nonpharmacological as well as pharmacological methods.

Nonpharmacological Methods

Various nonpharmacological ways are available such as transcutaneous electrical nerve stimulation (TENS), massage, acupuncture, water

Table 24.12 Advantages and disadvantages of GA

Advantages	Disadvantages
• Immediate onset • Better control of hemodynamics • Fast onset • Controlled airway	• Difficult intubation • Mendelson's syndrome/pulmonary aspiration risk • Neonatal depression • Maternal awareness • Intubation/extubation response

Abbreviation: GA, general anesthesia.

blocks, continuous support, and hypnosis. These are described in brief in **Table 24.13**.

Pharmacological Methods

1. **Parenteral analgesia: Table 24.14** summarizes commonly used parenteral analgesics in labor.

2. **Inhaled analgesia:** This includes entonox and volatile anesthetics.

- Entonox
  It is a 50% mixture of nitrous oxide and oxygen. It can be used as a sole analgesic or as an adjuvant. It should be used by

Table 24.13 Nonpharmacological techniques of labor analgesia

Technique	Mechanism	Advantages	Disadvantages
TENS	Based on the "gate" theory	• Noninvasive • Easy to use • Good for back pain	• Useful only in early labor • Cost implications
Massage	• Inhibits pain transmission • Provides support and distraction	Perceived as highly effective by those using it	Labor-intensive
Acupuncture (acupressure, laser acupuncture)	• Stimulates specific points on the body with fine needles (or pressure or laser) • May inhibit pain transmission or produce natural endorphins	"Drug-free"	• Invasive • Need a trained therapist • Can take 30 mins for effect
Water blocks	• Injection of 0.1 mL sterile water in four spots over the sacrum. Action similar to TENS	• Easy to perform • Good for back pain	• Provides temporary relief only (45–90 mins) • Initial burning sensation
Continuous support	Presence of a trained support person can improve the physiological and psychological aspects of labor	• Popular • Useful at any stage	None
Hypnosis	Entering of a hypnotic state to have better control over the pain	Noninvasive	• Not all women susceptible (10–20% are not) • Time-consuming • Can be harmful

Abbreviation: TENS, transcutaneous electrical nerve stimulation.

Table 24.14 Parenteral analgesics in labor

Drug	Dose	Side effects	Comments
Meperidine	50–100 mg IM, 25–50 mg IV	*Loss of beat to beat variability in fetal heart rate tracing*	Lesser respiratory depression
Fentanyl	25–30 µg IV	Maternal sedation, fetal respiratory depression	
Ketamine	0.25–1 mg/kg IV		
Tramadol	1–2 mg/kg IM or IV	Nausea, vomiting	Lesser respiratory depression
Benzodiazepines			Not routinely given
Promethazine	25–50 mg IV	Nausea, vomiting	Potentiates analgesic effect of opioids

inhaling it at the rate of about 10 breaths at the early onset of contraction, and its use is discontinued after the peak of the contraction. Side effects include nausea, dizziness, dysphoria, and lack of cooperation. It is not commonly used anymore due to inadequate analgesia and OT pollution.

- Volatile anesthetics

  Not routinely used; the most commonly used is sevoflurane (0.8%). Isoflurane, enflurane, and desflurane can also be used (0.2%). They may cause profound sedation, unpleasant smell, OT pollution, and loss of consciousness sometimes.

3. **Regional analgesia (RA):** It is the most effective technique of labor analgesia with minimal depressant effects on mother and fetus. Methods include epidural, spinal, and CSE. Paracervical block, pudendal, saddle block, and perineal infiltration also come under RA.

- Epidural analgesia

  Indicated when a patient is in active labor: 5 to 6 cm of cervical dilatation in primigravida and 3 to 4 cm in multigravida. **Table 24.15** enlists commonly used epidural drug regimens. However, it is noteworthy that even maternal request is a sufficient criterion for epidural analgesia.

  Ropivacaine is preferred over bupivacaine, as it gives differential blockade of the denser sensory blockade with relative sparing of motor blocking.

  With a bolus dose, analgesia lasts for a longer time than a single shot subarachnoid block. With the catheter in situ, prolonged analgesia can be given. Epidural analgesia causes no change in the duration of the first stage of labor. The second stage of labor may be prolonged and sometimes leads to instrumental delivery.

- Spinal analgesia

  Has a faster onset than epidural analgesia. The subarachnoid block is used for:

  ▶ Multiparous women in active labor (6–9 cm dilated).

  ▶ Primipara fully dilated with significant pain.

  ▶ Patients in early labor, 2 to 4 cm dilated, before the active phase.

  Saddle block is used in cases like:

  ▶ Forceps delivery.

  ▶ Repair of vaginal/rectal tears postpartum.

  ▶ Removal of placenta.

  If there is accidental dural puncture during epidural placement, then the catheter can be left in subarachnoid space, and continuous spinal analgesia can be given.

  Disadvantages: Short duration of action and PDPH.

- Combined spinal-epidural analgesia:

  Initially, a subarachnoid block of very low volume is given, followed by the placement of the epidural catheter and starting an infusion. It has the advantages of both spinal and epidural analgesia, early onset of analgesia, and prolonged duration with the

Table 24.15 Epidural analgesia regimens for labor analgesia

Drug in epidural for labor analgesia	Initial injection	Continuous infusion
Bupivacaine	10–15 mL of 0.125% solution	0.0625–0.125% at 8–15 mL/h
Ropivacaine	10–15 mL of 0.1-0.2% solution	0.2–0.5% at 8–15 mL/h
Fentanyl	50–100 µg in 10 mL solution	1–4 µg/mL

epidural catheter in situ. In case operative delivery (cesarean section) is required, analgesia can be converted to anesthesia by giving more concentrated LA solution via the epidural catheter.

It also has the advantage of more ability— walking epidural, reducing complications of epidural like patchy block, and poor sacral spread.

- Paracervical block, pudendal, saddle block, perineal infiltration:

  ▶ **Paracervical**: Paracervical block can be given by obstetricians also. It provides relief for the first stage of labor and does not adversely affect the progress of labor. Sensory nerve fibers from uterus fuse bilaterally at 4 to 6 o'clock positions and 6 to 8 o'clock positions around the cervix at the vaginocervical junction, which is blocked using 5 to 10 mL 1% lignocaine injection. It relieves the pain of uterine contractions along with the upper one-third vagina. It is not useful for episiotomy. It causes fetal bradycardia, so unsafe for fetus.

  ▶ **Pudendal**: It is suitable for vaginal as well as forceps delivery, as it provides perineal analgesia and relaxation but not helpful for labor analgesia. LAs, usually 20 mL lignocaine 1%, are given

either through transvaginal or perineal route to block S2, S3, and S4 nerves.

- ▶ **Saddle block**: Lower spinal anesthesia confined to the vagina and perineum; useful in midcavity forceps.

- ▶ **Perineal infiltration**: Useful for stitching of episiotomy.

Anesthesia for Manual Removal of Placenta

If the placenta is not delivered within 30 minutes of active management and within 1 hour of birth with physiological management, it is considered retained. Manual removal of the placenta is an emergency procedure to control PPH and puerperal sepsis. Retained placenta is one of the most important causes of PPH and the requirement of blood transfusion in obstetrics.

Manual removal of the placenta is an invasive procedure and requires adequate anesthesia and analgesia for sedation and pain control. A variety of anesthesia/analgesia or combinations can be used, as described in **Table 24.16**.

GA, with a volatile agent, is anesthesia choice. Desflurane is the inhalational agent of choice, as it gives brief but intense uterine relaxation. Previously, halothane was the agent of choice. Amongst the IV agents, etomidate and ketamine are preferred.

Table 24.16 Anesthesia techniques for manual removal of placenta

Technique	Advantages	Disadvantages
GA	• Dose-dependent uterine relaxation by volatile agents	• Risks of GA like airway compromise, failed intubation, aspiration risk
Spinal	• Rapid establishment of analgesia • Avoid risks of GA	• Potential for sudden hypotension if hemorrhaging severely
Epidural	• Good if catheter already in situ • Avoid risks of GA	• It takes time to establish the required level of surgical anesthesia
Sedation	• Quick and easy	• Poor uterine relaxation • Unprotected airway

Abbreviation: GA, general anesthesia.

Anesthesia for Nonobstetric Surgeries

In total, 2% of pregnant women require non-obstetric surgery. Common indications include:

- Appendicitis.
- Ovarian disorders (torsion or neoplasm).
- Trauma.

Elective surgery should be delayed until as late as 6 weeks postpartum, and *anesthesia is safest in the second trimester.* Several concerns need to be addressed, as highlighted in **Table 24.17**.

Avoidance of potentially dangerous drugs at critical times during fetal development and maintenance of adequate uteroplacental perfusion is imperative for fetal safety. Although no anesthetic drug is known to be teratogenic, except nitrous oxide, caution must be executed during administration. Some teratogenic effects of drugs are mentioned in **Table 24.18**.

Conduct of Anesthesia

RA or GA, depending on surgery to be performed, although the former should be preferred if there is a choice. **Table 24.19** compares the advantages of GA versus RA for nonobstetric surgeries:

- *General anesthesia*

  After a rapid preoperative assessment and preparation with aspiration prophylaxis beyond 14 weeks, for GA, rapid-sequence IV induction and intubation, with adequate cricoid pressure, should be preceded by preoxygenation with 100% oxygen for 5 minutes. Precautions to avoid supine hypotension syndrome (beyond 18 weeks

Table 24.17 Anesthetic concerns in nonobstetric surgeries in pregnancy

Maternal concerns	Fetal concerns
• Physiological changes in pregnancy • Conditions compelling surgery during pregnancy • Avoidance and treatment of preterm labor	• Placental transfer of drugs • Teratogenicity (timing of exposure, duration/dosage of exposure) • Maternal factors leading to fetal compromise (maternal hypoxia, hypo/hypercarbia)

Table 24.18 Teratogenic effects of drug

Drug	Teratogenic effect
Opioids	Neonatal jaundice, neonatal respiratory depression if used during labor, withdrawal symptoms with chronic use
Paracetamol	Safe
NSAIDs	Premature PDA closure
Aspirin	IUGR, stillbirth
Warfarin	Contradi syndrome, fetal hemorrhage
Phenytoin	Fetal hydantoin syndrome
Carbamazepine	Craniofacial defects and developmental defect
Benzodiazepines	Cleft lip/palate, *floppy infant syndrome*
Promethazine	Fetal platelet aggregation
Nitrous oxide	Congenital disabilities, bone marrow suppression *Should be avoided in early pregnancy*

Abbreviations: IUGR, intrauterine growth retardation; NSAIDs, nonsteroidal anti-inflammatory drugs; PDA, patent ductus arteriosus.

Table 24.19 Advantages of regional anesthesia versus general anesthesia for nonobstetric surgeries

Regional anesthesia	General anesthesia
• Reduces the exposure of fetuses to potential teratogens • Avoids the potential risk of failed intubation and aspiration • Provides excellent postoperative analgesia	• Volatile anesthetics such as halothane, sevoflurane, desflurane, and isoflurane are shown to inhibit the uterine contractility, which may prove beneficial in preventing preterm contractions

by wedge placement) and preterm labor should be taken. Prophylactic tocolytics may be considered in the third trimester for lower abdominal or pelvic surgery for inflammatory conditions. Volatile anesthetic agents may help to relax the uterus, although high concentrations can cause undesirable hypotension. Catecholamine surges should be avoided as they impair uteroplacental perfusion. *Fetal monitoring and uterine contraction monitoring should be done when possible.* Adequate fetal perfusion and oxygenation is the ultimate goal.

• *Regional anesthesia*

Management of neuraxial anesthesia for nonobstetric surgery in the pregnant patient is no different than its management for cesarean delivery. The primary concern with neuraxial anesthesia is maternal hypotension, which may reduce placental perfusion.

Conclusion

Pregnancy is unique in terms of the deviation of physiology from a nonpregnant woman. There is an alteration in the pharmacodynamics and pharmacokinetics of anesthetic agents; also, there is a selective transfer of anesthetic agents across the placenta. Pregnant patients are at risk of aspiration due to a full stomach condition (because of the gravid uterus). Tracheal intubation requires rapid sequence intubation and a smaller size endotracheal tube due to glottic edema. Needling during subarachnoid block may also be difficult due to decreased space between spinous processes. Labor pain pathways should be understood clearly to provide adequate labor analgesia.

CHAPTER 25

Pediatric Anesthesia

Anju Gupta

Introduction

Many significant changes occur as a newborn baby grows and develops into an adolescent and then an adult. All the physiological and psychological changes are unique to children and have a considerable impact while anesthetizing them. This chapter will help anesthetists to acquaint physiological changes in children along with their anesthetic implications.

Definitions: Pediatric age group ranges from neonate to adolescent as shown in **Table 25.1**.

Normal physiological values according to age are as follows:

1. Weight (kg) = (age + 4) × 2; accurate till 10 years of age.

2. Total body water (TBW): term neonate = 75%; estimated blood volume (EBV) = 85 mL/kg.

3. Preterm infants = TBW > 80% with >50% as extracellular fluid (ECF) and EBV = 90 to 100 mL/kg.

4. Respiratory rate = 24 – age/2; tidal volume = 6 to 8 mL/kg.

5. Cardiac output = 300 to 400 mL/kg/min at birth; 200 mL/kg/min within a few months.

6. Circulatory parameters (heart rate and systolic blood pressure [SBP]) are listed in **Table 25.2**.

Anatomical/Physiological Considerations

Children are not a smaller version of adults. There are a host of anatomical and physiological differences.

Table 25.1 Pediatric age group classification

Age group	Definition
Neonates	From birth till 44 weeks of postconceptional age
Infants	Up to 12 months of age
Child	1–12 years
Adolescents	13–16 years
Postterm infant	An infant born after 42 completed weeks of POG
Term infant	One born after 37 and before 42 completed weeks of POG
Preterm infant	One born before 37 completed weeks of POG
Preterm infant subgroups (based on actual weight)	
LBW infant	Weighs < 2,500 g regardless of the POG
VLBW infant	Weighs < 1,500 g
ELBW infant	Weighs < 1,000 g
Micropreemies	Infants weighing less than 750 g

Abbreviations: ELBW, extremely low birth weight; LBW, low birth weight; POG, period of gestation; VLBW, very low birth weight.

Table 25.2 Circulatory parameters in pediatrics

Age (years)	Heart rate (per min)	Systolic BP (mm Hg)
Preterm	120–170	40–55
Newborn	100–170	50–90
<1	110–160	80–90
1–2	100–150	85–95
2–5	95–140	85–100
5–12	80–120	90–110
>12	60–100	100–120

Airway

- They have a large head and large tongue with a short neck.

- The tongue is relatively large.

- Neonates are obligate/preferential nasal breathers (till 5 months of age).

- The larynx is high (C3–C4) and anterior. The epiglottis is long, floppy, and U-shaped. It tends to fall posteriorly in the supine position. *Unlike the "sniffing" position, the head needs to be in a neutral position to improve the glottic view.*

- The airway is funnel-shaped with the narrowest part at the level of the cricoid cartilage.

- The trachea is short (4–5 cm in the neonate). *There is a high chance of endotracheal tube (ETT) dislodgement or endobronchial migration of ETT with head movement.*

Respiratory System

- Limited respiratory reserve, absent "bucket handle" action of ribs, diaphragmatic breathing, and low functional residual capacity (FRC) due to highly compliant chest wall.

- FRC further decreases with apnea and anesthesia, causing lung collapse.

- The closing volume is larger than the FRC until 6 to 8 years of age. This causes an increased tendency for airway closure at end-expiration. Thus, neonates and infants generally need positive pressure ventilation (PPV) with positive end-expiratory pressure (PEEP) during anesthesia.

- The diaphragm has a lower percentage of type I muscle fibers and therefore easily subject to fatigue.

- The development of alveoli occurs over the first 8 years of life.

- Premature infants are at risk of apneas in the postoperative period.

- Respiratory distress syndrome (RDS) is frequent at <28 weeks due to reduced surfactant.

Cardiovascular System

- Patent ductus arteriosus (PDA) more common in premature infants; it closes typically 10 days to 2 weeks after birth but may reopen in the first few weeks after birth whenever pulmonary arterial pressure rises (hypoxemia, hypercarbia, acidosis, etc.), which is known as transitional circulation.

- The neonatal heart is poorly compliant and has reduced contractile force due to disorganized intracellular contractile proteins and immature sarcoplasmic reticulum.

- The *cardiac output is rate-dependent in neonates and children with reduced capacity to increase stroke volume by premature heart*. Therefore, bradycardia is poorly tolerated, and cardiac compression should be provided in the neonate with a heart rate < 60 bpm.

- The dominant vagal tone makes neonates and infants prone to bradycardia.

Renal System

- The glomerular function and tubular function mature by 2 years and 8 months of life, respectively.
- Normal urine output ranges between 1 and 2 mL/kg/h.

Hepatic System

- Liver cytochrome P-450 enzymes achieve maturity at the adult level by 6 months.
- Premature infants are prone to hypoglycemia because of hepatic glycogen storage development in the last few weeks of gestation.

Hematology

- The hemoglobin is around 18 to 20 g/dL at the time of birth, which decreases to 9 to 12 g/dL over the next 3 to 6 months.
- At birth, HbF is the predominant hemoglobin (70–80%), the levels of which drop to around 5% within 3 months.
- The deficiency of vitamin K-dependent clotting factors and platelets during the first few months of life puts neonates at risk of intracranial bleed. Therefore, *vitamin K is given at birth to prevent hemorrhagic disease of the newborn.*

Temperature Control

- Neonates and preterms are more prone to heat loss due to:
  - Relatively larger body surface-to-body weight ratio.
  - Poorly developed subcutaneous tissue.

- Inability to use shivering thermogenesis.
- These are partially compensated for by nonshivering thermogenesis via brown fat, which is inhibited by volatile and intravenous anesthetics.
- Hypothermia leads to cardiovascular stress, delays emergence from anesthesia.

Central Nervous System

- In infants, cerebral perfusion pressure varies directly with arterial blood pressure and, therefore, are at *risk of both intraventricular hemorrhage and inadequate cerebral perfusion with fluctuating blood pressure.*
- Pain pathways in neonates are fully developed early in gestation.
- The blood–brain barrier (BBB) is poorly formed.

Blood Volume and Pharmacokinetics

- Children have high ECF volume as well as increased volume of distribution and hence require a larger loading dose of drugs.
- *Reduced binding to albumin and α-acid-glycoprotein leads to increased free drug concentration.*
- Immature enzyme systems, impaired renal excretion, and hypothermia can prolong drug action.

Psychology

- *Infants less than 6 months*: Do not have stranger anxiety or separation anxiety.
- *Children < 4 years*: Upset by parental separation and unfamiliar surroundings. They have unpredictable behavior and are difficult to rationalize.
- *4 to 12 years*: Fear the mutilating effects of surgical procedure and the possibility of pain.

- Fear of loss of control and not being able to cope up with the pain associated with surgery is common in adolescents.

Anesthetic Management

Preoperative Evaluation

The preoperative evaluation provides an appropriate window to gain the trust of the child as well as the parent, obtain consent and assent, address fears and queries, and explain the anesthetic plan. The child's fears and queries should be addressed while involving the parents in the discussion. Discuss postoperative pain management. Preoperative evaluation should focus on history, including any allergy, previous history of anesthetic complications in family, medical problems, recent upper/lower respiratory tract illness (URTI/LRTI), congenital anomalies, current medications, recent immunizations, fasting times, loose teeth, etc.

The elective surgery should be postponed for at least 4 weeks in the presence of an active URTI.

Physical examination: Airway and cardiorespiratory systems should be examined. Nutritional status and sites for intravenous (IV) access should be assessed. Children must be weighed.

Investigations include the following:

- Hemoglobin: Premature infants, large expected blood loss, cardiorespiratory illness.
- Electrolytes: Renal/endocrine/metabolic disease, patient on IV fluids.
- Chest X-ray: Active cardiorespiratory disease, scoliosis, etc.

Preoperative Preparation

Psychological preparation in the form of role-play, operation theater (OT) trips, and cognitive behavioral therapy is very effective in gaining a child's confidence, reducing anxiety, and helping to reduce the need for premedicant drugs. However, in a combative child, sedative premedicant is useful to produce a calm or cooperative child. Drugs commonly prescribed are midazolam (0.5 mg/kg orally, maximum: 15 mg, 15–30 min prior); chloral hydrate (50 mg/kg orally, maximum: 1 g); and ketamine (3–8 mg/kg orally, 30–60 min prior).

Fasting times to be followed are as follow:

- Clear fluids: 2 hours.
- Breast milk: 4 hours.
- Solids (including formula and nonhuman milk): 6 hours.
- Solid (fatty or fried) foods: 8 hours.

The dose of anesthesia drugs, including emergency drugs (atropine, adrenaline, and suxamethonium), should be precalculated, displayed, and loaded in an appropriate dose and dilution. Airway and monitoring equipment should be checked and kept ready.

WETFLAG mnemonic is useful to estimate drugs and endotracheal tube (uncuffed) size for a child in an emergency (**Table 25.3a**).

Anesthesia Induction

The presence of parents at the time of induction makes the child calm and cooperative. Maintaining perioperative normothermia is of paramount importance in children. OT should be prewarmed to 29°C for neonates and 27°C for older infants. Use bandages to wrap the limbs and head. Head and extremities should be wrapped in cotton padding or plastic cover to prevent radiant heat loss.

A gaseous induction is preferred for the child that fears needles or has difficult venous access. A correctly sized oropharyngeal airway may be used. *Halothane and sevoflurane are the agents of choice for gaseous induction.* Sevoflurane is nonirritant and has a more rapid onset and offset. It has improved hemodynamic stability but is associated with emergence delirium. MAC values

Table 25.3a WETFLAG mnemonic

Parameter	Calculation
W = weight (kg)	(Age + 4) × 2
E = Energy (J) for defibrillation	4 J/kg
T = Tube (mm)	(Age/4) + 4.5
Fl = Fluid bolus (mL)	20 mL/kg
A = Adrenaline (µg)	10 µg/kg (0.1 mL/kg of 1:10,000)
G = Glucose 10% solution (mL)	2 mL/kg

are 3.3 in infants and 2.5 in children. Halothane is now outdated in most places because of slow induction, delayed recovery, and with the potential for arrhythmias.

Intubation

- Straight Miller blades are useful in neonates and infants. A size 0 blade is used for neonates and infants < 4 kg.

- Uncuffed tubes are used until around 8 years of age, and a small leak should be present.

- ETT size = age/4 + 4.5.

- Tube length in cm = age/2 +12 (or internal diameter [ID] × 3) for an oral ETT, and adding 2 cm for a nasal tube is easier to remember.

- Size 1 LMA up to 5 kg; 1.5 LMA 5 to 10 kg; 2 LMA 10 to 20 kg; 2.5 LMA 20 to 30 kg; 3 LMA for over 30 kg.

Intravenous Fluids

Choice of Fluid

Resuscitation fluid: Balanced salt solution (Ringer's lactate/plasmalyte). Fluid bolus for resuscitation = 10 – 20 mL/kg. 5% dextrose is contraindicated as a resuscitation fluid, as it may worsen the underlying hyponatremia. Blood bolus = 8 mL/kg (increases Hb by approximately 1 g/dL) of whole blood (or 5 mL/kg of packed cells).

Maintenance fluids: Balanced salt solution with 1% dextrose.

Holiday and Segar formula (4-2-1 rule) for calculating hourly maintenance fluid requirement:

- First 10 kg: 4 mL/kg/h.

- 10–20 kg: 2 mL/kg/h.

- For every additional kg: 1 mL/kg/h.

Maintenance

- Add regional analgesia where necessary and appropriate.

- Cautious use of narcotics in infancy, especially ex-premature infants and neonates.

- Use IV fluids to replace loss during surgical procedures.

- Anticipate laryngospasm at the time of extubation if the child is not fully awake.

- Monitor child in recovery until complete awakening.

Extubation

Extubation should be attempted once the child has spontaneous respiratory efforts, opening eyes spontaneously and showing power in the limbs. Children have a high incidence of postanesthesia complications. Provide supplemental oxygen when saturation falls below 93%.

The common causes of postoperative hypoxemia and their management are mentioned in **Table 25.3b**.

Postoperative Pain Management

Optimal pain management depends on regular pain assessment. Age-appropriate pain assessment tools (**Table 25.4**) should be used for children to know the severity of pain. Moderate or severe pain should be treated according to the WHO analgesic ladder.

Pain management strategies can be non-pharmacological, for example, hypnosis, transcutaneous electric nerve stimulation, acupuncture,

Table 25.3b Causes and treatment of postoperative hypoxemia in children

Cause	Management
Airway obstruction	• Neck extension • Jaw thrust • Lateral position
Laryngospasm	• 100% oxygen, continuous positive airway pressure • Subhypnotic dose of propofol (0.8 mg/kg) • IV succinylcholine 1 mg/kg with atropine 0.2 mg/kg
Laryngeal edema/croup	• High flow nebulized oxygen • 0.5 mL of 2% racemic epinephrine (diluted to 2–4 mL) given every 4 h • Dexamethasone 0.5 mg/kg 6 hourly for 4–6 doses
Respiratory depression	• Naloxone 0.01 mg/kg every 2–3 min
Postoperative apnea (premature infant)	• Caffeine 10 mg/kg
Postoperative pulmonary edema	• Positive pressure ventilation with PEEP • Diuretics and fluid restriction

Abbreviations: IV, intravenous; PEEP, positive end-expiratory pressure.

Table 25.4 Age-specific pain assessment score in pediatrics

Age (years)	Pain scale	Type	Score
0–5	FLACC scale	Observational or behavioral scale	0–10
4–12	Faces pain scale	Self-report	0–10
6 and above	NRS and VAS	Self-report	0–10

Abbreviations: FLACC, face, legs, activity, cry, consolability; NRS, numeric rating scale; VAS, visual analog score.
Score: 1 to 3 = mild; 4 to 7 = moderate; and 8 to 10 = severe.

cold therapy, localized heat, and immobilization. *For pharmacological pain management, multimodal analgesia approach is the best.* The rationale is combining different classes of analgesia achieves effective pain relief with minimal side effects. Analgesics should be prescribed regularly instead of on a need basis, using the least invasive route, preferably oral. All opioids can cause respiratory depression and require careful observation. Opioid-sparing analgesics like paracetamol, nonsteroidal anti-inflammatory drugs (NSAIDs), alpha-2 agonist drugs (clonidine, dexmedetomidine), ketamine, local anesthetics (LA), etc., should be employed judiciously. Paracetamol is the most common analgesic used for infants, the doses are as follows:

- IV: 15 mg/kg (6 hourly).
- Oral dose: 15 to 20 mg/kg (4 hourly).
- Per rectal: 30 to 45 mg/kg.

The upper limit of dose per day is 75 mg/kg in children, 60 mg/kg in neonates, and 45 mg/kg for premature infants. In higher doses, hepatotoxicity can occur due to its oxidized metabolite and N-acetyl-p-benzoquinone imine (NAPQI). Codeine and tramadol are weak opioid analgesics commonly used to treat mild-to-moderate postoperative pain. Severe postoperative pain can be treated with IV bolus or infusions of potent opioids like morphine and fentanyl. Regional anesthesia is known to be opioid-sparing, improve recovery, and postoperative outcomes.

Regional Anesthesia in the Pediatric Population

Placement of a block before the surgery provides the following:

- Excellent analgesia.
- Decreases anesthetic drug requirements.
- Ensures pain-free rapid emergence from anesthesia.
- Decreases stress response.
- Avoids the harmful effects of opioids.

The topical anesthesia, infiltration, regional nerve blocks, and neuraxial analgesia are common techniques of regional anesthesia and can be used alone or to supplement general anesthesia.

Neuraxial analgesia: It includes caudal, epidural, and spinal blocks. Caudal block is indicated for surgery below the umbilicus (e.g., inguinal hernia, club foot repair). The caudal space can be located by the anatomical landmarks (the sacral hiatus, found at the apex of an equilateral triangle, where the posterior superior iliac spines form the other two corners). Armitage formula (**Table 25.5**) is commonly used to calculate the LA dosage for various surgeries.

Continuous caudal catheters can be inserted through the sacral hiatus into the lumbar or thoracic vertebral level for continuous infusion in the postoperative period. Lumbar and thoracic continuous epidurals are indicated for major orthopedic, abdominal, and thoracic surgeries. The suggested maximum doses of local anesthetics such as bupivacaine, ropivacaine, and levobupivacaine recommended for neonates and children are similar. Various adjuvants to local anesthetics have been found to prolong the duration of analgesia significantly, for example, clonidine (mean 10 h), dexmedetomidine (mean 10 h), morphine (mean 15 h), and fentanyl (mean 6 h). *Clonidine and fentanyl should be avoided in infants < 6 months. The commonly used drugs for regional anesthesia are highlighted in Table 25.6.*

Contrary to local anesthetics, epidural opioids provide postoperative analgesia without motor

Table 25.5 Armitage formula for calculation of LA volume for caudal block

LA volume	Dermatomal level	Surgeries
0.5 mL/kg	Sacral	Perineal, penile
1 mL/kg	Lumbosacral	Inguinal hernia, orchidopexy
1.25 mL/kg	Midthoracic	Thoracotomies

Abbreviation: LA, local anesthetic.

Table 25.6 Epidural doses of bupivacaine, levobupivacaine, and ropivacaine in neonates and children

Drug	Bolus dose	Infusion dose
Bupivacaine, ropivacaine, levobupivacaine (0.2–0.25%)	Neonates 2 mg/kg Children 2.5 mg/kg	Neonates 0.2 mg/kg/h Children 0.4 mg/kg/h
Fentanyl	2 mg/kg	2–5 mg/mL of LA solution
Morphine	30 mg/kg	10 mg/mL
Clonidine	1–2 mg/kg	0.3–1 mg/mL of LA solution

Abbreviation: LA, local anesthetic.

and sensory block, but at the cost of respiratory depression, itching, nausea and vomiting, urinary retention, and decreased gastrointestinal motility.

Peripheral nerve block: Commonly used blocks such as brachial plexus block, lumbar plexus block, femoral nerve block, sciatic nerve block, fascia iliaca block, penile block, and peribulbar block provide excellent postoperative analgesia and patient comfort.

Management of Neonatal Surgical Emergencies

The general principles of management of neonatal emergencies are summarized in **Box 25.1**.

To summarize, children are not miniature adults. They differ from adults both anatomically as well as physiologically and require special attention during perioperative period as far as anesthetic management is concerned.

Conclusion

Children are not miniature adults. They deviate from adults both in terms of anatomy and physiological characteristics.

The alteration in pharmacokinetics and pharmacodynamics of anesthetic agents mandate choosing appropriate drugs with appropriate dosages and dilutions. Their body surface area is much larger than the body's size and hence prone to losing heat and at risk of hypothermia. Making the child calm and gaining confidence are pivotal during preoperative assessment, smooth induction, and smooth recovery after the surgery. Pain assessment during the postoperative course may be difficult to recognize because crying can be due to hunger, pain, and unfamiliar surroundings. Thus, preoperative assessment, provision of anesthesia, and postoperative care of children are tasks that every anesthetist should practice and master.

Box 25.1 Practical considerations for neonatal surgeries

Preoperative assessment: Check the following:
- Body weight, gestational age at birth, and postconceptual age.
- Birth history.
- Maternal illness during pregnancy.
- Vitamin K injection received.
- Any congenital abnormalities.
- Any cyanotic spell/feeding difficulties.

Operation room preparation:
- Drug doses based on body weight calculated and drawn up before induction.
- Appropriate airway equipment for neonate (Miller blade size 0, 1; endotracheal tube [ETT] size 2 to 4 mm ID).
- Monitoring (two pulse-oximeter probes, small ECG electrodes, noninvasive [NIBP cuff]).
- OT warmed to 27 to 29°C.

Anesthesia and postoperative:
- Use the nasogastric tube to decompress the stomach.
- Keep baby warm (cover head, heated intravenous [IV] fluid, warming devices).
- Check blood glucose and prevent hypo/hyperglycemia.
- Regular paracetamol, avoid nonsteroidal anti-inflammatory drugs (NSAIDs).
- Close postoperative monitoring in the first 24 h.
- Cautious use of opioids, regional anesthesia (RA) preferred.
- Higher risk of postoperative apnea especially in preterms.

CHAPTER 26

Geriatric Anesthesia

Ganasekran Srinivasan

Introduction

The term "geriatrics" was coined in English by Ignatz L. Nascher in 1909 from the Greek words *gêras*, meaning "old age" and *atrós*, meaning "physician." Aging is a normal physiological process which is associated with progressive fall in the function of all end organs, and these changes are highly variable between person to person. The prevalence of chronic health conditions increases with age. The physiological changes and their anesthetic considerations in each organ system require a proper understanding.

Physiological Changes in Old Age

Physiological changes in various organ systems are briefly discussed below:

1. Central nervous system (CNS):
   - A decrease in the volume of white matter and gray matter due to neuronal loss.
   - A decrease in the cerebral blood flow by up to 10 to 20%.
   - Reduction in the levels of neurotransmitters such as serotonin, dopamine, acetylcholine, and norepinephrine.
   - A decrease in the minimum alveolar requirement (MAC) of general anesthetics.
   - Neuraxial system: Shrinkage of epidural space, diminished cerebrospinal fluid (CSF) volume, and reduced diameter of myelinated fibers: *These physiological changes make aged individuals more sensitive to neuraxial blocks.*

2. Cardiovascular system:
   - Diminished arterial elasticity due to media fibrosis, leading to an increase in systolic pressure and afterload.
   - A decrease in the number of myocytes and an increase in left ventricular (LV) wall thickness, leading to a reduction in myocardial contractility.
   - Diminished beta-adrenergic activity, leading to a decrease in heart rate and baroreceptor reflex.
   - Sclerosis of aortic valves and calcification of mitral valves.

3. Respiratory system:
   - A decrease in the lung tissue elasticity, leading to an increase in closing capacity and residual volume.
   - Ventilation/perfusion mismatch, leading to decrease in PaO_2.
   - A decrease in chest wall compliance and respiratory muscle function, causing increased work of breathing.
   - Impaired ventilatory response to hypercapnia and hypoxia.

4. Renal function:
   - A decrease in the number of glomeruli and renal perfusion.
   - A decrease in glomerular filtration rate (GFR) and creatinine clearance.
   - A gradual increase in blood urea nitrogen (BUN) with aging.
   - Relatively unchanged serum creatinine due to a decrease in muscle mass. *Hence, serum creatinine levels poorly predict renal function in geriatric individuals.*

- Impairment in sodium conservation, concentrating ability, and thirst response predispose aged to dehydration and hyponatremia.
- A decrease in drug excretion.

5. Gastrointestinal system:
   - A decrease in hepatic volume by up to 20 to 40% and a reduction in hepatic blood flow.
   - Decrease in phase I metabolism of drugs.
   - A decrease in levels of albumin and plasma cholinesterase.

6. Endocrine system and metabolic function:
   - A decrease in oxygen consumption with age.
   - Impaired thermoregulation and decrease in heat production predispose the aged to hypothermia.
   - Decreased total body water due to reduced muscle mass and increased body fat.

7. Musculoskeletal system:
   - Reduction in muscle mass and skin atrophy.
   - Frail skin may cause damage to veins during cannulation.
   - Arthritis of various joints causing difficulty in positioning the patients.
   - Degenerative changes in the cervical spine, causing restriction of neck extension and complicating airway management.

8. Pharmacological changes:
   - Decreased clearance of drugs metabolized by the liver and eliminated by the kidneys.
   - The volume of distribution:
     - Reduced for water soluble drugs.
     - Increased for lipid soluble drugs.

- Alterations in plasma protein levels affecting drug distribution and elimination.
- The anesthetic requirement is reduced as evident by reduced MAC.

Anesthetic Considerations

Preoperative Evaluation

Look for chronic health diseases which may have significant anesthetic implications. **Table 26.1** summarizes the major system-wise comorbid illnesses encountered in the elderly.

The following preoperative tests are recommended for geriatric patients scheduled for elective surgical procedures.

1. Complete hemogram: Hemoglobin, total leucocyte count (TLC), differential count, platelet count, and erythrocyte sedimentation rate (ESR).

2. Renal function test: BUN, serum creatinine, and serum electrolytes.

Table 26.1 Chronic health conditions associated with the geriatric age group

System	Chronic disease
Cardiovascular	• Coronary artery disease • Essential hypertension • Atherosclerosis • Arrhythmias • Congestive heart failure • Valvular heart disease: Aortic stenosis, calcific mitral stenosis
Pulmonary	• Pneumonia • Emphysema • Chronic bronchitis
Endocrine	• Diabetes mellitus
Renal	• Obstructive uropathy • Nephropathy (diabetic/ hypertensive)
Central nervous system	• Dementia • Depression
Metabolic	• Malnutrition • Dehydration

3. Serum albumin.

4. Fasting blood glucose.

5. 12-lead ECG, echocardiography.

6. Chest X-ray.

General Anesthesia

Table 26.2 enlists anesthetic consideration of commonly used drugs for general anesthesia. Other considerations are as follows:

- Titrated boluses of induction agents to be administered.

- Shorter acting opioids like remifentanil are preferred.

- Cisatracurium is eliminated by Hofmann degradation, which is not influenced by age.

- Hypotension due to fall in systemic vascular resistance is more pronounced in geriatric age and can be treated with α adrenergic agonists.

- Care to be taken to prevent hypothermia.

Neuraxial Block

- Faster onset and more extensive spread with hyperbaric bupivacaine during subarachnoid block; no effect on the motor block.

- More profound hypotension can be observed.

- Technically difficult due to degenerative changes in the vertebral column; also, difficulty in positioning the patient.

- Advantages: The lesser the incidence of thromboembolism, the more preserved is the respiratory function.

Postoperative Cognitive Dysfunction

- It is defined as the "*objective decline in cognitive function, persisting beyond the period of expected normal recovery from the pharmacological effects of anesthesia and surgery.*"

- Risk factors include the following:

  ▶ Geriatric age.

  ▶ Previous history of delirium.

  ▶ Drugs: Psychotropics, anticholinergics, opioids, alcoholism.

  ▶ Pain, deprivation of sleep.

  ▶ Preoperative cognitive assessment in high-risk individuals.

In people with pre-existing cognitive deficits, the preoperative assessment and cooperation for anesthesia becomes difficult. In addition, the postoperative care also becomes challenging.

Table 26.2 Clinical pharmacology of general anesthetic agents in geriatric individuals

Anesthetic agent	Pharmacologic changes in aged
Inhalational agents	• ↓ MAC by 4% per decade of age above 40 years • ↑ V_d • ↓ Pulmonary exchange • Prolonged recovery
IV induction agents, benzodiazepines, and opioids	• ↑ Sensitivity • ↓ Clearance • ↓ Dose requirement
Neuromuscular blockers	• Pancuronium and vecuronium: ↓ Clearance • Atracurium and cisatracurium: Unaffected • Succinylcholine: Slower onset

Abbreviations: IV, intravenous; MAC, minimum alveolar concentration; V_d, volume of distribution.

Perioperative management to minimize the risk of postoperative cognitive dysfunction (POCD) includes the following:

- Regional anesthesia to be preferred whenever possible.
- Maintenance of optimum blood pressure preoperatively.
- Opioid-sparing techniques for management of pain.
- Identify and treat the cause of postoperative delirium.

Conclusion

With aging, there is a progressive decline in the functional reserve of organs, leading to the decreased vital capacity of lungs, decreased cardiorespiratory system's ability to tolerate surgical stress, and decreased ability to metabolize and excrete the anesthetic agents by the liver and kidneys. Preoperative assessment may be challenging due to cognitive decline. The cognitive decline also complicates the assessment of pain in the postoperative period. The chance of difficult bag and mask ventilation is high (due to loss of cheek fat and loss of teeth). Geriatric patients often have multiple comorbid illnesses and are on multiple drugs; the interaction with anesthetic agents requires choosing an appropriate anesthetic agent. These patients are very sensitive to opioids; hence, minimal dosage should be used to avoid respiratory complications.

CHAPTER 27

Anesthesia for Obese Patients

Ganasekran Srinivasan

Introduction

The word obesity is coined from a Latin word *obesus,* which means fattened by overeating. Body mass index (BMI) is the most commonly used epidemiological tool to assess obesity, which is obtained as follows:

BMI = body weight (kg)/height (metre^2).

Other useful terms are as follows:

- Ideal body weight (IBW) in kg = height (cm) – 100 in males and 105 in females.

- Lean body weight (LBW) = total body weight, excluding body fat.

The WHO classification of obesity is summarized in **Table 27.1.**

The number of obese individuals is on the rise worldwide, and so is the number of patients reaching to the operation theater. An obese patient may come for weight-reduction surgery (bariatric surgery) or nonbariatric surgery. The anesthetic management of obese individuals is often challenging and complicated because of multiple comorbidities and associated difficult

Table 27.1 WHO classification of obesity according to BMI

Classification	BMI (kg/m^2)
Underweight	<18.5
Normal weight	18.5–24.9
Overweight	25.0–29.9
Obese	
• Class I	30.0–34.9
• Class II	35.0–39.9
• Class III	40.0–49.9
Superobese	≥50

Abbreviation: BMI, body mass index.

airway. The various medical and surgical diseases related to obesity are mentioned in **Table 27.2.**

Anesthetic Management of Obese Patients

Minimally invasive surgical treatment (bariatric surgery) is increasingly popular worldwide. The surgical procedure can be classified into the following:

- Restrictive type (sleeve gastrectomy, laparoscopic adjustable gastric banding).

- Malabsorptive type (jejunoileal bypass, biliopancreatic diversion).

The goal of surgery is to reduce the volume of the stomach in order to achieve desired weight loss. A thorough preoperative evaluation of the obese patient with a focus on cardiovascular system, respiratory system, and airway is necessary.

Table 27.2 Medical/surgical conditions associated with obesity

Organ system	Disorders
Cardiovascular	• Coronary heart disease • Cardiomyopathy • Hypertension
Respiratory	• Restrictive lung disease • Obstructive sleep apnea • Obesity hypoventilation syndrome
Nervous system	• Cerebrovascular disease
Endocrine	• Diabetes mellitus • Hypothyroidism • Cushing's syndrome • Metabolic syndrome
Musculoskeletal	• Osteoarthritis
Malignancy	• Carcinoma of endometrium, cervix, prostate, breast, colon

Preoperative Assessment

It is important to assess the patient, taking into account his general and systemic well-being.

General Assessment

Height and weight should be measured to calculate BMI. The LBW and adjusted body weight to be calculated for accurate dosing of drugs.

Cardiovascular Assessment

History of chest pain, dyspnea on exertion, and palpitations should be asked to evaluate the cardiovascular system. The level of physical activity should be quantified into a number of metabolic equivalents (METs). The presence of fatigue, dyspnoea, and syncope may suggest pulmonary hypertension and must be ruled out.

Respiratory Assessment

The symptoms of obstructive sleep apnoea should be assessed using the STOP-BANG questionnaire (**Table 27.3**). *The STOP-BANG score of ≥5 indicates significant sleep apnea, and polysomnography is warranted.* The patients with substantial obstructive sleep apnea (OSA) may be on bilevel positive airway pressure (BiPAP) device to relieve the upper airway obstruction and prevent hypoxia.

Table 27.3 STOP-BANG questionnaire to screen OSA

Snoring: Do you **snore** loudly? (Loud enough to be heard through closed doors)	Yes/No
Tired: Do you feel **tired**/sleepy during the daytime often?	Yes/No
Observed: Has anyone **observed** you stop breathing/choking during sleep?	Yes/No
Pressure: Do you have/on treatment for high blood **pressure**?	Yes/No
BMI: BMI > 35 kg/m^2	Yes/No
Age: Age > 50 years	Yes/No
Neck: Neck circumference > 40 cm	Yes/No
Gender: Male	Yes/No

Abbreviations: BMI, body mass index; OSA, obstructive sleep apnea.

Notes: Risk of OSA is categorized as follows:

- High: Yes to 5 to 8 questions.
- Intermediate: Yes to 3 to 4 questions.
- Low: Yes to 0 to 2 questions.

Gastrointestinal Tract

Obese patients have delayed gastric emptying. Inability to lie supine without coughing and symptoms of heartburn may suggest gastroesophageal reflux disease (GERD), and therefore prolonged fasting (8–12 h) is prudent to minimize the risk of aspiration.

Airway

The detailed airway should focus on the following features:

- Facial features (fat cheeks).
- Presence of short neck and large tongue.
- Size of tonsils.
- Neck movement.
- Size of the breasts.
- Neck circumference at the level of thyroid cartilage (>60 cm is associated with difficult laryngoscopy).
- Mallampatti score.

Investigations

The routine blood investigations are not required in all obese patients; however, it depends on the obesity class, associated organ comorbidity, and the type of surgery. The role of investigations can be summarized as below:

- A 12-lead ECG: It is done to rule out cardiac arrhythmias, ventricular hypertrophy, and myocardial infarction.
- 2D-Echo: It may be required in patients with suspected pulmonary hypertension to identify ventricular dysfunction.
- Blood glucose: In diabetic patients.
- Pulmonary function testing including spirometry: For patients with obstructive and restrictive lung disease.

- Blood gas analysis: In patients with severe OSA to guide perioperative ventilatory management.

Premedication

- Avoid sedative premedication.
- Antiaspiration prophylaxis with H_2 blockers and a prokinetic (metoclopramide).
- Antisialogogue (glycopyrrolate) if awake fiberoptic intubation is planned.
- Deep vein thrombosis (DVT) prophylaxis with low-molecular weight heparin.

Choice of Anesthesia

Regional Anesthesia

As per the American Society of Anesthesiologists (ASA) practice recommendations, regional anesthesia (spinal, epidural) and peripheral nerve blocks should be preferred in obese individuals whenever possible. The regional anesthesia may be technically challenging due to difficulty in identifying bony landmarks. The use of ultrasound can increase the success of peripheral nerve blocks. The use of regional anesthesia decreases the need for analgesics, especially opioids, and hence decrease the risk of respiratory depression.

- Neuraxial blocks: Sitting position is preferred, and use extra-long spinal and epidural needles, with reduced volume of local anesthetics.
- Concerns with peripheral nerve blocks:
  ‣ Difficulty in positioning.
  ‣ Anatomic landmarks are difficult to identify.
  ‣ Needle length not adequate.
  ‣ The local anesthetic dose should be as per IBW.

General Anesthesia

General anesthesia in obese patients is complicated by the presence of difficult airway and risk of opioid-related respiratory depression.

Intraoperative Management

1. **Positioning:** The specially designed table with more weight-bearing capacity and extra width is required for the obese patients. Extra care is taken during positioning to avoid rhabdomyolysis. Pressure points should be protected to prevent necrosis. Arms should be well-supported and in neutral position to prevent brachial plexus injury.

2. **Airway management:** It is the most challenging component of anesthetic care in obese patients. The below-mentioned concerns are noteworthy:

   - The airway in obese patients should be anticipated as difficult, and the difficult airway cart with laryngeal mask airway (LMA), bougie, video laryngoscopes, fiberoptic bronchoscopes should be available.
   - OSA increases the risk of difficult mask ventilation and intubation; hence, awake fiberoptic intubation is preferred in severe OSA.
   - Ramp position: This is achieved with commercially available ready-made pillows or by placing folded towels beneath the head and shoulder, thereby placing the tip of chin above the level of the chest. The ramping aligns the oral, pharyngeal, and the laryngeal axes and therefore improves the laryngoscopic view.
   - Obese patients desaturate rapidly due to decreased functional residual capacity (FRC) and elevated O_2 consumption. Adequate preoxygenation in a head-up position is essential to avoid hypoxia during airway management. *The addition of continuous positive airway pressure (CPAP) of around 10 cm of H_2O during*

preoxygenation helps in maintaining oxygenation.

3. **Induction and maintenance of anesthesia:** The change in volume of distribution due to an increase in adipose tissue, increased cardiac output, and variable protein binding makes drug dosing difficult in obese patients. *The LBW correlates well with the cardiac output and the drug clearance and should be used for initial dosing.* The important considerations are summarized below:

- Rapid sequence induction (RSI) can be considered due to the increased risk of gastric aspiration.

- Fat-soluble drugs have increased volume of distribution; dosage should be calculated according to IBW; less fat-soluble drug dosage should be based on LBW.

- *Desflurane is the inhaled anesthetic of choice (poor lipophilicity results in rapid onset and recovery).*

- The muscle relaxants (nondepolarizing) should be given according to the LBW. *The addition of neuromuscular monitoring helps in accurate dosing and prevents postoperative residual paralysis.*

- The dosing of succinylcholine should be based on total body weight (*because of increased plasma pseudocholinesterase and volume of distribution*).

- The recent literature suggests the superiority of sugammadex over neostigmine in preventing postoperative recurarization.

- Invasive arterial pressure monitoring is indicated if appropriate-sized cuffs are not available.

- Intraoperative positive end-expiratory pressure (PEEP) improves oxygenation and prevents atelectasis.

- The fluid administration should be LBW-based with the target of euvolemia. In patients with preexisting cardiac disease, the administration of excess fluid can cause pulmonary edema.

- Tracheal extubation should be done when the patient is fully awake and alert. The head-up position (>30 degrees), application of PEEP/CPAP, and continued oxygen supplementation after extubation prevents atelectasis and hypoxemia.

Postoperative Management

These patients are at risk of postoperative hypoxemia, and therefore, careful monitoring is warranted to prevent respiratory complications. The postoperative care can be summarized as follows:

- Monitoring should be continued in a high-dependency unit (HDU) setup.

- Noninvasive CPAP can be given with O_2 supplementation (especially in patients with severe OSA).

- Nonopioid-based analgesia with nonsteroidal anti-inflammatory drug (NSAID) is preferred in the postoperative period.

- Early mobilization is preferred, although it is difficult.

- DVT prophylaxis should be instituted if early mobilization is not possible.

- Adequate pain relief and a completely alert state should be ensured before shifting the patient to unmonitored settings.

Conclusion

Obese patients have higher fat mass compared to lean individuals. Deposition of excess fat on the floor of the mouth makes the airway difficult. Similarly, the deposition of fat in the skin makes intravenous access challenging. The higher adipose tissue content accumulates lipophilic anesthetic agents (e.g., isoflurane and fentanyl); hence, recovery gets delayed after prolonged exposure to such agents. The dosing of individual anesthetic agents should be guided by the type of bodyweight appropriate for the particular drug. These patients are at increased risk of deep venous thrombosis, and adequate measures must be taken during the perioperative period to minimize the same. Securing the airway safely, avoiding overdosing on lipophilic drugs, and preventing airway complications during the perioperative course are the cornerstones of anesthetic management in such patients.

CHAPTER 28

Anesthesia for Laparoscopy

Ajisha Aravindan and Avishek Roy

Introduction

Laparoscopic surgeries have become the standard of care for modern practice by surgeons. The word *laparoscopy* means the visualization of the abdominal cavity via an endoscope. Surgeries are performed after lifting the anterior abdominal wall and creating space by inflating the abdomen with the help of gases, most commonly carbon dioxide (CO_2). It has become the preferred mode of many surgeries like cholecystectomy, hysterectomy, splenectomy, bariatric procedures, and even cancer surgeries. In the 1980s, it did not show better outcomes, as often the intra-abdominal pressure (IAP) used was more than 20 mm Hg. Modern-day laparoscopic surgeries are performed at IAP between 12 and 14 mm Hg with better anesthesia techniques and advanced monitoring, leading to better outcomes.

The advantages of laparoscopy over laparotomy are as follows:

- *Reduction of the stress response and pain due to surgery*: Laparoscopy is less invasive, and incisions are smaller and less painful.

- *Early wound healing*: Due to the reduced stress response, plasma levels of proinflammatory cytokines like IL-6, CRP, and intraoperative glucose levels during laparoscopy are lesser than open surgery. Elevated levels of the above are associated with delayed wound healing and delayed return of gastrointestinal (GI) functions. The reduced stress response also negates the negative nitrogen balance, thus promoting wound healing.

- *Improved postoperative function*: Patients become ambulatory early with laparoscopy than with open surgery because of the reduced pain.

- *Better cosmetic appearance*: Smaller size of incision gives a better cosmetic appearance.

The Technique of Laparoscopy

A pneumoperitoneum (air-filled peritoneal cavity) is created by inserting a "Veress" needle either blindly or under camera vision through a small incision in the abdominal wall and connecting it to the gas insufflator. *The abdomen is filled with the gas, starting with 1 to 2 L/min flow and then slowly increasing to not more than 4 to 5 L/min of flows with pressure not exceeding 15 mm Hg, after which a constant flow of 200 to 400 mL/min is maintained to perform surgeries.* One has to be careful during this step as cardiac arrhythmias can occur at this step, due to a sudden stretch of the peritoneum, causing vagal stimulation. To prevent the insufflation-related bradycardia, the upper limit of IAP, especially for patients with cardiovascular disease (discussed later separately) should not exceed 15 mm Hg. The patients are placed in different positions, for example, head up (reverse Trendelenburg) during cholecystectomy and upper abdominal surgery, head down (Trendelenburg) during gynecological/pelvic surgery, etc. The implications of these positions are also important (described later).

Pathophysiological Effects of Laparoscopy

All changes are described with respect to CO_2, which is used most commonly for laparoscopy.

- **Effect of increased IAP pressure:** *Raised IAP pushes the diaphragm upward, causing a reduction of functional residual capacity (FRC) by almost 30 to 50%.* Lung compliance is reduced, peak, and plateau pressure increases, leading to increased work of breathing (WOB). *These changes are marked in patients with chronic obstructive pulmonary disorder (COPD), obesity, and other pulmonary diseases.* Raised IAP reduces venous return to the heart and increases the arteriolar resistance, all of which may reduce the cardiac output. It also decreases renal blood flow and glomerular filtration rate (GFR). The rise in IAP > 20 mm Hg may cause reduced splanchnic blood flow and acidosis. Raised IAP and peritoneal stretch, along with surgical stress, increase blood levels of catecholamines, glucose, and vasopressin.

- **Effect of hypercapnia:** CO_2 is a pulmonary vasoconstrictor and a systemic vasodilator. The combination of the above effect with its permissive effect on the sympathetic nervous system can cause a variable impact on the vasculature. *$PaCO_2$ (partial pressure of CO_2) in the blood begins to rise almost immediately after pneumoperitoneum by nearly 15 to 20% of baseline levels until 20 to 30 minutes after surgery, after which it plateaus.* The main mechanism of the rise in $PaCO_2$ is absorption through the peritoneum, but hypoventilation and increased WOB in a spontaneously breathing patient may also contribute to it. *Minute ventilation (MV) should be increased by 10 to 20% in order to maintain normocarbia.* Although the difference between arterial and expired CO_2 ($PaCO_2$–$EtCO_2$) remains constant for healthy individuals, it might increase in patients with cardiopulmonary disease, probably because of increased dead space and shunt. Due to raised IAP, venous return and blood flow through pulmonary vasculature are reduced, and pulmonary resistance is increased, leading to increased dead space. In obese individuals, the loss of FRC increases the amount of nonventilated alveoli at the bases (atelectasis), causing an increase in the shunt fraction. *In COPD patients, this $PaCO_2$–$EtCO_2$ gap increases quite significantly, and hence, $EtCO_2$ tracing becomes unreliable in predicting arterial CO_2 levels in this subset of patients.* A lower $EtCO_2$ level of 35 to 40 mm Hg should be kept as a target, or $PaCO_2$ monitoring should be done by arterial blood gas analysis. CO_2 also stimulates the sympathetic nervous system, causing a rise in heart rate and blood pressure intraoperatively.

- **Effect on the cardiovascular system:** Due to pneumoperitoneum-induced compression of the inferior vena cava (IVC), preload to the heart reduces. Intermittent positive pressure ventilation leads to a rise in intrathoracic pressure (ITP) and central venous pressure (CVP), further reducing the preload. A combination of aortic compression and sympathetic stimulation increases systemic vascular resistance (SVR). In head-elevated positions, venous pooling in lower extremities further reduces preload, while in head-down posture, preload increases. These factors reduce cardiac output, whereas stimulation of the sympathetic nervous system tends to increase it. The net effect is determined by the interplay between the above factors. In patients with fixed low cardiac output states like valvular stenosis and heart failure with reduced ejection fraction

(EF), it may lead to hypotension. The rise in PaCO$_2$ and catecholamines may lead to arrhythmias intraoperatively. *During pneumo-insufflation, peritoneal stretch leads to intense vagal stimulation and bradyar-rhythmias, especially in patients with higher vagal tone. Among the various cardiac indices, mean arterial pressure (MAP), CVP, and pulmonary artery occlusion pressure (PAOP) rises, and measurement of right atrial pressure (RAP) and PAOP becomes unreliable during laparoscopy.*

- **Effect on respiratory system:** Raised IAP increases ITP and pulmonary vascular resist-ance, and the cranial shift of diaphragm decreases FRC, causing atelectasis. Due to the reduction of pulmonary blood flow, dead space ventilation increases, and the reduction of FRC increases the shunt fraction. This induces ventilation-perfusion (V/Q) mismatch and hypoxia. These changes may be more marked in obese individuals and COPD patients. Keeping IAP below 15 mm Hg, increasing minute ventilation, and application of positive end-expiratory pressure (PEEP) may attenuate these changes. Head elevation and descent up to 10° are well-tolerated. Anesthesia induced hypoventilation in a spontane-ously breathing patient may increase PaCO$_2$ further, which needs controlled ventilation and an increase in minute ventilation.

- **Effect on kidney, liver, and splanchnic bed:** Raised IAP decreases renal blood flow (RBF) and raises efferent arteriolar resistance, reducing the gradient of glomerular filtration. As much as a 50% reduction of RBF and GFR ensuing pneumoperitoneum, along with increased vasopressin levels, can lead to temporary oliguria. In otherwise healthy individuals, the renal function returns to normal once the CO$_2$ washes off, and IAP becomes normal. *Giving a small dose of a diuretic may also increase urine output by anti-ADH mediated activity.* IAP > 20 mm Hg may reduce hepatic and GI blood flow. But clinically, these events are rare, as CO$_2$ has a vasodilator effect.

- **Effect on the central nervous system (CNS) and eyes:** The rise in PaCO$_2$ leads to vasodilatation of the cerebral vessels and a rise in intracranial pressure (ICP). This vasodilator effect is noticed at PaCO$_2$ levels from 25 up to 80 mm Hg. A transient rise in intraocular pressure (IOP) is also seen with pneumoperitoneum. This rise in ICP and IOP is worsened by steep head low positions used in pelvic surgeries. Therefore, laparoscopy is not recommended for patients with intracranial lesions with features of raised ICP.

Gases Used in Laparoscopy

The ideal gas used in laparoscopy should have no physiological effect, should be rapidly excreted, be noncombustible (as cautery used in laparoscopy cause fire), and should be highly soluble.

The most commonly used gas is CO$_2$ as it is noncombustible, easily available, soluble in the blood (Ostwald's blood-gas solubility constant 0.49), and easily excreted. *But hypercapnia (excess CO$_2$ in blood) can cause acidosis by combining with water, and vasodilation of all vascular beds except pulmonary vessels, where it causes vasoconstriction.* CO$_2$ also causes activation of the sympathetic nervous system. Nitrogen and air are cheap and easily available, noncombustible, and have low Ostwald's blood-gas solubility (0.017), which might lead to an increased chance of gas embolism. Although inert gases like helium and argon are noncombustible, their cost and lesser blood solubility preclude their use, as they might expand and cause an air embolism. In addition, argon can reduce hepatic blood flow. N$_2$O supports combustion, and despite the fact that it is soluble (0.42), it might diffuse into air bubbles and cause their expansion and embolism. The individual gases and their properties are enlisted in **Table 28.1**.

Anesthesia Management

Laparoscopy is preferably performed under general anesthesia (GA) with a muscle relaxant; anesthesia-induced hypoventilation can lead to hypercapnia in spontaneously breathing patients. It can be performed under regional anesthesia (RA) with sedation as well, but the requirement of the high level of the block (up to T4–T5) and diaphragmatic irritation (due to fluids or blood under diaphragm) make it an inconvenient choice. RA (spinal block) can be used for a short duration with slightly lower IAP values of 10 to 12 mm Hg in patients with significant pulmonary disease, for example, COPD, bullae, which precludes positive pressure ventilation (PPV). The proposed advantages of RA over GA include effective

postoperative pain relief, no airway manipulation, shorter postoperative stay, cost-effectiveness, and reduced incidence of postoperative nausea and vomiting (PONV).

Important aspects of anesthesia management include:

- **Choice of airway device:** Endotracheal tube (ETT) is the standard of choice, which is combined with a separate gastric tube (Ryles'/suction catheter) that is inserted after intubation to deflate the stomach contents. Second-generation supraglottic airway (SGA) devices with gastric channel have been used with success in many surgeries. The need for higher airway pressures for ventilation, especially in obese individuals and in head low positions, can cause SGA dislodgement and leak. Hence, it may be used only by experienced anesthesiologists with utmost caution in select cases.

Table 28.1 Gases used in laparoscopy

Gases	Advantages	Disadvantages
CO_2	• Noncombustible • Highly soluble • Easily available • Cheap • Easily excreted	• Physiological changes due to hypercapnia
Air, oxygen	• Cheap, easily available	• Combustion • Air embolism
Nitrogen	• Cheap, easily available	• Gas embolism
Helium	• No physiological changes • Non-combustible	• Costly • Gas embolism
Argon	• No physiological changes • Non-combustible	• Costly • Gas embolism • Decrease hepatic blood flow
Nitrous oxide	• May be used for high-risk patients undergoing laparoscopy under regional anesthesia	• Supports combustion • May expand into air-filled cavities, cause an air embolism, bowel distension, etc

- **Monitoring:** Standard American Society of Anesthesiologists (ASA) monitors like EtCO$_2$, NIBP, SpO$_2$, ECG, and temperature suffice for most of the cases. Patients with poor ASA category (ASA class 3/4) and cardiovascular disease may need invasive (intra-arterial) blood pressure (IBP) monitoring.

- **Pneumo-insufflation:** During this step, bradyarrhythmias can occur due to sudden peritoneal stretch, which requires vigilant attention and management. Settings of the IAP should always be closely monitored by the anesthesiologist. A moderate IAP 12 to 15 mm Hg is advised for most surgeries to limit significant changes in splanchnic circulation and its associated cardiovascular complications. The proper anesthetic depth and use of muscle relaxants help to keep the IAP < 15 mm Hg.

- **Choice of anesthetic agents:** Inhalational agents (isoflurane, desflurane, and sevoflurane) are most commonly used in combination with opioids and muscle relaxants. N$_2$O is generally avoided because it can expand into air-filled spaces, leading to gas embolism, pneumothorax, bowel distension, etc. However, clinically it has been used without any significant side effects for short duration surgeries of less than 2 hours. Total intravenous anesthesia using propofol and fentanyl infusion can also be used to provide optimal surgical conditions for laparoscopy. Total intravenous anesthesia (TIVA) may be associated with a slight reduction in PONV due to propofol, but the evidence for this is lacking. Patient comorbidities must be kept in mind while choosing the anesthetic agents.

- **Patient position:** Implications of head up and head down position have been described. In addition to that, steep head down needed during robotic prostatectomy can cause laryngeal, cerebral edema, and raised IOP. Strapping around legs should be done gently to avoid common peroneal nerve injury, and careful padding of other bony prominences should be done to prevent pressure ulcers and stretch on other nerve plexuses, especially in obese patients. Many surgical positions require both arms to be strapped by the side of the patient, which limits the access to the intravenous (IV) line. In such situations, IV line extensions must be used after proper de-airing.

- **Fluid management:** Restrictive or goal-directed fluid strategy can be applied. During head down position, special care must be taken to avoid fluid overload, which may lead to cerebral, orbital, and laryngeal edema.

- **Analgesia:** Skin and the peritoneal incision can cause somatic pain, while peritoneal stretch and visceral handling cause dull aching visceral pain. Options for analgesia include IV and intrathecal opioids, local port-site infiltration, epidural analgesia, and truncal blocks like transversus abdominis plane (TAP) block and quadratus lumborum (QL) block. In most cases, IV opioids, nonsteroidal anti-inflammatory drugs (NSAIDs), paracetamol, and local infiltration provide satisfactory analgesia.

- **PONV:** Laparoscopy evokes PONV. Prophylactic administration of a combination of dexamethasone and 5-HT$_3$ antagonists is routinely practiced for most cases. The addition of metoclopramide to the combination may be beneficial in patients with a high risk of PONV.

Special Scenarios

Pregnancy: Physiological changes like the reduction of FRC and ensuing hypoxia during pregnancy can be accentuated during laparoscopy. Due to the compensated respiratory alkalosis seen in a pregnant patient, targeting a lower PaCO$_2$ of 30 to 35 mm Hg is advisable. *Surgeries are preferred during the second trimester, as any intra-abdominal surgery under anesthesia has the inherent risk of damage to fetal organogenesis during the first trimester, and during the third trimester, there is less room for surgery due to gravid uterus and high risk of premature labor.* Pregnancy being a prothrombotic state, application of pneumatic compression device (PCD) to the lower limbs is a must for deep venous thrombosis (DVT) prophylaxis.

Pediatric patients: The physiological effects of pneumoperitoneum and extremes positions are exaggerated in children. *IAP has to be kept at a lower level of 5 to 10 mm Hg for infants and 10 to 12 mm Hg for small children, and the rate of insufflation should be reduced to <1 L/min.* The absorptive surface area per body weight for CO$_2$ is more in children, so there is rapid systemic absorption of CO$_2$, leading to early hypercapnia and its associated adverse effects.

Patients with cardiovascular disease: Slow pneumo-insufflation (at 1–2 L/min), IBP monitoring, preload optimization to maintain cardiac output, and good analgesia are sine-qua-non (meaning absolutely necessary) for cardiac patients undergoing laparoscopy. The rest of the management depends on case-to-case basis, for example, inotropic support for low cardiac output states, beta-blockers to reduce heart rate in coronary artery disease (CAD) patients, monitoring urine output, and keeping postoperative monitored bed.

Patients with intracranial pathology: Laparoscopy is generally avoided due to hypercapnia-induced raised ICP secondary to cerebral vasodilation.

Complications of Laparoscopy

Mortality after laparoscopy ranges from 0.1 to 1 per 1,000 patients. The noteworthy complications are as follows:

- **Surgical emphysema (SE):** Egress of gas into the subcutaneous space causes surgical emphysema. It is diagnosed by the presence of subcutaneous swelling and crepitus on the skin. Risk factors of SE include age > 65 years, >200-minute surgery, *and Nissens fundoplication (here the peritoneum is cut near its diaphragmatic attachment, permitting air entry into the mediastinum and subcutaneous tissue).* In the presence of cervical emphysema, it is recommended to keep the patient intubated until it subsides, in order to avoid airway obstruction. SE generally is self-limiting and resolves once CO$_2$ is absorbed.

- **Pneumothorax, pneumo-mediastinum, and pneumopericardium:** Extension of emphysema into the thorax and mediastinum or congenital defects in the diaphragm can cause pneumothorax and pneumo-mediastinum during laparoscopy. Although rare, a pneumothorax can evoke massive hemodynamic perturbations and has been reported mostly with fundoplication (along with surgical emphysema). It presents with an increase in EtCO$_2$ and reduced breath sounds on the side of pneumothorax, and is associated with desaturation and paradoxical ballooning of the hemidiaphragm on the affected side. The important steps of management include the release of pneumoperitoneum, which helps in the reduction of IAP, stopping N$_2$O, and the addition of PEEP. Most of the cases do not need any intervention, as they are mild and self-limiting. But the presence of tension pneumothorax may necessitate immediate placement of a chest drain. *When CO₂ is present inside the pleural cavity, it is called "capnothorax."* Capnothorax can be dangerous as CO_2 rapidly gets absorbed from the larger surface area of both the peritoneum and pleural cavity.

- **Endobronchial intubation:** Frequently seen with laparoscopy in a head-down position, as the tube migrates into one of the bronchi, more commonly the right bronchus. This complication should be suspected with raised P_{PEAK} (peak airway pressure) and raised P_{PLAT} (plateau pressure), absence of breath sound on one side of the chest, and desaturation. Treatment involves pulling the tube out (preferably under laryngoscopy guidance) until breath sounds are heard equally on both sides of the chest.

- **Hypercapnia:** Systemic CO_2 absorption, V/Q mismatch, and hypoventilation in a spontaneously breathing patient under anesthesia all lead to hypercapnia. CO_2 levels peak within 30 minutes and can usually be managed by increasing minute ventilation by 15 to 20%. Any rise in $PaCO_2$ beyond this time point should raise the suspicion of other complications like capnothorax, CO_2 emphysema, etc. At the end of the surgery, CO_2 diffuses back into the blood, causing temporary hypercapnia and can remain elevated in the postoperative period.

- **Atelectasis:** In obese patients, basal atelectasis is a real concern. The performance of the periodic recruitment maneuver, along with the application of optimal PEEP, can ameliorate this problem.

- **Gas embolism (GE):** Inadvertent entry of air into a vessel can occur during the insertion of the Veress needle or from cut vessels during surgery. *Expansion of gas bubbles inside a vessel, seen more commonly with gases with low solubility*, can cause catastrophic consequences like obstructive shock, right ventricular failure, and pulmonary edema. *A transient rise in right ventricular pressure can open up foramen ovale (FO), even in healthy individuals (incidence of patent FO in a healthy individual is around 20–30%) and cause a paradoxical embolism.* GE is diagnosed with a sudden drop in EtCO₂, desaturation, and hypotension. If massive, it can lead to cardiac arrest. Echocardiography may show the presence of a gas bubble or dilated right atrium/right ventricle. Treatment includes supportive management including fluid resuscitation and vasopressor support, avoiding N_2O, giving 100% O_2, *putting the patient in head down left lateral (Durant position)*, and placement of central venous line to facilitate aspiration of the gas/air.

- **DVT:** Increased femoral venous pressure and pooling of blood in lower limbs can cause thrombosis of deep veins of legs, especially during prolonged surgeries in the presence of some other prothrombotic state like pregnancy or malignancy. The use of mechanical and/or pharmacological thromboprophylaxis is advisable in such conditions.

- **Gastric aspiration:** Theoretically raised IAP can cause gastric aspiration. However, this raised IAP also gets transmitted to the lower esophageal tone (LES), which prevents aspiration of gastric contents.

Contraindications of Laparoscopy

Although there are no absolute contraindications, the benefit of laparoscopy has to be weighed against its risk in patients with severe cardiovascular and pulmonary disorders. Hemodynamic instability can be further exacerbated with laparoscopy; so it is best avoided in patients with hemodynamic instability and severe hypovolemia. It is also avoided in patients with raised ICP (brain tumor, bleeding, etc.).

Conclusion

Laparoscopy surgeries are associated with significant cardiorespiratory stress to the patient. The Trendelenburg position can further add to cardiorespiratory stress. In addition, it also affects splanchnic and renal perfusion. An anesthetist must be aware of the adverse systemic effects of laparoscopy surgeries (related to pneumoperitoneum, patient positioning) and should set appropriate goals for each organ. There should be clear communication between the surgeon and the anesthesia provider to minimize complications related to laparoscopy surgeries.

CHAPTER 29

Anesthesia for Ophthalmic Surgeries

Ankur Sharma

Introduction

The aims of anesthetic management during eye surgery are pain-free procedures, quick recovery, and reducing complications. Patients who undergo eye surgery are mostly at the extreme end of their age and require vigilant intraoperative and postoperative monitoring and care.

Anatomy of the Eye

The eye and orbit can be viewed as a pyramid-shaped structure, whose base faces anteriorly and apex posteriorly. The eye's motor nerves consist of the 3rd, 4th, and 6th cranial nerves that are responsible for eye motility and the 7th cranial nerve for the frontalis and orbicularis oculi movement. The 3rd cranial nerve (oculomotor) supplies the medial, inferior, and superior recti and the inferior oblique muscles. The superior oblique is innervated by the 4th cranial nerve (trochlear), and the lateral rectus is innervated by the 6th cranial nerve (abducens). The facial nerve is split into the upper zygomatic branch, which supplies the upper lid's frontalis muscle and orbicularis oculi. The lower zygomatic branch supplies the orbicularis oculi of the lower eyelid. The 5th cranial nerve covers the sensory nerve supply of the eye and its adnexa.

Preoperative Evaluation

The preoperative medical assessment involves an examination of comorbid conditions and perioperative decision-making about prescribed medications to continue or not. People with diabetes should check blood sugar levels the day before surgery. On the morning of surgery, all diabetic medicine should be omitted. Hypertensive patients must get their blood pressure (BP) checked preoperatively.

All patients receiving regional anesthesia fasted from midnight of the day before surgery. Regular airway inspection should always be done. Detection of specific irregularities, including those symptoms that intervene with comfortable supine lying (e.g., congestive heart failure, chronic obstructive pulmonary disease [COPD], back pain, or claustrophobia), should be undertaken cautiously during preanesthetic evaluation.

Besides observing the patient's oral drugs, the anesthesiologist should be cautious of possible systemic consequences of these chronically administered ophthalmic solutions. Timolol eye drop, nonselective beta-adrenoreceptor antagonists, can decrease heart rate and increase systemic vascular resistance. Some ophthalmic solutions' systemic effects include increased heart rate (HR) or BP with muscarinic agonists like pilocarpine, increased blood pressure by phenylephrine, etc.

Choice of Anesthetic Technique

The type of operation, the estimated length, age, and fitness of the patient can affect the anesthetic technique. It can be done under topical, local, or regional and general anesthesia (**Fig. 29.1**).

1. Topical anesthesia

Topical anesthesia is a safe option in situations where the surgeon may not need full akinesia. It is the most common anesthesia technique for

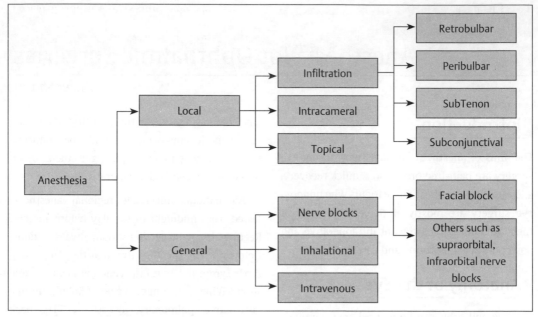

Fig. 29.1 Different techniques of ophthalmic anesthesia.

cataract and intraocular glaucoma surgery. Other applications include:

- Eye examination to allay pain.
- Tonometry.
- Gonioscopy.
- Corneal and conjunctival foreign body removal.
- Fundoscopy.
- Laser procedures.

The anesthesiologist applies a local anesthetic eye drop to the cornea and conjunctiva (e.g., 2% lidocaine, 0.5% proparacaine). It is rapid-acting (within 20 s) and lasts between 15 and 20 minutes. It is contraindicated in the presence of penetrating eye injury. It is the simplest method for anesthesia for the anterior eye chamber and can be employed as the sole anesthetic technique. Complication risk is minimal relative to other anesthetic techniques as no needle is used. It cannot provide eye akinesia. As the patient must remain motionless for the whole process, the proper patient selection is critical.

2. Intracameral anesthesia

Topical anesthesia can be combined with 1% lignocaine solution injection into the anterior chamber through paracentesis or side-port incision. This gives iris and ciliary body anesthesia.

3. Regional anesthesia

Regional anesthesia is more widely employed for cataract and glaucoma surgeries and less often for vitreoretinal surgery. It can be helpful in patients unable to tolerate general anesthesia. The objective of regional anesthesia is twofold. First, it achieves lid and eye muscle akinesia. Second, it provides analgesia to the eye. Lignocaine hydrochloride or bupivacaine with or without 1:1000 adrenaline and hyaluronidase are usually used in regional anesthesia. The incorporation of hyaluronidase enhances tissue permeability of the local drug and helps diffuse local anesthetic. Epinephrine is sometimes used to increase the anesthesia duration.

In regional anesthesia, facial nerve blocks are performed to obtain lids akinesia. Retrobulbar and peribulbar blocks are administered for both akinesia and globe analgesia.

- **Facial nerve block**

  It prevents squinting of the eyelids during operation and enables the speculation of the lid to be put. There are four techniques of facial block: Van Lint's block, Atkinson block, O' Brien block, and Nadbath block.

  ▶ **Van Lint's block:** The peripheral divisions of the facial nerve are blocked in van Lint's block. This procedure induces orbicularis oculi muscle akinesia without facial paralysis. A total of 2.5 mL of anesthetic agent is administered at the proximity of the orbital rim; the injection site is 1 cm lateral from the lower outer edge of the orbit, at the crossing of lines drawn parallel to the lower and temporal rim of the orbit.

  ▶ **O' Brien's block:** It is also known as the trunk block of the facial nerve. The block is done at the mandible neck in front of the tragus of the ear and near the condyloid process. The needle is placed at this level, and around 4 mL of local anesthetic is injected while removing the needle.

  ▶ **Atkinson's block:** The facial nerve's superior branch is blocked by administering anesthetic solution at the lower zygomatic bone margin.

  ▶ **Nadbath block:** In this block, the facial nerve is blocked at the stylomastoid foramen. It can cause vocal cord paralysis, laryngospasm, dysphagia, and respiratory distress.

- **Retrobulbar block (intraconal block)**

  Herman Knapp first described this method in 1884. A local anesthetic is injected behind the eye into the cone formed by extraocular muscles (**Fig. 29.2**). A blunt-tipped 25-gauge needle penetrates the lower lid at the junction of the middle and lateral one-third of the orbit (usually 0.5 cm

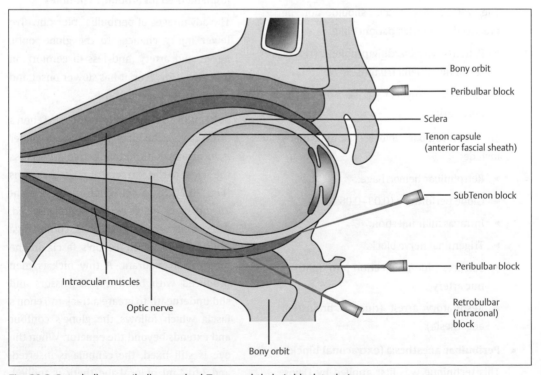

Bony orbit

Peribulbar block

Sclera

Tenon capsule (anterior fascial sheath)

SubTenon block

Peribulbar block

Retrobulbar (intraconal) block

Intraocular muscles

Optic nerve

Bony orbit

Fig. 29.2 Retrobulbar, peribulbar, and subTenon ophthalmic block techniques.

medial to the lateral canthus). Awake patients are told to gaze supranasally when the needle is advanced 3.5 cm to the muscle cone apex. Patients receiving this eye block would usually receive brief sedation during the block. After aspiration to avoid intravascular injection, 2 to 5 mL of local anesthetic is injected. Local anesthetic choices vary, although lidocaine 2% or bupivacaine 0.75% is more commonly used. The addition of epinephrine (1:200,000) can minimize bleeding and prolong anesthesia. Hyaluronidase (3–7 U/mL) is also applied to improve local anesthetic retrobulbar distribution. A retrobulbar block is followed by anesthesia, akinesia, and oculocephalic reflex abolition. Typically, the superior oblique muscle outside the muscle cone is not paralyzed. The retrobulbar block has a quicker onset than a peribulbar block, which is associated with less chemosis (i.e., conjunctiva swelling).

The retrobulbar block should not be practiced in selected patients like:

▸ Patients with bleeding problems (risk of retrobulbar hemorrhage).

▸ Excessive myopia (risk of globe perforation).

The retrobulbar block complications include:

▸ Retrobulbar hemorrhage.

▸ Globe perforation (0.03–0.08%).

▸ Intravascular injection.

▸ Trigeminal nerve block.

▸ Seizures (due to injection into ophthalmic artery).

▸ Respiratory arrest (due to brainstem anesthesia).

• **Peribulbar anesthesia (extraconal block)**

This technique was first applied by Davis. Unlike the retrobulbar blockade, the needle in the peribulbar blockade technique does not penetrate the cone formed by extraocular muscles. In peribulbar block, 6 to 12 mL of local anesthetic is administered into the orbit's peripheral spaces. The anesthetic agent diffuses through the muscle cone and eyelids, inducing global and orbicular akinesia and anesthesia. After topical conjunctiva anesthesia (**Fig. 29.2**), an inferotemporal injection is given halfway between the lateral canthus and the lateral limbus. The needle is progressed under the globe, parallel to the orbital floor; after reaching the eye equator, it is guided slightly medial (20°) and cephalad (10°), and 5 mL of local anesthetic is administered. A second 5-mL injection can be delivered through the conjunctiva on the nasal side, medial to the caruncle, and directed straight back parallel to the medial orbital wall, pointing slightly cephalad (20°). After injection, orbital compression is implemented for around 15 minutes.

The advantages of peribulbar block involve fewer injury chances to the globe, optic nerve, and artery, and less discomfort on injection. However, it has slower onset and a higher risk of ecchymosis.

• **SubTenon (episcleral) block:** Tenon's fascia covers the globe and muscles. Under it, local anesthetic extends circularly across the sclera to the extraocular muscle sheaths (**Fig. 29.2**). For a subTenon block, a blunt 25-mm or 19-gauge curved cannula is used. After topical anesthesia, the conjunctiva is lifted along with Tenon's fascia in the inferonasal quadrant. A tiny nick is then produced with blunt-tipped scissors and slid underneath to create a track in Tenon's fascia which follows the globe's contour and extends beyond the equator. When the eye is still fixed, the cannula is inserted, and 3 to 4 mL of local anesthetic is applied. Complications of subTenon blocks are much less than those of retrobulbar and peribulbar techniques.

A comparison of retrobulbar, peribulbar, and subTenon blocks are shown in **Table 29.1**.

4. Sedation and monitored anesthesia care (MAC)

Many intravenous (IV) sedation techniques are employed for eye surgery. An intraoperative light sedation regimen can be administered, containing midazolam (1–2 mg), either with or without fentanyl (25–50 µg). Doses vary considerably between patients but should be given in small increments. More than one category of medication (benzodiazepine, hypnotic, and opioid) may likely be used in a combination, and the dosage of other agents should be minimized accordingly. American Society of Anesthesiologists (ASA) standard monitors (including capnography for moderate or deep sedation) should be used during the procedure.

5. General anesthesia

General anesthesia is suitable for patients such as:

- Inability to communicate or cooperate.
- Patients with distress or claustrophobia.
- Inability to lie supine.
- Children.

Either endotracheal intubation with a non-depolarizing neuromuscular blocker or laryngeal mask airway (LMA) may be used. Maintaining a deep anesthesia plane is essential to prevent laryngospasm and coughing. Anesthetic agents usually lower intraocular pressure. *The exception to this includes ketamine hydrochloride and succinylcholine, which can elicit intraocular pressure transient elevation.* This should be kept in mind when intraocular pressure is examined under anesthesia (EUA) in children. Also, succinylcholine is not used in penetrating injuries since it increases intraocular pressure.

Table 29.1 Comparison of retrobulbar, peribulbar, and subTenon blocks

Name of block	Advantages	Disadvantages
Retrobulbar	<ul><li>Low volume</li><li>Rapid onset</li><li>Low pressure in orbit (but intraocular pressure may rise)</li><li>Minimum anterior hemorrhage</li></ul>	<ul><li>Skill required</li><li>Risk of damage to the globe and major structures</li><li>Retrobulbar hemorrhage</li><li>Globe perforation</li></ul>
Peribulbar	<ul><li>Reasonable akinesia</li><li>Reliable anesthesia</li><li>Injection away from the key structures of the apex</li><li>Minimum anterior hemorrhage</li></ul>	<ul><li>Skill required</li><li>Although the needle remains tangential to the globe, key structures may be damaged</li><li>Chemosis due to anterior spread of higher volume of local anesthetic agent</li><li>Risks of damage to the globe and major structures less frequent</li><li>Multiple injections required or outside the cone</li></ul>
SubTenon	<ul><li>Simple</li><li>Fast onset</li><li>Reliable anesthesia</li><li>Relatively safe</li><li>The minimum risk to the globe</li></ul>	<ul><li>Skill required</li><li>Chemosis</li><li>Conjunctival hemorrhage</li><li>Serious life-threatening complications are less frequent</li><li>Difficult to perform in patients who had previous and repeated eye surgery</li></ul>

Premedication

Premedication must be offered with caution, and thorough knowledge of the patient's medical condition is necessary. Adult patients are often older patients with various underlying disorders such as arthritis, diabetes mellitus, and coronary artery disease. Pediatric patients can present with congenital conditions.

Induction

Typically, the option of induction for eye surgery relies more on the patient's medical conditions than on the patient's eye disease or the particular operation envisaged. One exception is the patient with a ruptured globe. The key to inducing anesthesia in an open-eye injury patient is to avoid an increase in intraocular pressure with smooth induction. Coughing should be avoided during intubation with a deeper plane of anesthesia and paralysis. Intraocular pressure response to laryngoscopy and endotracheal intubation can be mitigated by IV lidocaine or opioid. Many patients with open globe injuries come with a full stomach and need rapid-sequence induction due to aspiration risk.

Monitoring and Maintenance

Eye surgery pushes the anesthesiologists away from the patient's airway, necessitating pulse oximetry and capnograph monitoring attentively. Endotracheal tube kinking, breathing circuit disconnection, and accidental extubation could be possible. Wire-reinforced or preformed oral RAE (Ring-Adair-Elwyn) endotracheal tube can minimize kinking. The risk of arrhythmias triggered by oculocardiac reflex increases the importance of continuously checking the electrocardiogram (ECG) and ensuring that the pulse sound is audible.

Emesis induced by vagal stimulation is a frequent postoperative problem after eye surgery, particularly with strabismus repair.

Intraoperative IV treatment of a 5-HT3 antagonist (e.g., ondansetron) reduces postoperative nausea and vomiting (PONV). IV dexamethasone (6–8 mg in adults) can also be administered to patients with a strong history of PONV.

Extubation and Emergence

A smooth emergence from general anesthesia is very important to minimize postoperative wound dehiscence. Coughing or gagging from the endotracheal tube stimulation may be reduced by extubating the patient at a reasonably deep level of anesthesia.

Oculocardiac reflex: It is the appearance of cardiac arrhythmias resulting from eye manipulation, specifically during pulling of extraocular muscles. This reflex's afferent and efferent pathways are mediated by trigeminal (V1) and vagus nerve, respectively. It is most often seen in pediatric patients undergoing squint operation, but it may be evoked in all different ages and in any ocular surgery, including cataract extraction, enucleation, and retinal detachment repair.

Oculocardial reflex occurs when traction is applied to extraocular muscles during the surgery. The manifestations include bradycardia (a 10–20% reduction in basal heart rate), junctional rhythms, hypotension, and occasionally asystole. Oculocardial reflex management includes:

- Prompt notification to the surgeon and temporary suspension of surgical stimulation until heart rate increases.

- Ensuring adequate breathing, oxygenation, and anesthesia depth.

- IV atropine (10 µg/kg) if bradycardia persists.

Intraocular Gas Expansion Considerations

During vitreous surgery, an ophthalmologist can inject a gas bubble into the posterior chamber. Intravitreal air injection helps to flatten a detached retina and facilitates healing. The air bubble is dissolved into the bloodstream within 5 days through diffusion into adjacent tissue.

If nitrous oxide is given during anesthesia, the bubble will increase in size, as nitrous oxide is 35 times more soluble in blood than nitrogen. It helps to diffuse into the air bubble faster than nitrogen (the main component of air). If the bubble expands after the eye is closed, intraocular pressure will rise.

Sulfur hexafluoride (SF6) is an inert gas, less soluble in blood than nitrogen. Compared to an air bubble, its longer action time (up to 10 days) will have a therapeutic advantage. Bubble size rises within 24 hours of application, as inhaled air nitrogen reaches the bubble quicker than the sulfur hexafluoride diffuses into the bloodstream. If the patient breathes nitrous oxide, the bubble grows exponentially in size and can contribute to intraocular hypertension.

Complications related to the intraocular expansion of gas bubbles can be minimized with the following measures:

- Avoid nitrous oxide during vitreoretinal surgeries.
- Discontinue nitrous oxide at least 15 minutes before injection of air or sulfur hexafluoride.
- Avoid nitrous oxide use until the bubble is absorbed (5 days after air and 10 days after sulfur hexafluoride injection).

Considerations for Specific Surgical Procedures

1. Cataract surgery

Many cataract procedures are conducted under MAC and topical or regional anesthetic techniques. Topical analgesia is the most common technique, followed by peribulbar (extraconal) block or, less frequently, retrobulbar (intraconal) block. General anesthesia is usually reserved for adults who cannot communicate, comply, or stay stationary during eye surgery and for children.

2. Intraocular glaucoma surgery

Topical anesthesia could be the choice for patients with glaucoma surgery to prevent intraocular pressure's transient rise during local anesthetic injections with regional anesthesia. The outcomes of glaucoma surgery tend to be similar, regardless of the anesthetic procedure used.

However, some surgeons favor general anesthesia in patients undergoing trabeculectomy due to particular issues about the increased possibility of injury to the optic nerve during injections of local anesthesia in patients with glaucoma and problems in relation to inadequate healing following administration of subconjunctival lidocaine. During the induction of general anesthesia, the goal is to prevent an increase in intraocular pressure during laryngoscopy and endotracheal intubation. Complete akinesia is required during intraocular glaucoma surgery. A nondepolarizing neuromuscular blocking agent is administered, and a deeper plane of anesthesia is maintained.

3. Vitreoretinal surgery

Topical anesthesia is not suitable for vitreoretinal surgeries because of the longer duration of surgery and increased chances of retinal injuries if the patient moves during the procedure. General anesthesia without nitrous oxide or regional anesthesia is the preferred modality. Nitrous oxide should not be used if sulfur hexafluoride injection is planned.

4. Squint surgery

Children undergoing repair of squint are at higher risk of oculocardiac reflex intraoperatively and PONV. The risk of malignant hyperthermia is also high in such a group of patients.

Conclusion

Most ophthalmic surgeries can be performed under topical anesthesia and ocular nerve blocks in a cooperative patient. However, general anesthesia is required in children, uncooperative patients, and in cases where ocular nerve blocks cannot be performed. Oculocardiac reflex is an important complication associated with squint surgery. Proper communication between surgeon and anesthetist is paramount in preventing it. Releasing surgical traction and deepening the plane of anesthesia are often enough if it occurs. However, IV atropine has to be given if bradycardia does not resolve with the above measures.

CHAPTER 30

Anesthesia for ENT Surgery

Ajisha Aravindan and Avishek Roy

Introduction

Anesthesia for ENT procedure varies from simple daycare procedure to complex airway reconstruction procedure. Massive bleeding conditions like juvenile nasal angiofibroma (JNA) and carotid body tumors require hypotensive anesthesia as a well multidisciplinary approach. ENT surgeries are versatile in the context of age group, sex, airway, position during operation, bleeding, and need for postoperative ventilation. This chapter will overview the anesthetic considerations for common ENT procedures that include:

- Anesthesia for adenoidectomy/ tonsillectomy.
- Anesthesia for ear surgeries.
- Anesthesia for nasal surgeries.
- Anesthesia for panendoscopy.
- Anesthesia for bronchoscopy.
- Anesthesia for obstructive sleep apnea (OSA) surgeries.
- Anesthesia for parotid surgeries.
- Anesthesia for peritonsillar abscess (PTA) and Ludwig's angina.
- Anesthesia for temporomandibular joint (TMJ) surgeries.
- Laser surgeries and airway fire.

Anesthesia for Adenoidectomy/ Tonsillectomy

Tonsillectomy is a frequently performed surgical process with or without adenoidectomy. The procedure entails significant surgical as well as anesthetic challenges with substantial morbidity and mortality. Important clinical features are respiratory difficulty due to nasal obstruction, frequent infections, otitis media, decreased hearing (due to Eustachian tube obstruction), and OSA.

Indications

- Features of upper airway obstruction, dysphagia, and sleep disorders.
- PTA not adequately responding to medical management.
- Febrile seizures due to tonsillitis.
- Tonsillar pathology requiring biopsy for a definitive diagnosis.
- Chronic infectious adenotonsillitis.
- Obstructive sleep apnea syndrome (OSAS).

Anesthetic Considerations

Preoperative

Preoperative evaluation should focus on age group, associated comorbidities (such as Downs syndrome), OSA, and upper respiratory tract infection. These are the main factors in stratifying perioperative complications, including post-extubation laryngospasm and bronchospasm. Important points of consideration are listed below:

- Polysomnography (PSG) is the gold standard to diagnose OSAS in children, but it is not possible in all children.
- Electrocardiogram (ECG) in patients with OSA (to exclude right heart involvement secondary to pulmonary artery hypertension).

- Hemoglobin and hematocrit should be done to rule out anemia and polycythemia (in patients with OSA), respectively.

- Total leucocyte counts and a chest X-ray if respiratory tract infection is present.

- Coagulopathy should be excluded, as adenoidectomy/tonsillectomy may lead to massive bleeding during the perioperative period.

- Cautious use of premedication because of risk of upper airway obstruction.

Intraoperative

- The choice of anesthetic technique matters mainly in the presence of upper respiratory tract infections (URTI). Even though the laryngeal mask airway (LMA) is not used frequently for adenotonsillectomy, the evidence suggests that it may have advantages over the tracheal tube.

- The endotracheal tube (ETT) is the gold standard of airway management. A preformed south pole-facing tube (oral Ring–Adair–Elwyn [RAE]) is preferable. LMA, especially reinforced one, can be used for airway management but with adequate training and experience.

- End-tidal CO_2 monitoring is vital to detect early ETT tube kinking, due to placement of mouth gag as well as displacement.

- The eye should be well taped and protected from direct pressure and corneal injury. After positioning and Boyle–Davis gag placement, ETT should be examined for obvious kinking and any airway pressure.

- Anesthetic medications with lower potency of airway irritation such as propofol, sevoflurane, and halothane are preferred over thiopental and desflurane, which cause airway irritation.

- The choice for the neuromuscular blocking agent for intubation is suxamethonium, if not contraindicated.

- In a child with URTI, deep extubation is preferable.

- Patients must be extubated in lateral and head low position (*posttonsillectomy position*) after the surgery, and it should also be maintained in the postoperative period.

- Before extubation hemostasis, throat free of any secretion or any gauze must be established.

- Patients must be shifted to the recovery room in the lateral position and monitored for bleeding as well as any decrease of consciousness.

Coroner's Clot

It is an occult clot of blood left behind the nasopharynx posterior till the soft palate. It usually occurs in surgeries in areas of nasopharynx or trauma, mainly due to adenotonsillectomy. It has the potential to cause fatal airway obstruction following extubation.

Postoperative Management

The following should be taken into consideration while managing the patient postoperatively:

- Keep the child in the recovery position.

- Constant monitoring for bleeding.

- Pain control with multimodal analgesia.

- Postoperative nausea and vomiting (PONV) prophylaxis with dexamethasone and ondansetron.

Complications

- Posttonsillectomy bleeding

  The worst complication is bleeding tonsil in this group of patients. It is an emergency and, if not mediated in time, can lead to rapid deterioration of hemodynamics and airway compromise.

- Laryngospasm

At the beginning of the postoperative period, tonsillectomy and adenoidectomy have the highest incidence of laryngospasm (21–26%). Laryngospasm is preventive but can have damaging and life-threatening consequences like negative-pressure pulmonary edema, pulmonary aspiration, bradycardia, oxygen desaturation, and cardiac arrest.

Anesthesia for Ear Surgery

Common surgery of the ear includes otitis media and its related complications. Otitis media is very common in children. The common ear surgery includes:

- Myringotomy.
- Mastoidectomy.

Myringotomy

In this surgical procedure, a small incision is made in the tympanic membrane. Myringotomy and insertion of tympanostomy (grommet tube) are used to improve middle-ear aeration for a prolonged period and to also prevent the accumulation of fluid. It is a daycare procedure of a short duration.

Anesthetic Considerations

- The preoperative examination should be focused to elicit features of URTI and OSA secondary to adenotonsillar enlargement. Due to URTI, the airway becomes hyper-reactive, which leads to perioperative airway complications like laryngospasm and bronchospasm.
- Anesthesia for myringotomy can be given through facemask or LMA by maintaining spontaneous breathing and with the head rotated to one side.

- For analgesia, paracetamol and nonsteroidal anti-inflammatory drug (NSAID) can be given preoperatively.

Mastoidectomy

Mastoidectomy is a surgical procedure that is used for the removal of chronic suppurative middle-ear disease. The most common indication is the treatment of cholesteatoma and the associated infection.

Anesthetic Considerations

- The important anesthetic concerns are the usage of nitrous oxide in middle-ear surgery. The solubility of nitrous oxide in the blood is around 34 times higher than nitrogen. It easily diffuses in the middle-ear cavity, which leads to very high pressure within 30 minutes of use. The raised middle-ear pressures can lead to:
  - ▶ Dislodgment of tympanoplasty grafts.
  - ▶ Deterioration of deafness and rupture of the tympanic membrane.
  - ▶ High incidence of PONV.
- During discontinuation, the rapid reabsorption of nitrous oxide gas can result in negative pressure in the middle ear, which can cause dislodgment of the underlay tympanic membrane graft.
- For the bloodless surgical field, various methods can be used, such as head-up elevation of around 10 to 15° to reduce venous ooze, vasoconstrictor-like adrenaline infiltration, and maintaining low blood pressure (up to 20% of mean arterial pressure [MAP]).
- The use of muscle relaxants should be properly timed if facial nerve monitoring is used.

- Total intravenous (IV) anesthesia is an attractive substitute for general anesthesia (GA) with a lesser incidence of PONV.

- Anesthesia can be maintained with propofol, short-acting opioids, and inhalational agent like sevoflurane. It also allows maintenance of anesthesia without muscle relaxant and unobstructed facial nerve monitoring.

- For airway, ETT and reinforced LMA can be used. The reinforced LMA is a good option for airway management due to less airway stimulation and smooth emergence.

Analgesia and Antiemesis

- Multimodal analgesia should be given to minimize opioid dose. Analgesia with paracetamol and NSAIDs can be given through oral, IV, and rectally in the perioperative period.

- Opioids like remifentanil, fentanyl, and morphine, providing adequate analgesia, should be given in a low dose with strict postoperative monitoring. A greater auricular nerve block has shown to reduce the postoperative opioid requirement.

- For PONV, measures like prevention of long preoperative fasting, good hydration with IV fluids, no nitrous oxide, the practice of total intravenous anesthesia (TIVA), and multimodal analgesia to reduce opioid dose are very helpful.

Anesthesia for Nasal Surgery

The nasal surgeries are performed to relieve upper airway obstruction. The common nasal surgeries are:

- Septoplasty.
- Endoscopic sinus surgery.
- Rhinoplasty.
- Dacryocystorhinostomy.

Anesthetic Considerations

Preoperative

- Rule out OSA by history, examination, and PSG (if needed).

- Exclude systemic illness, especially coronary artery disease (CAD) and cardiac arrhythmia; in that case, surgeon should cautiously use local vasoconstriction.

- If the patient has a history of chronic use of steroids, they should receive daily maintenance dose perioperatively.

- History of the use of anticoagulant and recent nasal bleeding is also important.

Intraoperative

- For minor procedures or in a patient who cannot tolerate GA, it can be done under local anesthesia (LA).

- For complicated surgical procedures, GA is the anesthesia of choice.

- ETT seems to be the prime option for endoscopic sinus surgeries, because of its superior protection against aspiration compared to supraglottic airway (SGA) devices. Blood can still sip through the outer surface of the ETT to vocal cord and trachea. Therefore, throat pack is necessary in case of ETT too, in order to prevent blood aspiration.

- The oral RAE tube is better due to its preformed shape, and due to that, less kinking intraoperatively. Fixation of ETT should be done in midline.

- Patient head (airway) is away from anesthesiologists; hence, EtCO$_2$ and airway pressure monitoring is prudent to diagnose any kinking or disconnection.

- Throat pack should be removed before extubation, and for that, checklist should be followed, because if left, then catastrophic consequences can occur.

- Throat pack removal should be followed by a careful examination of the oral cavity and nasopharynx for any clot.

- For maintenance, TIVA is an ideal anesthetic technique. It has certain advantages like less bleeding due to low blood pressure, better surgical field, and reduction in the incidence of PONV.

- The position of the patient in reverse Trendelenburg with 15° head up helps in decreasing blood loss. This positioning should be done slowly to avoid hypotension.

- The patients who are on steroids pre-operatively should continue perioperatively to reduce edema and inflammation.

- Vasoconstrictor (epinephrine, pheny-lephrine) topical and injection applied on nasal mucosa helps to decrease congestion and hemostasis. Vasoconstrictor should be used with caution, especially in a patient with a history of CAD, cardiac arrhythmia, or myocardial infarction (MI).

- There are certain advantages of awake extubation like less chance of aspiration of blood or secretion due to the full return of laryngeal reflex. Drawbacks of this technique are coughing, bucking, and laryngospasm.

- Additional suctioning and laryngoscopy should be done to reduce chances of aspiration of blood or secretions during deep extubation.

Postoperative Care

- Multimodal analgesia for pain control.
- PONV can be prevented by:
  - ▶ Use of TIVA.
  - ▶ Liberal IV fluid.
  - ▶ Use of dexamethasone, ondansetron.
  - ▶ Judicious use of opioid.

Anesthesia for Panendoscopy

Panendoscopy is also called "triple endoscopy," which includes rigid laryngoscopy, bronchoscopy, and esophagoscopy.

Indications

- Evaluation of head and neck cancer for documentation of the extent of tumor.

- Biopsy for tissue diagnosis.

- Search for primary tumor and any recurrence after treatment.

- Evaluation of vocal cord lesions and pathology involving the pharynx, larynx, or tongue.

Anesthesia Considerations

Panendoscopy is a short but highly stimulating procedure requiring deep anesthesia, obtunded hemodynamic reflexes, immobile surgical field, and rapid emergence with early return of protective airway reflexes. An antisialogogue (i.e., glycopyrrolate 0.2 mg IV or intramuscular [IM]) can be given to minimize secretions prior to induction. Usually, a routine IV anesthetic induction is preferred along with the application of LA (i.e., lidocaine 4%) to the vocal cords prior to further airway manipulation. It should be corroborated with the surgeon whether LA will interfere with their planned procedure.

Preoperative

- A proper evaluation of pathology and its impact on ventilation, intubation, and cricothyroid access is essential.

- The surgeon's preference for airway management should be given consideration.

- The cardiovascular and pulmonary comorbidities must be evaluated and optimized before the surgery.

- Reflux history and potential for aspiration should be noted carefully.

Intraoperative

- Prior detailed discussion and close communication with the surgeon and sharing the airway during the procedure.

- The eyes should be covered and well-padded. Upper dentition should be protected with a mouth guard or folded gauze.

- The regular ETT, which is used for GA, is not suitable for this procedure as it will compromise vision due to its bigger size. LMA/tubeless technique/microlaryngeal surgery (MLS) tube is used to secure the airway for this procedure.

  ▶ LMA: It is used at the beginning of the procedure and also at the end to secure the airway for sedated patients and for smooth emergence.

  ▶ Tubeless technique: The technique involves either apnea bag-mask ventilation or ventilation through rigid bronchoscope.

- For known or suspected difficult airway, the procedure can be done either by awake intubation, prophylactic placement of a cricothyroid cannula, or awake tracheostomy. A discussion with the ENT surgeon and a preoperative nasal endoscopic examination of the upper airway may aid in the decision-making.

- For maintenance, TIVA is useful in this procedure and decrease the chances of OT pollution.

- The emergence phase can be managed by many techniques. At the completion of panendoscopy, the muscle relaxation is reversed if nondepolarizing agents are used, and the IV or volatile anesthetic is stopped. The patient management can be done with bag/mask ventilation or by insertion of a SGA device until spontaneous ventilation is resumed.

Postoperative

- The patient should be kept in the recovery position.

- Pain control with multimodal analgesia.

- Watchful monitoring for respiratory distress and stridor.

Complications

- Hypercarbia due to inadequate ventilation.

- Direct trauma to the tracheobronchial tree, including lacerations, hemorrhage, or arytenoid dislocation.

- There can be a dental injury, eye trauma, and injury to the lips and tongue.

- Surgical manipulation can result in edema or bleeding, causing laryngospasm or airway obstruction.

- Neurological injury related to neck extension, if a patient has atlantoaxial instability, is a disastrous consequence.

A postoperative chest X-ray should be done in case of any suspicion of pneumothorax or pneumomediastinum.

Anesthesia for Bronchoscopy

Bronchoscopy is a technique used to visualize the airways and have access to diagnostic and therapeutic purposes. It poses distinctive challenges for anesthesiologists, such as the sharing of the airway and the working place.

Indications

- Management of pulmonary hemorrhage.

- Removal of foreign body in children.

- Laser debulking or stenting in case of obstructive endobronchial lesions.

- To relieve airway obstruction due to malignancy.

- For optimization of respiratory condition before surgery.

- Iatrogenic stenosis (including postintubation fibrosis and posttransplant stenosis).
- Extrinsic compression due to tumors of the mediastinum.
- Intraluminal tracheobronchial repair of sealing defects.

Contraindications

- Arrhythmias.
- Uncooperative patient.
- Recent CAD.
- Coagulopathy.
- Recent unstable angina.
- Uremia.
- Significant debilitation or malnutrition.

Anesthesia Considerations

Preoperative

- Apart from the routine preanesthetic examination, emphasis should be on comorbidities, condition of the patient (oxygen requirement), any predicted difficult airway, and difficulty of procedures. Accordingly, anesthesia support (the type of sedation) and place (OT or bronchoscopy room facility) will be decided.
- Important preoperative investigations required are routine blood investigations and coagulation profiles if the patient is on anticoagulants.
- Pulmonary function test if any symptoms suggestive of airway obstruction.
- Computed axial tomography scan along with angiography to know the feeding artery if patients have a history of hemoptysis and clinical suspicion of tumor.
- An arterial blood gas is also helpful to know baseline hypoxemia and hypercarbia.

- Patients with multiple comorbidities may require multidisciplinary involvement. Periprocedural complications like delayed recovery, postprocedure requirement for mechanical ventilation, and ICU care should be explained in detail before the procedure.
- The complex procedure may require help from a cardiac and thoracic surgeon.

Intraoperative

- Patients generally tolerate this procedure under sedation after premedication with short-acting benzodiazepines, opioids, or both. In some center, clinician prefer to give antisialogogue (glycopyrrolate) before the procedure to dry secretions.
- The pharynx and vocal cords are locally anesthetized by nebulization of lidocaine (1 or 2%) after the calculation of a safe toxic dose. Bronchodilators may be used in some patients to relieve bronchospasm.
- Rigid bronchoscopy: It requires general anesthesia, including analgesia and muscle relaxation.
- Flexible bronchoscopy: In most of the cases, flexible bronchoscopy is done under conscious sedation, usually provided by bronchoscopist.
- Standard monitoring is a must to detect hypotension, bradycardia, and respiratory depression.
- Ventilation strategies in bronchoscopy: The different techniques of ventilation are:
  ► Apneic ventilation.
  ► Spontaneous ventilation with assistance.
  ► Controlled ventilation.
  ► Manual jet ventilation.
  ► High-frequency jet ventilation.

- Topical anesthesia: Topical anesthesia makes patients more comfortable for bronchoscopy along with sedation. It is generally indicated when anesthesia for nostrils, oropharynx, and hypopharynx is required. It also decreases the cough reflex and allows bronchoscope to pass the glottis. It can be done with the help of 2% viscous lignocaine on the nasal mucosa and spraying with 10% lignocaine orally.

Postoperative Care

Patients should be monitored for complications.

Complications

- Hypoxia due to inadequate ventilation, hemorrhage, and bronchospasm due to bronchial secretions or tissue fragments.
- Pneumothorax.
- Hemodynamic instability.
- Laryngospasm.
- Cardiac arrhythmias may occur secondary to hypoxia and hypercarbia.
- Local anesthetic systemic toxicity (LAST) due to local anesthetic overdose toxicity, especially in elderly.
- Repeated maneuverings can cause trauma to teeth, gum, vocal cords, and pyriform sinus.
- Airway perforation.
- Laser-associated complications.

Anesthesia for Obstructive Sleep Apnea Surgery

OSA is a disorder defined by a repeated episode of cessation of respiration during sleep due to upper airway collapse. Important symptoms are snoring, sleep disturbances, and daytime somnolence. The management of OSA requires a multidisciplinary approach. Continuous positive airway pressure (CPAP) is one of the effective treatment modalities used to improve symptoms as well as the quality of life. CPAP also improved cardiac and neurocognitive symptoms.

The role of surgery for the management of OSA is controversial. When CPAP therapy fails, or the patient is noncompliant, then surgery like uvulopalatopharyngoplasty is effective. In craniofacial malformation, maxillary–mandibular advancement surgery can be helpful. Weight loss and bariatric surgery are effective in morbidly obese patients. If the OSA is due obstructive pathology, then surgery to relieve obstruction like inferior turbinate reduction and tonsillectomy alone or in combination is used to improve the effect of CPAP and reduce CPAP pressure requirements.

Anesthesia Considerations

Preoperative

- Preoperative assessment should focus on the severity of OSA, any associated complications, and CPAP requirement as well as compliance to it at home.
- Instructions to bring the CPAP machine should be given, and its need in the postoperative period should be explained to the patient.
- The routine anesthetic preoperative examination should focus on identifying patients with a difficult airway. Modified neck circumference is also a good predictor for the screening of OSA. A modified neck circumference of 43 to 48 cm indicates an intermediate probability of OSA and >48 cm indicates a high probability of difficult airway.
- PSG can be used for assessment of the severity of OSA and the success of the surgery.
- OSA is generally associated with multiple comorbidities like hypertension, diabetes mellitus (DM), CAD, metabolic syndrome,

and in severe cases, unexplained respiratory or right heart failure and pulmonary hypertension.

- All coexisting diseases should be properly evaluated by respective specialists and optimized before surgery.

- Echocardiography and stress tests may be useful in selective cases. Patients with multiple comorbidities generally are on various medications and should be continued in the perioperative period.

- Discontinuation of anticoagulant and anti-platelet drugs should be discussed with cardiologists and surgeons.

- Premedication should be avoided, and if needed, it should be given in an area where observation and monitoring are possible. These patients are very prone to respiratory depression after premedication. No hypnotic should be administered at night before the operation.

Intraoperative

- In morbidly obese patients, ramping with the help of pillow or ramp increase intubation success.

- If the airway is difficult, then intubation may require fiberoptic bronchoscopy (FOB)-guided intubation.

- The choice of the ETT (standard ETT, RAE tube) depends upon availability. Packing with saline-soaked gauze should be done to protect from possible blood aspiration, and the pack must be removed before extubation.

- Anesthesiologists should be cautious when self-retaining mouth gag (Crowe–Davis) is placed by the surgeon for possible injury to teeth and tongue and also examine ETT for possible kinking and increased airway pressure.

- Before incision, the surgeon infiltrates the palate with 1% lidocaine along with epinephrine 1:1,00,000 for hemostasis. An inadvertent intravascular injection and arrhythmia, especially in patients with cardiac disease, should be monitored.

- Before extubation, nasopharynx, hypo-pharynx, and esophagus should be irrigated and suctioned to remove accumulated blood with a soft catheter.

- At the end of the surgery, the insertion of a nasopharyngeal airway helps in the prevention of airway obstruction.

- IV dexamethasone is useful to reduce pharyngeal edema during the perioperative period.

- The trachea should be extubated when the patient is fully awake and following command.

Postoperative Care

- Patients should be closely monitored with continuous pulse oximetry in post-anesthesia care unit (PACU). Patients with body mass index (BMI) $\geq$ 30 and/or apnea hypopnea index (AHI) $\geq$ 22 are more likely to require oxygen in the post-PACU setting and should be monitored overnight.

- The patient with comorbidities like significant underlying cardiac or pulmonary disease and extensive surgery like concomitant nasal surgery may require intensive care unit admission.

- For analgesia, opioids should be avoided to prevent postoperative respiratory depression.

- To avoid airway edema, a short course of steroid (dexamethasone) is helpful.

- Some patients may require CPAP in the postoperative period, and patients' own machine is more helpful with increased compliance.

Complications

The common complications are:

- Airway obstruction.
- Hemorrhage.
- Fall in SpO$_2$, and pulmonary edema.

Anesthesia for Parotid Surgeries

Anesthetic Considerations

Preoperative

- The focus is on the tumor displacement of the airway as well as TMJ mobility.
- The mouth opening, submandibular space compliance, thyromental distance, neck diameter, and neck range of motion must be assessed.
- Any previous radiation is taken as an independent factor for difficult mask ventilation.

Intraoperative

- GA with ETT is a must to ensure a calm patient.
- Whenever facial nerve monitoring is planned, the timing of the use of muscle relaxants is of vital concern. The train of four (TOF) monitoring is useful to guide the maintenance dose of relaxant.
- Achieving immobility is quite challenging in the absence of muscle relaxants. It requires a balanced anesthetic technique, employing a relatively large dose of opioid and inhalational agents.
- TIVA is also a good alternative maintenance technique, especially in a patient with a history of malignant hyperthermia.
- After completion of identification and dissection of the facial nerve, nerve monitoring can be stopped, and muscle relaxants can be given.

Postoperative Care

- Keep patient in the recovery position.
- Multimodal analgesia for pain control.

Complications

- Airway edema.
- Expanding hematoma may cause an immediate airway threat and respiratory failure; that is why extubation should be attempted after ensuring airway patency.
- Other complications are transient facial paresis or permanent facial paralysis, due to unintentional iatrogenic facial nerve injury, and ear lobe dysesthesia, due to damage to greater auricular nerve (GAN) branches.
- Frey's syndrome is another common complication, also known as "gustatory sweating," as the patient sweats on affected side during eating food.

Anesthesia for Peritonsillar Abscess and Ludwig's Angina

Peritonsillar Abscess

PTA is one of the most common deep cervical fascial plane infections of the neck, occurs mainly in young patients, and is fatal if not managed timely. Adequate hydration, drainage of the abscess, and the broad-spectrum antibiotic is the key to management. The incidence is highest among adults in 20 to 40 years of age.

Common organisms isolated in PTA are group A streptococcus, *Staphylococcus aureus*, and *Hemophilus influenza*.

Anesthetic Considerations

After diagnosis, there are three ways to drain this infection: incision and drainage of the abscess, tonsillectomy, or needle aspiration.

Drainage of the abscess is the initial approach in managing this infection. Important anesthetic considerations are:

- This procedure is generally performed under topical anesthesia.
- In children, conscious sedation or monitored anesthesia care is required.
- For GA airway, securing with a cuffed ETT and gentle packing with gauze is an ideal method.
- Video laryngoscope nowadays is a useful adjunct to secure airway, and accidental rupture is also avoided.
- Steroids help in faster recovery, thus decreasing hospital stay as well as pain.

Complications

- Airway compromise.
- Aspiration pneumonia.
- Spread of infection into the deep planes of the neck or superior mediastinum.
- Fatal hemorrhage due to erosion of carotid artery.
- Glomerulonephritis and rheumatic fever if causative organism of the abscess is group A streptococcus.

Ludwig's Angina

Ludwig's angina is characterized by a rapidly spreading cellulitis of the floor of the mouth, and its distinguishing features are brawny induration of the floor of the mouth and suprahyoid region (bilaterally). This swelling may push the tongue, resulting in airway obstruction. Earlier it was fatal, but due to antibiotics and surgical management, mortality has reduced.

Anesthetic Considerations

- Airway management depends on the case scenario, facility available, and expertise of the clinician.

- The airway can be managed by direct laryngoscopy, awake fiberoptic, video laryngoscopy, and tracheostomy, depending on reduction in mouth opening, due to the spread of abscess and protrusion of the tongue.
- In extreme life-threatening conditions under LA, cricothyrotomy can be done for securing the airway.
- If there is no intraoral extension, blind nasal can be used as an alternative, but nowadays, it is not much in practice and requires expertise.
- Airway maintenance is challenging in advanced cases. Awake fiberoptic nasal intubation should be done while the patient is in an upright position. Video laryngoscope is now a good alternative in case of reduced mouth opening.
- The last option for airway management is cricothyroidotomy or tracheostomy under LA.

The choice of airway management plans should be individualized, depending on the clinical scenario, availability of equipment, and experience of managing clinicians.

Complications

- Sepsis.
- Pneumonia.
- Asphyxia.
- Empyema.
- Pericarditis.
- Mediastinitis.
- Pneumothorax.

Anesthesia for TMJ Surgeries

TMJ ankylosis is a pathologic condition in which the mandibular condyles fuses with the base of the skull by bony or fibrous tissue. This results in difficulty in mastication, talking, and oral cleanliness.

Anesthetic Considerations

Preoperative

- Detail airway examination, any associated comorbidities, and previous anesthetic history, especially any record regarding airway management and postoperative complications.
- Detail history and investigation for OSA, room air saturation/arterial blood gas (ABG), and any use of CPAP.
- In the pediatric age group, association with adenotonsillar hypertrophy, craniofacial deformity, and syndromic association should be examined, and proper workup should be done preoperatively.
- Due to difficulty in eating, these children are malnourished; hence, routine hemogram and serum electrolyte should be done preoperatively.
- If there is bilateral pathology with severe retrognathia, then counseling and consent for the requirement of tracheostomy should be done beforehand.
- If you are planning awake FOB, then assurance and explanation of procedure with or without nerve block should also be done during the preanesthetic examination.
- Sedative premedication should be avoided in these patients because it may exacerbate airway obstruction. If premedication is needed, then patients should be monitored and only practiced in areas in which immediate help and resuscitation equipment are available.
- Antisialogogue, like glycopyrrolate, helps to dry oral and nasal secretion, which makes FOB easier.

- Nasal decongestant and vasoconstrictor drugs like xylometazoline and adrenaline-soaked gauze help in decreasing vascularity of nasal mucosa; hence, less bleeding during bronchoscopy and nasal intubation.

Airway Management

- Awake fiberoptic intubation is a gold standard for securing a difficult airway. In the pediatric age group, awake FOB is not possible; hence, FOB requires sedation (IV or inhalational), with the preservation of spontaneous breathing or GA.
- The best and safe way to secure the airway is FOB-guided intubation under sedation, with the preservation of spontaneous breathing.
- End-tidal CO_2-guided blind nasal intubation is another option, but it requires expertise and repeated attempts.
- Repeated attempts may cause bleeding, laryngeal edema, airway injury, and loss of airway.
- If there is severe retrognathia, then ENT standby availability for tracheostomy is also required.
- A difficult airway cart with a cricothyrotomy set should be available inside the operation room.

Intraoperative

- If a surgeon needs nerve monitoring till the exposure of the joint, then TIVA with propofol infusion (manual or target-controlled infusion [TCI]) may be used for maintenance of anesthesia in that period.
- If the patient airway is distant and there is a requirement of movement of the head in bilateral surgery, then the anesthetist must observe the $EtCO_2$ graph along with

airway pressure for early diagnosis of disconnection and kinking.

- The patient's eye should be taped and padded to prevent any corneal injury and inadvertent direct pressure on it.

- Generally, a nasal RAE tube is used as ETT and fixed, secured away from the head with the help of a catheter mount.

- Awake extubation (obeying command) is the gold standard in these patients with restricted mouth opening.

Postoperative Care

- Multimodal analgesia (paracetamol, NSAID).

- Opioid should be avoided in patients with OSA.

Laser Surgeries and Airway Fire

Nowadays, light amplification by stimulated emission of radiation (LASER) plays a significant role in ENT surgery. LASER is moreover used as a noun describing the actual device. Since their invention, laser use and applications have expanded rapidly. Laser surgery has many advantages like:

- Microscopic precision.

- A bloodless operative field.

- Complete sterility.

History

Theodore Maiman discovered the ruby laser in 1960. ENT specialists were first to use it as a surgical tool. In the beginning, lasers caused substantial tissue damage and were not able to achieve adequate wavelengths for tissue absorption. After the invention of the CO_2 laser, it became popular in medical use. The use of CO_2 laser on cadaveric larynx was first done by Jako and Polyani in 1967. Later in 1968, Bredemeier's developed an endoscopic delivery system and CO_2 delivery through a microscope. In the 1980s, different lasers were produced with a specific use (**Table 30.1**).

Table 30.1 Types of laser

Type	Wavelength (nm)	Tissue absorption	Tissue penetration	Coagulation	Cutting effect	Use
CO_2	10600	High	0.1	Low	High	Papilloma, Laryngectomy, Stapedectomy, Subglottic hemangioma
Nd:YAG	1060	Low	4	High	Low	Tracheobronchial surgeries
Argon	488–514	Selective high in blood	1	Medium	Low	Stapedectomy
KTP	532	Selective high in blood	1	Medium	Low	Stapedectomy, laryngeal, sinus surgeries
Holminium YAG	2100	-	3–5	-	-	Tonsillectomy, FESS, laryngeal surgeries

Abbreviation: FESS, functional endoscopic sinus surgery.

Indications

- Cordotomy, cordectomies.
- Management of tracheal stenosis.
- Resection of airway malignancies.
- Polyps and laryngeal papilloma (diffuse papillomatosis).
- Cordal nodules.
- Stapedectomies and myringotomies.

Anesthetic Consideration

1. General safety considerations

Education: All the OT personnel should be educated about the hazards of laser surgery. All staff must be familiar with laser surgery and local safety policies. Simulation classes and education to all OR personnel may help in better real-time crisis management.

Warning signs outside OT: Whenever laser surgery is going on, doors should be locked, and at the entrance, a warning sign should be displayed, preventing unwanted staff traffic inside OR.

Eye and skin protection: The laser absorbed through water (e.g., CO_2) can cause impairment to the anterior portions of the eye (cornea, lens). The laser wavelengths in the visible and near-infrared range such as argon and Nd:YAG can pass across optical media of the eye and damage the retina. Hence, throughout the procedure wavelength, specifically protected eyeglass with side protector along with double layer saline-moistened eye pad is a must. Also, the areas bordering the operative field like mucous membranes and teeth must be covered with saline-soaked gauze. The surgical drapes should be made of flame-resistant/waterproof material. CO_2 fire extinguisher and water should be ready to prevent any fire or explosion.

Smoke evacuation: A separate suction setup in the aerodigestive tract for smoke, steam evacuation from the operative field, and constant suctioning to avert inhalation by patient, surgeon, or personnel. It possesses a great risk of infection transmission in the operation theater personnel in case of resection of papillomata with laser, as there is an aerosol generation of viruses. Hence, for minimizing the risk, specifically designed masks are used.

Fire drill: The OT personnel should be alert for an airway fire, and a "fire drill" must be in place. Also, a 50-mL syringe filled with 0.9% saline must be kept at the time of surgery.

2. Airway fire

Airway fire and explosion is the major hazard in ENT laser surgery. The incidence occurrence rate is 0.5 to 1.5%. It occurs by direct laser illumination, reflecting laser light.

The airway fire causes thermal burns and chemical response to burns.

All OR personnel should be aware of the following situations in which airway fire might happen:

- Surgical site: Head neck procedure.
- Surgical tool: Electrocautery, laser, or FOB light source.
- Anesthetic factor: High FiO_2 and use of nitrous oxide (N_2O).

Prerequisite for airway fire: The three components for airway fire are fuel, oxidizing agent, and an ignition source.

Head, neck, and the ENT surgery has all the above; hence, the potential of fire is greater.

The oxygen and nitrous act as an oxidizing agent and support combustion; the ETT made of PVC, which is an inflammable material, acts as a fuel source; and the laser and electrocautery act as an ignition source.

Anesthetic Considerations to Reduce the Incidence of Airway Fire

- Use of ETT suited for laser surgery is more resistant to airway fire.

- If laser-compatible ETT is not available, then normal ETT can be used after wrapping aluminum foil. Cuff of ETT should be filled with saline and methylene blue.
- Ventilatory modes like apneic ventilation and jet ventilation (high-frequency jet ventilation) can be used to reduce fire incidence.
- Oxygen concentration (FiO_2) should be minimal < 40%, and N_2O should be avoided.
- For maintenance of anesthesia, TIVA can be used.
- If possible, avoid electrocautery use.

Endotracheal Tubes for Laser Surgery

There are several types of nonflammable ETTs available, which are used during laser surgery. These tubes are made up of laser resistant material, but none is completely safe from direct laser energy. They disintegrate energy of the laser and thus reduce the chances of airway fire. The common laser-compatible ETTs are:

- Bivona Fome-Cuff laser tube.
- Laser Flex.
- Laser-Shield tube.
- Metal tracheal tube.

Airway Fire Protocol

- Acknowledge and close communication with the surgeon.
- Immediately switch off the ventilation, remove ETT, and disconnect from breathing circuit.

- Flood the airway with preloaded saline (if the fire is not controlled).
- Start ventilation with the help of mask with FiO_2 of 100.
- After stabilization, assessment and removal of remains of fire along with damaged mucosa, with the help of direct laryngoscopy and rigid bronchoscopy.
- Continuous monitoring with SpO_2.
- An ABG analysis to obtain oxygenation status.
- If the patient deteriorates, then reintubation or tracheostomy can be considered on an individual case-to-case basis.
- Continue supportive care like ventilation, antimicrobial, analgesic, and NSAIDs.

▌Conclusion

Anesthesia for ENT surgeries is unique because of the common sharing of the airway between the surgeon and the anesthetist. The patients may come with a narrowed airway (e.g., subglottic stenosis) that mandates small-sized endotracheal tubes. A difficult airway may require awake intubation and surgeries on the vocal cords and in the subglottic region, leading to airway obstruction in the postoperative period. Thus, careful airway assessment and formulation of an appropriate airway management plan are crucial in such patients. The use of lasers adds to airway fire risk; therefore, airway fire protocol should be employed in all laser surgeries.

CHAPTER 31

Anesthesia in Trauma Patients

Ajit Kumar and Niyati Arora

Introduction

In the case of trauma, an anesthesiologist not only plays a role in operation theaters but also participates in the primary survey and resuscitation, airway protection, intubation, and other procedures in the emergency room.

Anesthesia care in cases of trauma requires complete knowledge of the advanced trauma life support (ATLS) guidelines. This chapter aims to deliver the most important information required for an undergraduate under the following headings:

- Evaluation of trauma patient by ATLS guidelines.
- Resuscitation goals.
- The blood component therapy.
- Special monitors and pharmacology in the treatment of trauma patients.
- Traumatic brain injury (TBI).
- Burns.

Evaluation of Patient

Clinicians rapidly assess injuries of injured patients and institute life-saving therapy. The initial assessment includes:

- Preparation including triage.
- Primary survey (airway, breathing, circulation, disability, exposure [ABCDE]).
- Consideration of the need for patient transfer.
- Secondary survey (head-to-toe evaluation and patient history).
- Adjuncts to the secondary survey.

- Continued postresuscitation monitoring and reevaluation.
- Definitive care.

The assessment of patients is not longitudinal, as mentioned above, in a clinical scenario, and primary as well as secondary survey should be done frequently to achieve optimal patient care.

Preparation

It has two phases, prehospital and the hospital phase.

Prehospital Phase

The prehospital system notifies the receiving hospital, which enables trauma members to do the required preparations, in order to receive patients. The trained members manage airway, control bleeding, immobilize the patient, and make necessary arrangements to transfer the patient to the nearest appropriate treatment facility (preferably a trauma center).

Hospital Phase

The hand over between prehospital providers and those at the receiving hospital should be a smooth process, which is directed by the trauma team leader. All health care workers should practice standard precautions during patient transfer due to the risk of transmitting infectious diseases through body fluids.

Primary Survey with Simultaneous Resuscitation

The primary survey encompasses the ABCDE of trauma care. It includes:

- A: Airway maintenance with restriction of cervical spine motion.

- B: Breathing and ventilation.
- C: Circulation with hemorrhage control.
- D: Disability (assessment of neurologic status).
- E: Exposure/environmental control.

Clinicians can quickly assess A, B, C, D, and E in a trauma patient by asking the patient for his or her name and asking what happened (*10-s assessment*). An appropriate response, that is, ability to speak clearly, ability to generate air movement to permit speech, and alertness to describe what happened, suggests that there is no significant airway compromise and breathing is not severely compromised.

Airway Maintenance with Restriction of Cervical Spine Motion

Securing a compromised airway, delivering oxygen, and supporting ventilation remain the cornerstone of care of trauma patients, and management of other conditions can be done later.

Supplemental oxygen with a tight-fitting mask (flow—10 L/min) should be administered to all trauma patients. Other vital steps are:

- Observe the patient for the sign of hypoxia (agitation) and hypercarbia (obtundation).
- Use of accessory muscles and retractions suggest respiratory distress.
- The presence of noisy breathing, snoring, gurgling, hoarseness, and stridor may indicate upper airway/vocal cord edema or narrowing.
- Pulse oximetry can detect inadequate oxygenation before cyanosis develops.
- Remove the foreign body from the oral cavity to clear the airway and identify any facial fracture as a culprit of airway obstruction.
- Neck trauma with compromised airway mandates early institution of definitive airway.

- Triad of hoarseness, subcutaneous emphysema, and a palpable fracture identifies a possible laryngeal trauma.

Trauma with life-endangering injuries compels trauma members to acquire skills to assess the airway rapidly in trauma patients. The mnemonic "LEMON" helps identify difficult airway in emergencies.

L—Look externally

- Presence of small mouth or jaw, large overbite, or facial trauma predicts difficult bag and mask ventilation.

E—Evaluate the 3-3-2 rule

- At least 3-finger breadths gap between patient's incisors (3).
- At least 3-finger breadths between hyoid bone and chin (3).
- A gap of at least 2-finger breadths between thyroid notch and floor of mouth (2).

M—Mallampati class

- Poor mallampati class (MPC) makes intubation difficult.

O—Obstruction

- Rule out culprits of airway obstruction (e.g., foreign body, facial trauma, etc.).

N—Neck mobility

- Restricted neck mobility is associated with difficult laryngoscopy.

Assume cervical spine injury in all trauma patients unless proven. The absence of neurological deficits does not rule out damage to the cervical spine. The cervical spine must be stabilized with a cervical collar in all patients, and extreme caution should be taken during transfer and airway handling. Head tilt and chin lift to keep the airway patent is contraindicated in trauma patients with a suspected cervical spine injury; however, jaw-thrust can be used to maintain patency of the airway, if required. In case of risk of aspiration and/or inability to keep airway patent, the airway should be secured with an endotracheal tube and with surgical techniques (tracheostomy or cricothyroidotomy) if endotracheal tube placement fails.

Breathing and Ventilation

A patent airway ensures the free movement of gases till alveoli. The presence of airway obstruction, central nervous system (CNS) depression, altered ventilatory mechanics, and chest trauma, along with paresis/paralysis of respiratory muscles, can compromise ventilation significantly. The entities like tension pneumothorax, open pneumothorax, massive hemothorax, and tracheal or bronchial injuries can cause mortality if not treated in time.

Circulation with Hemorrhage Control

Circulatory collapse due to excessive bleeding is a common cause of mortality. Death can also occur due to nonhemorrhagic reasons of circulatory collapse. All these need to be identified and should be treated in a timely fashion to save lives.

Identifying sources of bleeding, controlling it in a timely fashion, and adequate resuscitation can improve the patient's morbidity and mortality significantly. Hypotension due to bleeding should be the first differential of circulatory collapse after the exclusion of tension pneumothorax in trauma victims.

Clinical Evaluation

Clinical evaluation that yields essential information within seconds is:

- Deranged level of consciousness.
- Pale extremities showing poor skin perfusion.
- Rapid thread pulse.

Bleeding

The source of bleeding can be from either an external site or an internal organ.

External hemorrhage is addressed during the primary survey by direct manual pressure on the wound and application of tourniquets over bleeding sites at the extremities.

Internal hemorrhage: The physical examination and imaging (e.g., chest X-ray, pelvic X-ray, focused assessment with sonography for trauma [FAST], or diagnostic peritoneal lavage [DPL]) can identify the internal source of bleeding (chest, abdomen, pelvis, etc.). Immediate chest decompression, stabilization of pelvis, and application of splint on extremities are initial measures to control bleeding, followed by definitive management with interventional radiology and surgery.

Classification of Hemorrhage

Aggressive and continued volume resuscitation cannot replace for definitive control of bleeding. The hemorrhage can be categorized into four classes, based on severity (**Table 31.1**):

- Class I hemorrhage: For example, an individual who has donated one unit of blood.
- Class II hemorrhage: Uncomplicated hemorrhage which requires resuscitation crystalloid fluids.
- Class III hemorrhage: Complicated hemorrhagic state, which may require blood transfusion along with resuscitation with crystalloids.
- Class IV hemorrhage: The patient will die within minutes if not resuscitated in time; blood transfusion is required.

Management of Hemorrhagic Shock

Hemorrhagic shock is hypovolemic in nature, and resuscitation starts with crystalloid fluids along with simultaneous assessment of response to fluid therapy. Infused fluid should be warm, as massive volume resuscitation with cold fluids can cause dangerous hypothermia. Fluid administration in excess can cause dilutional thrombocytopenia and dilutional coagulopathy and add to further bleeding.

Early use of tranexamic acid has shown promising results in decreasing coagulopathy.

Table 31.1 Signs and symptoms of hemorrhage by class

Parameter	Class I	Class II	Class III (moderate)	Class IV (severe)
Approximate blood loss	<15%	15–30%	31–40%	>40%
Heart rate	↔	↔/↑	↑	↑/↑↑
Blood pressure	↔	↔	↔/↓	↓
Pulse pressure	↔	↓	↓	↓
Respiratory rate	↔	↔	↔/↑	↑
Urine output	↔	↔	↓	↓↓
GCS score	↔	↔	↓	↓
Base deficit	0 to –2 mEq/L	–2 to –6 mEq/L	–6 to –10 mEq/L	–10 mEq/L or less
Need for blood products	Monitor	Possible	Yes	MTC

Abbreviations: GCS, Glasgow coma scale; MTC, massive transfusion protocol.

Bolus should be administered within 3 hours and can be given by the paramedic team in the prehospital phase, followed by infusion in the hospital over 8 hours.

Causes and Management of Nonhemorrhagic Shock

The category of nonhemorrhagic shock includes tension pneumothorax, cardiogenic shock, cardiac tamponade, neurogenic shock, and septic shock.

Tension Pneumothorax

Tension pneumothorax is a reversible and life-threatening injury that should be treated by needle decompression in the second intercostal space in the midclavicular line, followed by chest tube insertion in the fifth intercostal space (anterior axillary line).

Cardiogenic Shock

Blunt cardiac injury, cardiac tamponade, an air embolus, or, rarely, myocardial infarction can cause fatal cardiac dysfunction. ECG is the most common investigation ordered in patients with blunt trauma to the chest in order to detect dysrhythmias.

Cardiac Tamponade

Cardiac tamponade can be caused due to blunt as well as penetrating injuries to the chest. The presence of tachycardia, muffled heart sounds, and dilated, engorged neck veins with hypotension and insufficient response to fluid therapy suggest cardiac tamponade. It can be diagnosed with FAST in emergency department (ED) and should be managed with the definitive operative intervention (pericardiocentesis is a temporary measure only). Transthoracic echocardiography can help in diagnosing cardiac tamponade but is often not available due to limited resources.

Neurogenic Shock

Neurogenic shock is uncommon in isolated intracranial injuries without injury to the brainstem. The classic presentation of neurogenic shock is hypotension without tachycardia or cutaneous vasoconstriction.

Septic Shock

It is a rare cause of hemodynamic instability in trauma patients. However, it can occur when the patient arrives at the ED after several hours of injury. Penetrating abdominal injuries and the contamination of peritoneal cavity by intestinal content are common culprits of septic shock in trauma patients. Normal circulating volume, modest tachycardia, warm skin, near-normal systolic blood pressure (BP), and wide pulse pressure characterizes the early phase of sepsis.

Measuring Patient Response to Fluid Therapy

The rise in pulse rate, pulse pressure, and BP suggests improving perfusion during the resuscitation phase. Urinary output of 0.5 and 1.0 mL/kg/h in children and adults, respectively, is an adequate and sensitive indicator of renal perfusion.

Patterns of Patient Response

The patient's response to initial fluid resuscitation is the key to determining subsequent therapy.

- Rapid response: "Rapid responders" quickly respond to the initial fluid bolus and become hemodynamically stable with no evidence of inadequate tissue perfusion. Usually, these patients come under class I hemorrhage and require no further fluid bolus or immediate blood administration.

- Transient response: "Transient responders" initially respond to resuscitative measures but later on deteriorate because of ongoing blood loss. Transient responders belong to class II/III hemorrhage and require blood transfusion. Also, identifying such a group of patients for the possible operative or angiographic intervention to control bleeding is very important.

- Minimal or no response: The trauma victims with class IV hemorrhage rarely respond to fluid and blood product administration. They require activation of massive blood transfusion protocol and immediate definitive operative intervention at the earliest.

Massive Blood Transfusion

In cases of blood loss, most deaths happen in the first 6 hours, and thus early blood transfusion initiation efforts are needed. The goal of massive transfusion is not just the replacement of intravascular volume, but the correction of trauma-induced coagulopathy, in an attempt to curb further blood loss. Massive transfusion definitions include:

- Replacement of whole blood volume in 24 hours (7% of ideal body weight in adults).

- Replacement of 50% of blood volume in 3 hours.

- Blood loss > 1,500 mL in 10 minutes.

Blood products in the ratio of 1:1:1 are widely followed. A fibrinogen level lower than 100 mg/dL substantially increases in-hospital mortality. With ongoing resuscitation, one should target to achieve the below-mentioned goals:

- Hematocrit > 30%.

- Platelets > 50,000/μL.

- Prothrombin time (PT) < 18 seconds (international normalized ratio [INR] < 1.5).

- Activated partial thromboplastin time (APTT) < 45 seconds.

- Fibrinogen > 150 mg/dL.

The massive transfusion of blood is not without complications and can lead to lung injury (in the form of transfusion-related acute lung injury [TRALI], transfusion-associated circulatory overload [TACO], infectious complications, hypothermia, and hypocalcemia).

Point of care is coagulation studies or thromboelastogram (TEG), which is now considered the gold standard for all massive transfusion protocol (MTP) monitoring. It is beyond the scope of this chapter to discuss TEG, but readers are encouraged to understand the use and functionality of TEG in a clinical scenario.

Disability (Neurologic Evaluation)

The Glasgow coma scale (GCS), supplemented by measurement of pupil size, is a rapid and sensitive tool for neurological evaluation in trauma victims. GCS is an objective method to determine the level of consciousness, with the motor component defining the outcome. A low GCS can be caused by the direct cerebral injury. Also, hypoglycemia, alcohol, narcotics, and sedatives can alter the patient's level of consciousness. It will be worth discussing the concept of primary and secondary brain injury:

- Primary brain injury occurs due to structural effect of injury to the brain. Once it has occurred, it needs to be managed medically or surgically.

- Secondary brain injury is the injury that occurs due to inadequate oxygenation and perfusion. As this is avoidable, our primary goal is to initiate management in order to prevent secondary brain injury.

Exposure and Environmental Control

Patients need to be undressed during the primary survey for the identification of all the injuries. Caution should be taken to keep the environment warm during this phase of assessment as heat loss from exposed body surfaces can lead to profound hypothermia. Patients should be covered with warm blankets as soon as the assessment is over.

Monitors and Tests in Trauma Patients

Continuous electrocardiography, pulse oximetry, end-tidal carbon dioxide (CO_2) monitoring, and assessment of ventilatory rate and arterial blood gas (ABG) measurement are commonly used during primary survey. Also, urinary catheters can be placed to monitor urine output and assess for hematuria. Gastric catheters decompress distention and evaluate for evidence of blood. Other helpful tests include blood lactate, X-ray examinations (e.g., chest and pelvis), FAST,

extended focused assessment with sonography for trauma (eFAST), and DPL.

Physiologic parameters such as pulse rate, BP, pulse pressure, ventilatory rate, ABG levels, body temperature, and urinary output are assessable measures that reflect the adequacy of resuscitation. Values for these parameters should be obtained as soon as possible during or after completing the primary survey and reevaluated periodically.

Need for Transfer

During the primary survey with resuscitation, the evaluating doctor frequently obtains sufficient information to determine the need to transfer the patient to another facility for definitive care. An in-depth assessment is not warranted at this stage as delay in transfer will worsen the patient's outcome.

Secondary Survey

The secondary survey is a head-to-toe evaluation of the trauma patient, that is, a complete history and physical examination, including the reassessment of all vital signs.

History

The prehospital personnel, with the help of family, can extract relevant history from a trauma victim. The AMPLE history is a useful mnemonic for this purpose:

- A: Allergies.
- M: Medications currently used.
- P: Past illnesses/pregnancy.
- L: Last meal.
- E: Events/environment related to the injury.

Physical Examination

During the secondary survey, physical examination follows the sequence of the head, maxillofacial structures, cervical spine and neck, chest, abdomen and pelvis, perineum/rectum/vagina, musculoskeletal system, and neurological system.

The examination in the secondary survey usually includes findings that were missed during resuscitation and primary survey. It focuses on investigations to confirm the diagnosis and then decide about the definitive treatment (conservative or operative).

It cannot be stressed enough that trauma guidelines are universal. It is beyond the scope of this chapter to go into any further details; thus, it is recommended for all anesthesiologists to acquaint themselves with the current ATLS guidelines.

Authors, thus, would be directing their discussion toward anesthesia management in operation theater in conditions like:

- TBI.
- Burns.

Anesthesia in TBI

Although the protocols for receiving of patient, evaluation, primary survey, resuscitation, and secondary survey are the same for all trauma patients, some critical points need to be highlighted in a patient of head injury.

Assessment

The assessment of CNS by the GCS has been mentioned in **Table 31.2**.

Alert verbal painful unresponsiveness (AVPU) score can also be used for CNS assessment (**Table 31.3**). This is easier to carry out and interpret. Patients who are not alert and are not responding to commands are equivalent to a GCS of around 8, which indicates a severe injury; a GCS of 8 or fewer warrants securing a definitive airway. The immobilization of the cervical spine is a must, as discussed in the primary survey.

Pathophysiology

Before planning the anesthesia management of such a patient, it is essential to understand the pathophysiology of brain injury.

Primary Brain Injury versus Secondary Brain Injury

Primary brain injuries result immediately from the initial trauma. The secondary injury to the

Table 31.2 GCS score

Best eye response (E)	Spontaneous eye-opening	4
	Open to verbal commands, speech, shout	3
	Open to pain	2
	None	1
Best verbal response (V)	Oriented	5
	Confused conversation, but able to answer questions	4
	Inappropriate words	3
	Incomprehensible speech	2
	None	1
Best motor response (M)	Obeys command for movement	6
	Purposeful movements to stimulus	5
	Withdraws from pain	4
	Abnormal flexion, decorticate posture	3
	Extensor response, decerebrate posture	2
	None	1

Abbreviation: GCS, Glasgow coma scale.

Table 31.3 AVPU score

A	Alert
V	Response to voice
P	Response to pain
U	Unresponsive

brain occurs due to ischemia as sequelae of hypoxia, hypercarbia, and a rise in intracranial pressure (ICP).

Excitotoxicity

Head injury leads to the release of glutamate from neuronal cells, which causes increased concentration of glutamate in the cerebrospinal fluid (CSF). This increased glutamate levels, and glutamate receptor stimulation leads to an increase in intracellular calcium ion. The raised intracellular calcium level activates several calcium-dependent enzymes, which ultimately damage lipids, proteins, and nucleic acid, resulting in free radical-mediated cellular damage.

Cerebral perfusion pressure (CPP) and the factors affecting it:

- The skull, a rigid box, contains the brain (80%), CSF (8%), and blood (12%). Monroe–Kellie hypothesis states that an increase in the amount of any of these will lead to increased ICP since the skull cannot expand. This, in turn, will affect the cerebral blood flow (CBF) as the CPP is dependent on the mean arterial pressure (MAP) and the ICP.
- Normal ICP is about 5 to 13 mm Hg.
- An increase in the ICP and/or a fall in MAP or a combination of both will ultimately lead to a situation where CPP becomes very low, leading to the progressive decrease in CBF, eventually causing brain death (CPP = MAP – ICP). Assessment of CPP is vital and possible either by measurement of both ICP and MAP or by measuring MAP and making a reasonable estimate of ICP.

- During anesthesia, therefore, if ICP is raised, a fall in BP must be avoided or treated quickly by volume replacement or vasopressors. When CPP is inadequate, the oxygen saturation of jugular venous blood falls (normal range 65–75%) because of increased oxygen extraction. Inadequate CPP (less than 70 mm Hg) has been shown to be a significant factor in the poor outcome of patients with raised ICP.

Cerebral Blood Flow

The normal CBF is 45 to 50 mL/100 g/min ranging from 20 mL/100 g/min in white matter to 70 mL/100 g/min in gray matter. There are two essential facts to understand about CBF:

- First, in normal circumstances, when the flow falls to less than 18 to 20 mL/100 g/min, the physiological electrical function of the neuronal cell begins to fail.
- Second, with raised ICP and loss of autoregulation, cerebral blood becomes BP-dependent.

Autoregulation:

- CBF is maintained at a constant level (MAP range, 50–150 mm Hg) in the normal brain in the face of the usual fluctuations in BP by the process of autoregulation.
- However, in the traumatized or ischemic brain with concomitant loss of autoregulation, CBF may become BP-dependent.
- CO_2 causes cerebral vasodilatation. As the arterial tension of CO_2 increases, CBF increases, and when CO_2 levels fall, vasoconstriction is induced.
- Hyperventilation can lead to a mean reduction in ICP of about 50% within 2 to 30 minutes; however, when $PaCO_2$ is < 25 mm Hg (3.3 kPa), there is no further reduction in CBF. Acute hypocapnic vasoconstriction will only last for a relatively short time (5 h).

Considering this, pathophysiology anesthesia plan is executed.

Anesthesia Targets

- Maintain MAP, that is, avoid hypotension.
- Avoid a precipitous increase in ICP and thus intracranial hypertension (ICH).
- Avoid secondary injuries by maintaining CPP > 70 mm Hg.

Anticonvulsant Use in TBI

Long-term anticonvulsants have no role in head trauma, but some patients may have seizures in the first week, which responds to phenytoin. The Brain Trauma Foundation (BTF) guidelines recommend short-term prophylaxis with phenytoin for head-injured patients.

Anesthesia Plan

Induction

Intravenous (IV) lignocaine may be administered before intubation to prevent a rise in the ICP.

The common drugs for induction include an IV narcotic (fentanyl 100–150 µg, pethidine 50 mg, or morphine 5 mg), followed by a slightly reduced dose of thiopentone 150 to 200 mg to ensure anesthesia, without causing hypotension. A reduced dose of propofol 90 to 100 mg can also be used for induction.

Ketamine, although believed to increase ICP, is believed to be neuroprotective due to N-methyl D-aspartate (NMDA) receptor blocker and thus is no longer contraindicated in head injury.

All intubations should be done as rapid sequence induction (RSI), and thus rocuronium should be used. Scoline is known to increase ICP and, therefore, should be avoided in cases of head injury.

Monitoring

Apart from electrocardiography, pulse oximetry, temperature, and end-tidal CO_2 monitoring is essential. Continuous invasive arterial BP monitoring is useful for monitoring CPP, titrating vasopressor infusion, and fluid therapy. Central venous access will help in assessing volume status as well as allow the infusion of vasopressor. *ICP monitoring is extremely useful, and an intraventricular drain* placed during the surgery can be used postoperatively for monitoring as well as CSF drainage as a temporizing measure to decrease ICP. Urine output needs to be monitored as a surrogate of perfusion and also because mannitol is used to control ICP.

Maintenance of Anesthesia

- Anesthesia can be maintained using narcotics (IV fentanyl 150 µg or morphine 10 mg given slowly), vecuronium 10 mg, and the patient ventilated with inhalational agents (isoflurane as the first choice) in oxygen-enriched air.
- Most IV drugs decrease metabolism and maintain coupling, excluding ketamine.
- While using inhalational agents, it is essential to remember that high inspired concentrations of inhalational agents (>1 minimum alveolar concentration [MAC]) will cause cerebral vasodilatation with increased cerebral blood volume, cerebral edema, and consequent rise in ICP. It decreases metabolism and changes metabolic coupling. At the same time, inhalational agents will cause a fall in BP. This combination of raised ICP and low BP is hazardous as it leads to a reduction in CPP, worsening neuronal damage, and may lead to adverse outcomes.
- Nitrous oxide is contraindicated in patients with raised ICP.

Ventilatory Strategy

Aim of ventilation in a head-injured patient is to provide adequate oxygenation in order to avoid hypoxemia and thus prevent a sudden increase in CBF and ICP. Intermittent positive pressure ventilation is given to achieve low normal arterial CO_2 ($PaCO_2$ 35 mm Hg), which will help reduce cerebral swelling and hence ICP. Severe hyperventilation is not recommended. Moderate hyperventilation to reduce intracranial hypotension is likely to work only for a short period (<5 h), and it just gives time before more definitive management can be undertaken.

Fluid

The free water can cross the blood–brain barrier easily. It is necessary, therefore, not to give hypotonic fluids such as dextrose solutions in water (5% dextrose) as dextrose metabolism will leave just the free water, which will be taken up by the brain, leading to further cerebral edema and an increase in ICP. Normal saline (0.9%) is the fluid of choice. Colloids, blood, and blood products can be used to treat hypovolemia due to significant blood loss.

Management of Intracranial Hypertension

The manifestations of the physiological effects of raised ICP are *hypertension, bradycardia, wide pulse pressure–the Cushing's triad and ventricular dysrhythmias*. ICH must be aggressively treated with immediate interventions aimed at lowering ICP and increasing CPP. *Sustained ICP ≥ 20 mm Hg for more than 10 minutes* is associated with poor outcomes, and prompt treatment is necessary. Important points of consideration here are as follows:

- *The use of therapeutic hyperventilation* reduces ICP through vasoconstriction. It is recommended to maintain the $PaCO_2$ at the low end of normal, while more definitive strategies for reducing ICP are attempted.

- *Maintain CPP*: This is done by reducing the ICP and ensuring adequate MAP to maintain CPP > 60 to 70 mm Hg with fluid resuscitation and vasopressor support. Vasodilators such as diazoxide, hydralazine, nitroglycerine, or nitroprusside should not be used.

- *Osmotic diuresis*: *Mannitol is given as a 0.5 to 1 g/kg bolus and repeated every 6 to 8 hours to maintain serum osmolarity at > 310 mOsm/L in order to cause* osmotic diuresis. The altered osmolar gradient facilitates fluid shifts and reduces cerebral edema.

- *Hypertonic saline*: Hyponatremia indicates worse outcomes, and serum sodium should be maintained at the upper limits of normal. Sodium chloride is the fluid of choice for resuscitation. The hypertonic saline solution increases serum osmolarity, which expands intravascular volume, improves CBF, and facilitates the removal of fluid in cerebral edema. It also affects microcirculation (Sr Na target: 150–155 mEq/L).

- *Hypothermia*: Hyperthermia increases ICP and should be prevented. Hypothermia reduces ICP and may mediate apoptosis, coagulopathy, and electrolyte abnormalities. Shivering may occur, which increases ICP.

- *Corticosteroids*: Previously, steroids were thought to be of help in reducing cerebral edema, but recent studies have shown increased mortality in patients receiving steroids when compared to placebo. Steroids also increase blood glucose levels, which can adversely affect the injured brain. So, according to the current evidence, there *is no role of steroids in the head-injured patient* and should not be used. Glycemic control is essential as hyperglycemia is likely to lead to poor outcomes in severely head-injured patients and, if present, should be aggressively treated.

- *Postural drainage*: 15 to 30° head elevation and neck maintained in a midline position facilitate the venous return and reduces ICP.

- *Sedation and analgesia*: The use of benzodiazepines and propofol can reduce agitation and decrease ICP.

- *Vasodilators* such as diazoxide, hydralazine, nitroglycerine, or nitroprusside may be catastrophic in this situation.

- *Neuromuscular blockade*: Therapeutic paralysis reduces ICP and prevents shivering if induced hypothermia is attempted with the disadvantage of masking the seizure activity.

- *Barbiturate coma*: This may be considered in patients with *refractory ICH or in those with uncontrolled seizures.* Continuous bedside EEG monitoring is necessary to monitor adequate burst suppression with barbiturate infusions.

- *CSF drainage*: Removal of CSF through an intraventricular catheter reduces ICP. Drainage should be continued to maintain the ICP between 5 and 15 mm Hg; however, the chances of infection are high.

- *Decompression craniectomy*: Decompression craniectomy can facilitate ICP reduction and may improve the patient's outcome. However, studies so far have failed to show an improvement in long-term neurological consequences.

Postoperative Care

- If the patient has undergone simply an evacuation of extradural hematoma, he can be extubated once wide awake.

- If additional injuries such as diffuse axonal injuries are present, then ventilation for a more extended period may be required.

- It is important to remember that peak brain edema can take 24 to 72 hours to occur. The care in postanesthetic care unit (PACU) aims at:

  ► Prevention of secondary injuries due to physiological factors, which may cause cerebral edema.

  ► Observation to detect any deterioration.

  ► Providing adequate analgesia.

► Any further insult can be detected by changes in the level of consciousness, development of focal neurodeficit, or unequal pupils.

► Prophylactic treatment with phenytoin should be initiated as soon as possible after the injury to decrease the risk of posttraumatic seizures and then stopped after 7 days.

In Case of Multiple Trauma

- Intra-abdominal and intrathoracic bleeding complication take precedence over intracranial injury.

- Limb-threatening injuries should be dealt with as a damage control operation rather than definitive repair.

- Trauma as well as neurosurgeons can perform surgeries simultaneously.

Anesthesia Management in Burns Patient

Most emergency medical services and hospitals will, from time to time, need to deal with the immediate management of patients with major burns. For most doctors, handling these patients will be a major challenge. Therefore, anesthetists, plastic surgeons, and general surgeons should be competent in the early assessment and management of burn patients, that is, burn depth evaluation, percentage of total body surface area (TBSA), identifying when an escharotomy is required, initial fluid therapy, airway management, intensive care issues, and wound care. Knowledge of pathophysiology and anatomy is advantageous.

This chapter aims to give clinical guidance on how to treat patients in the early phase of a major burn injury. To understand the whole picture, authors have systematically addressed all aspects of attending and treating burn patients.

Types of Burns

- Thermal burns—scald or flame.
- Electric burns include lightening burns.
- Chemical burns.
- Frostbite.

Depth of Burns

Assessment of the depth of the burn is essential for planning wound care and predicting functional and cosmetic results. Different types of wounds based on depth are as follows:

- *Superficial*: Only the epidermis is damaged. It heals spontaneously within 7 days with no scarring. There is erythema, no blisters, it blanches on pressure, and is painful.
- *Superficial partial thickness (superficial dermal)*: The complete destruction of epidermis along with the upper one-third of dermis but the preservation of the adnexal skin structures (hair follicles, sebaceous glands, sweat glands). However, the epithelium regenerates rapidly, and the wound heals within 10 to 14 days without any scarring. It has a red and mottled appearance with swelling and blanches on pressure. There is a blister formation and is painful.
- *Deep partial thickness (deep dermal)*: Loss of epidermis and a substantial part of the dermis along with adnexal structures. Healing may take several weeks or months as epithelialization is slow. There is scarring. It is pale in appearance with no blanching. There is no pain; only pressure sensation is felt. These burns require excision and grafting for the rapid return of function.
- *Full thickness*: It involves the destruction of all skin elements destroyed and may extend to include deep structures such as muscle, bone, and major neurovascular bundles. It appears dark, leathery with a dry surface.

It is painless and does not blanch on pressure. It requires excision and grafting.

Assessment of burn by BSA involved using formulae:

- *Wallace rule of nines*: It is used to assess the percentage of BSA burnt. Although it tends to overestimate the burned area, it is an excellent method for measuring medium to massive burns (**Table 31.4**).
- *Palmar surface*: The palmar surface of the patient's hand, with fingers very slightly spread, equates to approximately 1% of the patient's TBSA. This is a quick and reliable method of assessing patchy areas of burns up to 15% of TBSA. It is not very accurate in estimating moderate burns.
- *Lund and Browder chart*: It is used to assess the area of burns in children (**Fig. 31.1** and **Table 31.5**).

Definition of Major Burns

Having calculated the BSA and depth of burn, we need to define if the given burn is major or minor. The following categories are included in major burns:

- Third-degree (full thickness) burn injuries involving > 10% of TBSA.
- Second-degree (partial thickness) burn injuries involving > 20% TBSA at extremes of age and > 25% TBSA in adults.

Table 31.4 Wallace rule of nines

Part of the body	Percentage of burn area
Head and neck	9%
Upper extremities	9% each
Chest (anterior and posterior)	9% each
Abdomen	9%
Lower back	9%
Lower extremities	18% each
Perineum	1%

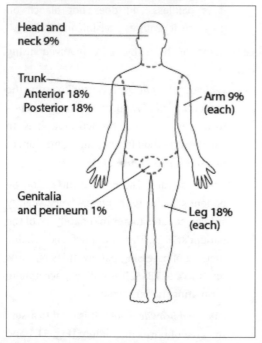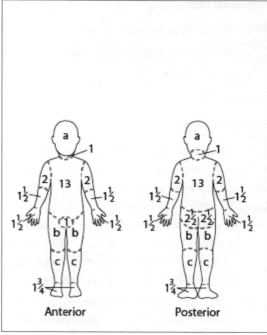

Fig. 31.1 Assessment of area of burns as per Lund and Browder's method.

Table 31.5 Relative %BSA affected by growth as per Lund and Browder's chart

Body part	Age				
	0 year	1 year	5 years	10 years	15 years
a = ½ of head	9 ½	8 ½	6 ½	5 ½	4 ½
b = ½ of 1 thigh	2 ¾	3 ¼	4	4 ¼	4 ½
c = ½ of 1 lower leg	2 ½	2 ½	2 ¾	3	3 ¼

Abbreviation: %BSA, percentage of burn surface area.

- Burns involving face, hands, feet, genitalia, perineum, and major joints.

- Inhalational injuries.

- Chemical burn injuries.

- Electrical burn injuries.

- Burn injuries in patients with coexisting medical disease.

- Burns associated with trauma.

Role of Anesthesiologists in a Burn Patient

Anesthesiologists role in a burn case is multifaceted in the following aspects:

- Initial resuscitation of the burn patient.

- Adequate fluid resuscitation and prevention and management of sepsis and multiorgan failure in ICU.

- Emergency for various surgical procedures like early excision of damaged tissues, removal of granulation tissue, and escharotomy under general anesthesia.

- Change of dressings or/and for skin grafting after the acute phase.

- Reconstructive plastic surgery procedures are done to relieve contractures, correct deformities, and restore limb function.

Pathophysiology of Burns

Burn injury affects all systems in the body. Depending on if the burn is major or minor, the systemic response will vary. Burns cause a local and systemic inflammatory reaction, which results in the release of various inflammatory mediators (oxygen radicals, histamine, prostaglandin, bradykinin, nitric oxide, serotonin and substance P and complement).

Hemodynamic Response

- The systemic inflammatory response causes an increase in capillary permeability, which results in the loss of large amounts of protein-rich fluids from the intravascular compartment to the interstitial compartment. As a result of this, there is *hypoalbuminemia*, which is further exacerbated by decreased hepatic albumin production in favor of acute-phase protein synthesis.

- There is decreased circulating blood volume because of the increased movement of fluid into the interstitial compartment.

- *Cell membrane* adenosine triphosphatase activity is reduced, leading to decreased functioning of cell surface transporters (e.g., Na-K ATPase).

- The fluid loss also continues by *evaporation and exudation* from the wound site, further causing intravascular depletion.

- Catecholamine surge during the initial 24 hours of burn causes peripheral and splanchnic vasoconstriction and decreased cardiac contractility. All this can result in the hypoperfusion of the end organs. This phase is known as *burn shock*. It is due to a combination of hypovolemia, cardiogenic, and distributive element.

- Excessive administration of fluids at this stage leads to generalized edema, which further compromises tissue oxygenation.

Reperfusion of the ischemic zone releases oxygen-free radicals, causing local cell membrane damage and immune response. After the patients are adequately fluid-resuscitated, there will be a phase of increased cardiac output and a marked reduction in systemic vascular resistance.

Respiratory Responses

- Release of inflammatory mediators can cause bronchoconstriction in the absence of inhalation injury.

- In patients with inhalational injury, the release of inflammatory mediators can lead to the development of acute respiratory distress syndrome (ARDS).

Metabolic Responses

- After major burns, there is a hypermetabolic response that lasts for up to 1 year after the burns injury. There is decreased protein synthesis and increased muscle breakdown.

- Increased circulating levels of catabolic hormones lead to increased gluconeogenesis, which is resistant to insulin infusion.

- Increased peripheral lipolysis leads to the rapid depletion of glycogen stores.

- All these changes lead to impaired wound healing, exposing patients to increased infection risk. Rehabilitation is often difficult in these patients.

Thermoregulation

- Due to the hypermetabolic responses, the metabolic *thermostat* is reset. Burns patients increase their skin and core temperatures somewhat above normal regardless of the environmental temperatures.

- Following thermal injury, *thermoregulatory functions of the skin* like vasoactivity, sweating, piloerection, and insulation are either abolished or diminished.

- Daily evaporative water loss is 2,500 mL/m² in adults and 4,000 mL/m² of BSA in children.

Immune System Responses

- Following severe burns, there is a loss of protective skin barrier and suppression of the immune system.
- Also, these patients need invasive lines and urinary catheters for monitoring.
- As a result of all this, burns patients are susceptible to increased risk of repeated episodes of infection.

Hematologic System

- Burns patients are usually *anemic* due to:
  - ▶ Loss of erythrocytes from the burn wound.
  - ▶ Bleeding during surgeries.
  - ▶ Hemolysis of erythrocytes due to thermal injury and suppression of erythrocyte production.
  - ▶ Decreased erythrocyte survival after burns.
  - ▶ The hematocrit is increased for at least 48 hours after burns due to hemoconcentration and may not be an appropriate guide for the need for transfusion.
- Platelet counts and coagulation factors are decreased due to dilution and consumption. There is the activation of thrombotic and fibrinolytic mechanisms.

Renal and Electrolytes

- Decrease in renal blood flow:
  - ▶ Secondary to hypovolemia and decreased cardiac output.
  - ▶ Systemic vasoconstriction due to circulating catecholamines.
  - ▶ Nephrotoxic effects of drugs.
  - ▶ Myoglobin.
  - ▶ Sepsis.

- Renin-angiotensin-aldosterone system gets activated due to decreased renal blood flow, resulting in the release of antidiuretic hormone.
- The net effect on the renal function is the retention of sodium and water and exaggerated losses of potassium, calcium, and magnesium.
- Hyperkalemia may occur due to tissue necrosis and hemolysis.

Gastrointestinal Tract

- Ileus is common in burns patients; hence, early decompression of the stomach through a nasogastric tube is indicated.
- Curling's ulcers are acute ulceration of the stomach or duodenum seen in patients with sepsis or extensive burn injuries. The exact etiology is unknown. Endotoxemia can result from the disruption of the gastric mucosal barrier. Gastric mucosal ulcerations can be minimized by proper hemodynamic resuscitation, early enteral feeding, and the use of antacids and H2 receptor blockers.

ABCDE of Burn

The resuscitation of a burn patient is in accordance with the same guidelines of ATLS as discussed above except for a few highlights:

A. First aid: In the initial first aid, one should try and stop the burning process and cool the burn wound. Chemical powders should be cleared from the wound. The burnt area should be rinsed with tepid water (at least 15°C for 20–30 min). Ice should never be used because it causes vasoconstriction, leading to further tissue damage and hypothermia. The patient should then be covered with warm, clean, and dry linens to prevent hypothermia.

B. Primary survey: All burns patients should receive 100% oxygen with a reservoir mask.

The threshold for intubation is kept very low because of intoxication, inhalational injury, alcohol, and carbon monoxide (CO) poisoning.

C. Breathing and ventilation: The chest should be exposed to ensure that chest expansion is adequate and equal. Look for signs of respiratory distress (increased respiratory rate, tracheal tug, and excessive use of accessory muscles). Circumferential burns to the chest may restrict breathing and impair gaseous exchange. An escharotomy may be required in circumferential burns that compromise breathing.

D. Circulation with hemorrhage control: Rapid assessment of the volume status should be done. Monitor the BP, pulse, and capillary refill in both burned and unburned limbs. Escharotomies may be required if there are isolated poor perfusion in a limb with circumferential full-thickness burns. Use of a BP cuff may be difficult in a burned patient, and invasive arterial monitoring may be needed.

E. Disability: Neurological status (as explained above).

F. Exposure and environmental control: Remove any jewelry and clothing and keep the patient warm.

ICU/Ward Care for a Burn Patient

Fluid resuscitation is the most crucial aspect and is proportional to burn size. This is because tissue burns cause massive fluid shifts due to increased capillary permeability. This results in edema formation, particularly during the first 36 hours. The resultant fluid depletion is most significant in the first few hours, and early fluid resuscitation is essential to avoid hypovolemic shock and acute renal failure (ARF). Adults with greater than 15% TBSA burns and children with greater than 10% TBSA burns will need fluid resuscitation. While resuscitating burns, a urinary catheter should be inserted to monitor urine output as a function of organ perfusion. One should aim for a urine output of at least 0.5 mL/kg/h in adults and 1 mL/kg/h in children who weigh less than 30 kg. Two large bore IV cannulas should be inserted, preferably in a nonburned area. Upper extremities are preferable to lower extremities for venous access because of the high incidence of phlebitis in the saphenous veins. Other options are saphenous cut-down, femoral cut-down, and intraosseous needles in children less than 6 years. Warmed Ringer lactate solution should be used for treating hypovolemic shock.

Parkland formula is widely used for burns resuscitation. The fluid requirement is 4 mL/kg/% BSA of burns; give half in first 8 hours and the remaining over the next 16 hours.

In children, it is necessary to administer maintenance IV fluids containing glucose in addition to the burn formula. These formulae are only a guide, and assessment of resuscitation should be based clinically on heart rate, BP, capillary refill, central venous pressure (CVP), urine output, peripheral and core temperature, and mental state of the patient.

The use of colloid for resuscitation is controversial, but few studies suggest the use of 4.5% albumin in fluid resuscitation.

Blood should be collected for grouping and cross-matching, complete blood count (CBC), blood glucose, serum electrolytes, serum urea and creatinine, COHb levels, and ABG analysis. Urine should be tested for myoglobin/hemoglobin. A chest X-ray should be done. Other X-rays may be indicated if there are associated injuries.

Pain management: A burn patient often requires long-term ICU stay with multiple sessions of dressing, debridement, and grafting procedures. Inadequate pain management during such procedures may lead to long-term anxiety and posttraumatic stress disorder. NSAIDs and oral acetaminophen provide mild analgesia. The use of opioids is associated with dependence tolerance and gastrointestinal side effects. Use of dexmedetomidine and clonidine can cause hypotension due to volume depletion in burn patients. Ketamine, because of its hemodynamic stability, ability to preserve airway reflexes, as well as hypoxic and hypercapnic responses, is always a preferred choice for pain management in such group of patients. A severely burned patient may be restless and anxious due to hypoxemia and hypovolemia rather than pain. Hence, these patients respond better to oxygen or increased fluid administration rather than narcotic analgesics or sedatives, which may mask the signs of hypoxemia or hypovolemia. Narcotic analgesics and sedatives should be administered in small frequent doses through IV route only. Intramuscular and subcutaneous injections should be avoided as absorption will be erratic and analgesia delayed.

After assessing the size and depth of burns, wash the burnt area and do the dressing. Use dressing (preferably transparent to facilitate wound inspection) to cover the burnt area as it protects the wound and reduces heat and evaporative losses.

Insert nasogastric tube and decompress the stomach if nausea and vomiting are present in patients with burns more than 20% TBSA and all intubated patients.

As patients with burns are in a highly catabolic state, establishing enteral feeding within 4 hours of admission helps improve the outcome. Early enteral nutrition promotes normal gut function and decreases the potential for bacterial translocation across the gastric mucosa. Antibiotics are reserved for the treatment of infection with no role of prophylactic antibiotics. Tetanus prophylaxis should be given. Early referral to a burn center would be appropriate.

Operation Theater for Escharotomy, Emergency Debridement/Amputation

It may sometimes be inevitable for a postburns patient to undergo an emergency escharotomy, especially in case of circumferential burns around the chest, causing decreased cardiac output/perfusion. This is in the early phase of 24 to 48 hours when the pathophysiological changes of burn shock are not stabilized, and the patient has a high risk of decompensating.

Emergency debridements are postponed up until 48 hours as this is the time of initial stabilization. However, in both the scenarios, patient has a high chance of systemic complications, and anesthesia management should be well executed.

History

A complete medical and surgical history should be taken, and a thorough physical examination should be done. A burns history would tell you about the possibility of inhalational injury.

Examination

In the preanesthetic evaluation, the age and the percentage of TBSA of burns will give an idea about the patient's physiologic condition. The adequacy of resuscitation should be assessed. In the airway assessment, one should check the MPC, thyromental distance, and head and neck mobility. The presence of facial burns can make mask ventilation difficult. Edema, scarring, or contracture formation may limit mouth opening and neck mobility. Traditional IV access sites may be unavailable.

Investigation

Blood grouping and cross-matching, CBC, blood glucose, serum electrolytes, serum urea and creatinine, and ABG analysis should be done to know COHb levels. A chest X-ray should be done. Adequate blood should be kept ready as blood loss has been estimated to range from 200 to 300 mL/% of body surface excised and grafted. ECG has to be done in patients above 40 years of age or if they have associated medical conditions.

Preoperative Optimization/Preparation

In major burns patients, it is challenging to achieve adequate nutritional status as they are in a hypercatabolic state. Therefore, avoiding prolonged periods of fasting before the surgery would be beneficial. These patients are many times on analgesics for pain relief and should be continued through the perioperative period. Depending on the extent of surgical excision, adequate-sized IV access should be taken. Location of burns and donor skin sites indicate the need for special positioning, for repositioning the patient during the operation, or both.

Monitoring

Intraoperative monitoring should include ECG, BP, $ETCO_2$, pulse oximetry, core temperature, neuromuscular, and urine output monitoring. Cutaneous burns may make the placement of conventional monitoring devices, such as ECG electrodes or BP cuff, difficult. Gel electrodes may not pick up ECG through damaged skin. Skin staples or subcutaneous needles attached to crocodile clips will give a good signal. Invasive BP monitoring would be preferable in patients requiring extensive debridement. It may be challenging to get the pulse oximetry trace due to peripheral burns or vasoconstriction. Alternative sites like ear, nose, or tongue can be used. Also, the cutaneous vessels in the burnt area cannot constrict and prevent heat loss by radiation. The operating room ambient temperature should be 28 to 32°C, and all topical and IV fluids should be warmed. When possible, nonoperative sites should be covered and forced-air warming devices used.

Induction of Anesthesia

General anesthesia with the combination of an opioid, muscle relaxant, and a volatile agent is the most widely used technique for burn excision and grafting. Laryngeal mask airway (LMA) is useful in maintaining the airway in both adults and children with burns. Consider awake fiberoptic intubation if mouth opening is restricted. Tracheostomy is generally undesirable because of the risk that infection may spread to the damaged skin. Various IV agents can be used successfully for induction.

Ketamine has a lot of advantages. It not only provides stable hemodynamics but also has analgesic properties. Hence, it has been used extensively as the primary agent for both general anesthesia and analgesia for burn dressing changes. Its major drawback is its tendency to produce dysphoric reactions. An antisialagogue premedication is a must. Etomidate can be an alternative to ketamine in the hemodynamically unstable patient. Thiopentone can be used as an induction agent in patients who are resuscitated and hemodynamically stable. Succinylcholine should be avoided 24 hours after burns injury due to hyperkalemia and the unpredictable response of muscle relaxation action. After burns, there is an increase in the number of postjunctional receptors, which cause prolonged depolarization and marked release of potassium. This process of receptor proliferation takes several days to develop, with an initial window of the safety of unknown duration. The most dangerous period is thought to be between 4 days and 10 weeks after thermal injury. Scoline is further avoided until 2 years postburns.

Maintenance of Anesthesia

If a laryngeal mask is used, the patient can be kept spontaneously breathing with O_2, nitrous, and inhalational agent. The choice of a volatile agent does not appear to influence outcomes from anesthesia for burn surgery. If the patient has been intubated, then nondepolarizing muscle relaxants (atracurium or vecuronium) can be used for controlled ventilation. The following should be kept in mind during maintenance of anesthesia:

- As these patients routinely receive opioids for various procedures or routine pain management, they develop tolerance and may need large doses of opioids in the perioperative period for pain relief.

- Epidural local anesthetic should be used cautiously in extensive debridements as there is a potential for massive blood loss and hypotension. However, epidural opioids can be safely used.

- For patients requiring burn dressings, usually IV ketamine and titrated opioids produce adequate pain relief.

- Patients needing skin grafting are electively posted after 3 weeks, and although the airway management is still challenging, the acute hemodynamic changes associated with burns have settled.

Now, sometimes patient with a previous history of burns is posted for postburn contracture release of face and neck. The main concerns here would be difficult airway, and thus knowledge of difficult airway intubation and extubation is indispensable for an anesthesiologist. A detailed airway examination is warranted to document MPC grading, thyrohyoid/thyrosternal distance, and temporomandibular (TM) joint movement. According to the airway findings, an airway plan is devised 1 day before surgery. All airway gadgets are kept ready in the operation theater on the day of surgery, including a rigid bronchoscope. Patients can have limited neck mobility and microstomia. Due to the facial scarring, it may not be possible to get a good mask seal, making mask ventilation difficult. Insertion of an LMA would be difficult due to microstomia. Blind nasotracheal intubation is unlikely to succeed if the neck movements are restricted, or it is fixed in a flexed position. Microstomia and distortion of the oral cavity make use of the LMA and oral fiberoptic intubation difficult. Retrograde intubation may not be possible because of extensive scarring on the anterior surface of the neck, which distorts the surface anatomy of the larynx. So, the technique of choice widely used is awake fiberoptic intubation; however, one has to check for patency of external nares. A proper airway preparation is mandatory for awake fiberoptic intubation.

IV access in the upper limbs will be difficult due to scarring. Since surgery does not require muscle relaxation, the patient can be maintained on spontaneous ventilation using inhalational agents.

Sometimes surgeons release neck contractures under local anesthesia known as tumescent local anesthesia. It is a type of infiltration anesthesia where a large volume of local anesthetic with adrenaline is infiltrated into the subcutaneous tissue. After a waiting period of 20 minutes, the neck contracture can be released.

One formula uses 25 mL of 2% lidocaine and 1 mL of 1:1000 adrenaline for each liter of sodium lactate IV infusion. Lignocaine doses of up to 35 mg/kg have been used without any side effects. This is because dilution of lidocaine and epinephrine-induced vasoconstriction diminishes and delays the peak plasma lidocaine concentrations, thereby reducing potential toxicity. Infiltrating a large volume of dilute epinephrine assures diffusion throughout the entire targeted area while avoiding tachycardia and hypertension. Clinical local anesthesia can last as long as 18 hours, obviating the need for postoperative analgesia.

If required, analgesic doses of ketamine 0.5 mg/kg can be given.

Conclusion

Trauma care and burn management constitute a significant part of anesthesia expertise and should be carried out efficiently. To do that, you must be well versed with the ATLS guidelines, airway techniques, airway management flow-charts, management of shock, and anesthesia management of these patients in operation room. Thorough reading and practical application of guidelines are advocated to improve patient management and outcome.

Patients of trauma, traumatic brain injuries, and burns have severely altered hemodynamics and require multidisciplinary assistance and care. A careful assessment of airway, volume status, and risk of perioperative complications is essential for managing such patients. Burn patients often require multiple surgeries and prolonged ICU stay.

CHAPTER 32

Anesthesia for Orthopedic Surgery

Ajit Kumar and Roshan

Introduction

Orthopedic diseases are common across all age groups and cause substantial disability and loss of quality of life. The treatment of orthopedic conditions is time-extensive and puts a huge burden on health care costs. The patients may come for the correction of joint and spine deformity, for removal of bone tumor, in addition to the traumatic injuries of bones and joints. The anesthetic management of such patients may be complicated by comorbid illness, large intraoperative blood loss, painful surgeries, and prolonged hospital stay with the risk of infections and deep vein thrombosis (DVT). This chapter is an overview of anesthetic care of common orthopedic diseases, which include the following:

- Arthroplasty.
- Anesthesia for orthopedic tumors.
- Anesthesia for scoliosis surgery.

Anesthesia for Arthroplasty

Arthroplasty is a surgical procedure in which a malformed or diseased joint is altered or completely replaced to restore optimal function or relieve pain. Worldwide, the most commonly performed arthroplasty is that of the knee joint and hip joint, followed by shoulder, wrist, ankle, and finger joints. The spectrum of patients ranges from a young, healthy trauma victim to an elderly patient with multiple comorbidities. *Therefore, preoperative assessment of patients at risk of mortality and morbidity, preparedness for the intraoperative and postoperative complications, and provision of postoperative care are the main areas of concern for an anesthesiologist.*

Preoperative Assessment

In recent times, joint replacement in the active aging population is increasing. *The advanced age and cardiopulmonary complications are the most common risk factors for perioperative mortality.* Therefore, patients must be evaluated for:

- Preexisting comorbidities including cardiovascular disease.
- Hypertension.
- Pulmonary disease.
- Diabetes.
- Obesity.
- Age-related concerns.

Underlying conditions like rheumatic arthritis, osteoarthritis, and diabetes mellitus pose challenges of a difficult airway, which should be carefully evaluated. Patient's medications, particularly antihypertensive medication, anticoagulant, steroids, and opioids, should be reviewed, and continuation or discontinuation of these medications should be guideline-adherent.

Technique of Anesthesia

Due to localized surgical sites, regional anesthesia is the preferred choice. Regional anesthesia technique offers several advantages over general anesthesia, including:

- Decreased incidence of nausea and vomiting.
- Less cardiorespiratory complication.
- Improved postoperative analgesia.
- Enhanced rehabilitation, early ambulation, and early hospital discharge.

For arthroplasty of lower extremity joints, especially knee and hip joints, central neuraxial blockade provides excellent intraoperative anesthesia and improved outcome. Based on current evidence, the International Consensus on Anaesthesia-Related Outcomes after Surgery (ICAROS) group recommends neuraxial over general anesthesia for hip/knee arthroplasty. *Combined spinal-epidural anesthesia (CSEA), along with sedation, is now considered as the technique of choice, where epidural catheter acts as a conduit for postoperative analgesia.*

Peripheral nerve blockade, although rarely used as the sole anesthetic, can be used with general anesthesia to reduce the requirement of anesthetic drugs and opioids or for postoperative pain management. The commonly used nerve blocks for knee and hip arthroplasty are listed in **Table 32.1**.

Perioperative Concerns

A few of the perioperative concerns which should be borne in mind are explained below.

1. Blood loss

Intraoperative blood loss is a major concern during arthroplasty. Total hip arthroplasty can cause significant blood loss up to 1 to 2 L. *Intraoperative and postoperative blood loss is less in regional anesthesia due to reductions in mean arterial pressure and venodilatation.* Intraoperative use of tranexamic acid or fibrin spray has also been shown to reduce blood loss. Deliberate, controlled hypotension can also be used as a means of reducing surgical blood loss and need for transfusion. A pneumatic tourniquet can be used to reduce blood loss and provide a bloodless field during surgery.

2. Fat embolism syndrome

It is a common occurrence during traumatic orthopedic injuries with fractures of long bones and pelvis being the commonest. The symptomatology usually starts between 24 and 72 hours of insult. The patient presents with dyspnea, chest discomfort, altered mental status, restlessness, hypotension, tachycardia, petechial rash (over conjunctiva, axilla, neck, and upper torso). The dyspnea, petechial rash, and confusion constitute a classical triad of fat embolism syndrome. Gurd and Schonfeld are the most common diagnostic criteria for fat embolism syndrome.

The fat embolism syndrome is hypothesized to occur due to fat emboli-mediated endothelial injury in lungs and brain, leading to acute respiratory distress syndrome (ARDS) and cerebral edema, respectively. The investigations which provide a clue to fat embolism syndrome are:

- Retinal examination: Fat globules in retinal vessels.
- Urine examination: Fat globules.
- Chest X-ray: Diffuse interstitial infiltrates.
- Abnormal coagulation studies.
- Thrombocytopenia.
- High serum lipase (but it does not correlate with disease severity).

Table 32.1 Peripheral nerve blocks for arthroplasty

Knee arthroplasty	Hip arthroplasty
• Posterior lumbar plexus (psoas compartment) block • Adductor canal block • Femoral nerve block • Sciatic nerve block • Obturator nerve block	• Posterior lumbar plexus block • Femoral nerve block • Sciatic block • Fascia iliac block

The patients with fat embolism syndrome require vigilant monitoring for mental status and respiratory difficulties, and they may need respiratory support with mechanical ventilation in case of respiratory failure. The management aspect includes:

- Early stabilization of the fracture.
- Oxygen therapy.
- Mechanical ventilation (noninvasive/invasive) for respiratory failure.
- A trial of glucocorticoids can be given (to decrease immune response to fat globules and halt the progression of disease).

3. Bone cement implantation syndrome

Methyl methacrylate cement fixation of the prosthesis can cause bone cement implantation syndrome, which is characterized by:

- Intraoperative hypotension.
- Hypoxia.
- Cardiac arrest.
- Fat embolism syndrome postoperatively.

Implementing "cement curfew" protocol can minimize chances of BCIS and help in timely management if it at all occurs. The patient, surgeon, anesthetist, and other team members of the operation theater are part of this protocol.

The patient must be informed about the risk of bone cement implantation syndrome. The surgeon should be wise in choosing the patient (based on comorbidities and risk of bone cement implantation syndrome) and type of prosthesis for the given patient. He must inform the anesthetist before inserting the prosthesis. The anesthetist must engage in adequate preparation, in order to manage if BCIS occurs. The other team members in the operation theater should be aware and ready to play their roles in case of occurrence of BCIS.

Several mechanisms have been postulated for these events, *including embolization of bone marrow debris to the circulation during pressurization of the long bone canal, toxic effects of circulating methyl methacrylate monomer, due to cytokines released during reaming of the femoral canal which promote the formation of microthrombi and subsequent pulmonary vasoconstriction.*

Management:

- For high-risk patients, consider strict hemodynamic monitoring including invasive arterial pressure and central venous pressure (CVP).
- At the time of cementation, FiO_2 should be increased.
- Intravascular fluid and vasopressors for hemodynamic instability.
- Advanced cardiac life support protocol in case of cardiac arrest.

4. Postoperative cardiopulmonary complication

The ACC/AHA classify orthopedic surgery as intermediate-risk surgery due to increased risk of perioperative myocardial morbidity and mortality. *Multiple medical comorbid conditions, age-related limited functional capacity, surgery-induced systemic inflammatory response syndrome, fluid shifts, and blood loss during surgery and postoperative pain can trigger a stress response, leading to tachycardia, hypertension, and increased oxygen demand which could lead to myocardial ischemia.*

Patients at risk of perioperative cardiac complications should be assessed postoperatively for myocardial ischemia. Age-related respiratory changes, embolization of bone marrow debris to the lungs during surgery, obesity, and obstructive sleep apnea can lead to respiratory complications.

5. Venous thromboembolism

The incidence of deep venous thrombosis (DVT) is quite high with arthroplasty surgeries. Anticoagulant prophylaxis or intermittent pneumatic compression should be considered in patients with a high risk of bleeding.

6. Postoperative pain management

Multimodal analgesia is essential for pain relief and minimize side-effects while maintaining rehabilitation and patient satisfaction.

Anesthesia for Orthopedic Tumors

Tumors encountered in orthopedic practice develop either within the bone or soft tissue. Metastatic tumors are more common than primary tumors. There are four most common types of primary bone cancer:

- Multiple myeloma.
- Osteosarcoma.
- Ewing's sarcoma.
- Chondrosarcoma.

Generally, surgical removal of the tumor is the preferred treatment. Often radiation therapy or systemic chemotherapy is used in combination with surgery (limb salvage surgery, amputation).

Preoperative Assessment

Patients should be assessed for comorbid conditions just like other surgeries. Special consideration is given to the type, size, tumor invasiveness, plan of surgical procedure, and current chemotherapy and radiotherapy treatment.

All possible side effects of chemotherapeutic agents should be investigated preoperatively. Table 32.2 highlights the important chemotherapeutic agents and their side effects.

Myelosuppressive effect of radiotherapy and chemotherapy could cause anemia. Therefore, iron therapy or erythropoietin therapy should be used to optimize the hemoglobin level.

Laboratory investigation for patients who received radiotherapy or chemotherapy should include hemogram, platelet count, coagulation profile, renal function test, and liver function test.

Anesthesia Technique

Either general or regional anesthesia can be used. *With regional techniques, the risk of intraoperative blood loss and DVT is reduced.* Caution should be taken before opting for regional anesthesia if patients have drug-induced neuropathy. Peripheral nerve blocks lessen the stress response to surgery as well as opioid and volatile requirements; therefore, they can be used along with general anesthesia.

Table 32.2 Chemotherapeutic agents and their side effects

Chemotherapeutic agent	Side effect	Investigation to be done
• Doxorubicin • Paclitaxel • Ifosfamide • Cyclophosphamide • Anthracycline • Methotrexate • Etoposide • Busulfan • Cyclophosphamide • Paclitaxel • Cisplatin • Vincristine, cisplatinum	• Cardiomyopathy • Diastolic dysfunction • Interstitial pneumonitis, pulmonary fibrosis, pulmonary veno-occlusive disease • Acute hypersensitivity pneumonitis • Acute chest pain syndrome • Acute renal failure • Peripheral neuropathies	• ECG • 2D Echo • Pulmonary function test • Arterial blood gas analysis • Renal function test • Nerve conduction studies

Intraoperative Considerations

Monitoring

Standard monitors, that is, pulse oximetry, non-invasive blood pressure monitor, ECG, and temperature monitoring, are mandatory for the intraoperative period. In addition:

- Invasive arterial blood pressure monitoring is appropriate in case of anticipated significant blood loss.

- Cardiac output monitoring should be considered in patients with cardiovascular comorbidities and in patients with chemotherapy-induced cardiotoxicity.

- Urine output monitoring is indicated in case of prolonged surgery or surgery with a major fluid shift.

- Chemotherapy and radiotherapy induce immune suppression; therefore, all aseptic precautions should be taken in the perioperative period to avoid iatrogenic infection.

Intraoperative Blood Loss

It is the major concern in the case of tumor surgery. *Tumor volume, invasive nature of the tumor, surgical approach, and extent of surgery are the significant factors affecting blood loss.* Blood loss can be mitigated with the help of:

- Tourniquet.
- Antifibrinolytic agent.
- Controlled hypotension.
- Preoperative embolization of the feeding vessel of tumors.
- Blood conservative strategies (preoperative optimization of hemoglobin, autologous blood donation, acute normovolemic hemodilution, and cell salvage).

In case of significant blood loss, careful fluid management and timely blood transfusion help to maintain hemodynamic stability. *A 1:1:1 strategy for packed red blood cells (PRBC), fresh frozen plasma (FFP), and platelet therapy during a massive transfusion can be adopted to avoid dilutional coagulopathy.* A point of care test, thromboelastography, can be used for goal-directed bleeding control and to avoid iatrogenic coagulopathy.

Bone Cement Implantation Syndrome

In some cases, bone cement is used, which carries the risk of bone cement implantation syndrome. The high-risk patients are:

- Patients with chronic obstructive pulmonary disease (COPD).
- Pulmonary or cardiac comorbidity.
- Metastatic bone tumors.
- Pathological fractures.
- High American Society of Anesthesiologists (ASA) scores.
- Those receiving diuretics or warfarin.

Sudden hypotension, desaturation, and arrhythmias are the hallmark features in this case. Management includes:

- Increased inspired oxygen concentration.
- Avoidance of intravascular volume depletion.
- Aggressive early management of hypotension, hypoxia, and arrhythmia.

Postoperative Concerns

Deep Venous Thrombosis

DVT is a major issue with bone or soft-tissue tumors. Cancer, major orthopedic surgery, and prosthetic reconstruction are factors are independently associated with a high risk of DVT. Pharmacologic anticoagulation with low-molecular weight heparin (LMWH) is a standard treatment. Mechanical prophylaxis should be applied when pharmacological anticoagulation is not possible. In major surgery, the risk of DVT is reduced with a combined approach of pharmacological anticoagulation, mechanical compression devices, and early mobilization.

Postoperative Care and Pain Management

- In view of the patient's clinical condition, comorbidities, and intraoperative blood loss, the patient should be cared for in a high-dependency unit.

- Acute postoperative pain management should be the primary concern as inadequate pain relief could lead to poor rehabilitation and development of chronic pain conditions.

- Multimodal analgesia, including opioids, nonsteroidal anti-inflammatory drugs (NSAIDs), paracetamol and peripheral nerve blocks, and the epidural catheter is widely used for postoperative pain management.

Anesthesia for Scoliosis Surgery

Scoliosis is a deformity of the spine, resulting in lateral curvature and rotation of the vertebrae as well as deformity of the rib cage. Anesthesia for scoliosis surgery is challenging as scoliosis surgery has its specific concerns along with concerns related to the involvement of the respiratory, cardiovascular, and neurologic systems.

Classification of Scoliosis

- *On the basis of the region involved:*
  - ▶ Cervicothoracic.
  - ▶ Thoracic.
  - ▶ Thoracolumbar.
  - ▶ Lumbar.
- *On the basis of etiology:*
  - ▶ Idiopathic scoliosis:
    - ○ Early-onset (infantile).
    - ○ Late-onset (juvenile or adolescent).
  - ▶ Neuromuscular scoliosis:
    - ○ Cerebral palsy.

- ○ Myopathies.
- ○ Poliomyelitis.
- ○ Syringomyelia.
- ○ Muscular dystrophy.
- ○ Friedrich's ataxia.
- ▶ Congenital scoliosis:
  - ○ Vertebral anomalies.
  - ○ Spinal dysraphism.
- ▶ Mesenchymal disorders:
  - ○ Marfan's syndrome.
  - ○ Amyoplasia congenita.
  - ○ Rheumatoid arthritis.
  - ○ Still's disease.
  - ○ Osteogenesis imperfecta.
- ▶ Traumatic.
- ▶ Neoplasms.
- ▶ Infection: Tuberculosis, osteomyelitis.

Epidemiology

The prevalence of scoliosis in the general population is 0.3 to 15.3%. As much as *75 to 90% of all scoliosis cases are of idiopathic type, out of which adolescent type is the most common.*

Assessment of Severity of Scoliosis

The severity of scoliosis is defined by the Cobb angle (**Table 32.3** and **Fig. 32.1**).

Preanesthesia Assessment

Preoperative assessment for scoliosis should be done meticulously as other systems are profoundly involved.

Airway Assessment

Upper thoracic or cervical spine scoliosis presents with difficult airway due to restriction of cervical movement. Tongue hypertrophy present in Duchenne muscular dystrophy results in difficult ventilation and laryngoscopy.

Table 32.3 Cobb angle and disease severity

Cobb angle (degree)	Disease severity
<10	Normal or postural
>10	Scoliosis definition
<25	Mild scoliosis
25–50	Moderate scoliosis
>50	Severe scoliosis
>45–50	Indication for surgery
>65	Significant decrease in lung volume
>100	Dyspnea on exertion, pulmonary hypertension
>120	Alveolar hypoventilation, chronic respiratory failure

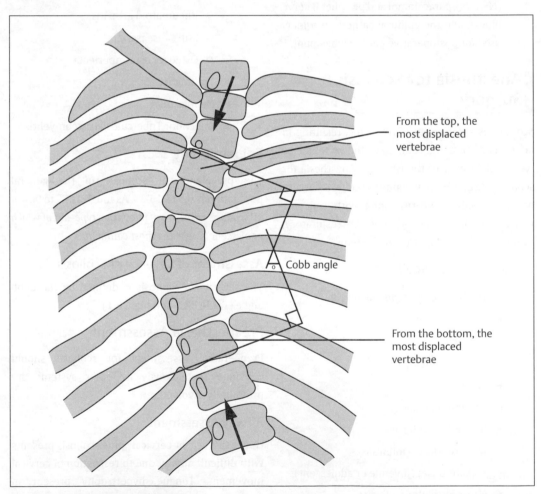

Fig. 32.1 Measurement of Cobb angle.

Respiratory System Assessment

- Scoliosis results in decreased lung volume (functional residual capacity and vital capacity) and restrictive lung disease pattern.

- Hypoxemia and alveolar hypoventilation can lead to pulmonary hypertension and chronic respiratory failure.

- Compliance of the respiratory system decreases due to thoracic cage deformity, thus increasing the work of breathing. With infantile and juvenile type of scoliosis, there is true lung hypoplasia and limited respiratory muscle function.

- Significant rotation or displacement of the trachea or main bronchi may cause airway obstruction.

- Assessment of exercise tolerance, pulmonary function test, and arterial blood gas analysis should be done preoperatively.

This information helps in deciding the extent of surgery permitted at one time and the requirement for postoperative ventilatory support. *Vital capacity of less than 40% of the normal range is predictive of the need for postoperative mechanical ventilation.*

Cardiovascular Assessment

Hypoventilation and ventilation-perfusion mismatch cause prolonged alveolar hypoxia, resulting in irreversible vasoconstriction and pulmonary hypertension, which eventually causes right ventricular hypertrophy, leading to cor pulmonale. An ECG and echocardiography should be done to assess the severity of involvement.

Neurological Assessment

Meticulous neurologic examination and documentation are important because of medicolegal issues. *Patients with preexisting neurologic dysfunction are at an increased risk of developing spinal cord injury during scoliosis surgery.* The risk of postoperative aspiration is increased in muscular dystrophy due to the involvement of bulbar muscle.

Other evaluations include coagulation profile assessment and preoperative vision checkup. Thromboembolic prophylaxis, by way of long duration of surgery, prone position, and prolonged periods of postoperative recumbency, put patients at risk of thromboembolism.

Anesthesia Technique

In recent years, usage of intraoperative neurophysiological monitoring (IONM), either somatosensory-evoked potential (SSEP) or transcranial motor-evoked potential (TcMEP) or both, has been increased in scoliosis surgeries as there is a risk of damage to the spinal cord during surgery.

SSEP monitors the spinothalamic pathway of the spinal cord, and TcMEP is for the corticospinal tract. Therefore, a preoperative discussion between anesthetists and the surgeons should focus on:

- The need for IONM.

- The approach of surgery (anterior or posterior).

- Need for double-lumen tube for lung isolation for anterior spine access.

- Anticipated blood loss.

- Postoperative pain management.

"Wake up test" can also be used to assess the integrity of motor function of the spinal cord during the surgery. In this test, volatile and/or intravenous (IV) anesthetics are switched off, and the patient is awakened. The motor function is assessed by asking the patient to move his limbs. After the assessment, the patient is again anesthetized. Care must be taken to avoid accidental extubation.

Premedication

- Avoid the use of narcotics or heavy sedation as premedication *in the presence of pulmonary impairment.*

- For preoperative optimization of lung function, nebulization with bronchodilators can be useful.

- To minimize secretion and to avoid loosening of tape securing the endotracheal tube, antisialogogues should be used.

- For aspiration prophylaxis, H2 blocking agents or proton-pump inhibitors may be given. Antibiotic prophylaxis and tranexamic acid loading dose should be given before incision.

Induction, Intubation, and Maintenance of Anesthesia

- IV induction by the routinely used anesthetic agent is common.

- Alternatively, an inhalational induction may be used, guided by the patient's condition.

- Nondepolarizing neuromuscular blocking agents should be preferred for intubation *as succinylcholine in the presence of myopathies or denervation can cause a hyperkalemic response or sudden cardiac arrest.*

- For maintenance of anesthesia, total IV anesthesia without nitrous oxide and neuromuscular blockage provide the optimal condition for TcMEP, and inhalational agent along with neuromuscular blockage can be used during SSEP monitoring.

- As massive blood loss is anticipated during surgery, large-bore peripheral IV cannula and central venous cannula as an additional route for IV infusions for fluid, blood, or vasopressor/ionotropic agents should be inserted.

- Urinary catheterization and urine output monitoring are required for all cases due to the long duration of surgery and major fluid shift.

- Monitoring should include ECG, invasive blood pressure, pulse oximetry, capnography, and temperature. *Minimally invasive monitors for cardiac output measurement using arterial waveform pulse contour analysis or transesophageal Doppler can be used to monitor hemodynamics in high-risk cases.*

Patient Positioning

The position of the patient depends on the surgical approach (anterior or posterior) and the level of the spine to be operated upon:

- The *anterior approach* to thoracic spine happens via thoracotomy, with the patient supported in the lateral position.

- The posterior approach needs prone positioning with the following concerns:

  ▶ Risk of brachial plexus injury.

  ▶ Risk of injury to the ulnar nerve.

  ▶ Excessive pressure over the abdomen causes venous engorgement and more bleeding from valveless epidural veins.

  ▶ Bony points and genitals should be padded and protected.

  ▶ Keep the head on headrests to avoid pressure on the eyes while maintaining the neck in a neutral position. Some include a mirror to facilitate easier intraoperative checking. Since imaging is often required during surgery, the surgical site is kept away from the table's central support area.

Perioperative Complications

- *Blood loss*:

  Intraoperative massive blood loss is a major concern during scoliosis surgery. The contributing factors are:

- Long incision.

- Wide exposure with stripping off of muscle from the bone.

- Long duration surgery.

- Wide decortications of osteoporotic bone with wide vascular channels.

- The number of levels that are operated on.

During posterior procedures, average per vertebrae level estimated blood loss was reported to be 65 to 280 mL in scoliosis patients.

Blood loss during surgery can be reduced by the following:

- Antifibrinolytics agents (aminocapronic and tranexamic acid).

- Avoiding any increase in intra-abdominal pressure, which can lead to a reduced epidural venous pressure and consequently venous surgical bleed.

- Blood conservative techniques.

- Controlled hypotension is an age-old practice not encouraged these days because of the risk of hypoperfusion/ ischemic spinal cord injury. *It is advisable to keep mean arterial pressure above 85 mm Hg to avoid any spinal cord injury.*

- *Intraoperative neurophysiological monitoring.*

A significant drop in evoked potentials' amplitude indicates impending nerve or spinal cord injury. *Before making any such assumption, it should be ensured that there is no hypotension, hypothermia, anemia, hypoxemia, or hypocarbia, or a bolus dose of anesthetic agents is not given.* If there is a significant change in amplitude, then:

- Ask the surgeon to stop the surgery.

- Irrigate the surgical area with warm saline.

- Increase blood pressure by 20%.

- Irrigate the surgical area with a local arteriolar dilator (papaverine).

If these maneuvers do not improve the signal, then there is a high chance of spinal cord or nerve injury.

- *Hypothermia*:

  Factors such as wide surgical exposure, prolonged surgery, blood loss, and cold ambient temperature contribute to hypothermia. The use of warm IV fluid and warm air blanket should be used to avoid hypothermia.

- *Postoperative ophthalmic complications*:

  The incidence of postoperative vision loss (POVL) in spine surgery is 0.028 to 0.2%. Causes of POVL are:

- Ischemic optic neuropathy.

- Central retinal artery occlusion.

- Ocular injury.

- Cortical blindness.

The most common type of POVL in spine surgery is ischemic optic neuropathy (ION). Risk factors are male gender, obesity, blood loss > 1,000 mL, >6 hours of surgery duration, anemia, and use of Wilson frame. ASA recommended a practice advisory for perioperative visual loss associated with spine surgery which includes:

- Maintenance of BP to ± 20% of the baseline.

- Avoid a large amount of crystalloid.

- Avoid direct pressure on the globe.

- Keep blood transfusion threshold > 30%.

- 10° of reverse Trendelenburg position during prone surgery.

- Staging of long-duration surgery.

Postoperative Care

- After the surgery, all patients should be managed in the intensive care unit in view of preexisting respiratory and cardiovascular dysfunction and surgery, which inflict several further stresses like significant blood loss, major fluid shifts, prolonged anesthesia, and hypothermia.

- In most of the cases, mechanical ventilation is provided for a few hours in the postoperative care unit until hypothermia and metabolic derangements have been corrected.

- After extubation, oxygen by the mask may be required for longer periods in those with preexisting pulmonary dysfunction.

- Pulmonary complications are the most common postoperative complications; vigilant monitoring, incentive spirometry, and chest physiotherapy are essential for reducing morbidity, particularly in patients with preexisting pulmonary dysfunction.

- Other complications which could occur after scoliosis surgery are neurologic injury, pneumothorax, dural tears, syndrome of inappropriate antidiuretic hormone (ADH) secretion, and ileus and urinary complications.

Postoperative Pain Management

Multimodal analgesia, which includes opioids, NSAIDs, paracetamol, epidural/spinal block and local wound infiltration, should be used to provide a pain-free postoperative period.

- IV opioids are associated with side-effects such as nausea, vomiting, respiratory depression, sedation, and gastrointestinal ileus.

- NSAIDs, despite having complications like increase bleeding, gastritis, and acute renal failure, particularly in the presence of hypovolemia and hypotension, are commonly used for their opioid-sparing effects.

- Epidural analgesia by local anesthetic agents, alone or in combination with opioids provide satisfactory pain relief, but it can make neurological assessment difficult.

- Intrathecal analgesia by morphine to be 2 to 5 µg/kg, which provides comparable analgesia for 24 hours but with fewer side-effects such as respiratory depression, nausea, and pruritus.

Given the complex nature of scoliosis surgery, a careful and meticulous discussion should be carried out between anesthesiologists and surgeons regarding perioperative management and rehabilitation of patients to improve surgical outcomes.

Conclusion

Orthopedic surgeries are associated with difficult patient positioning, moderate-to-severe blood loss, and significant postoperative pain. Wherever possible, regional anesthesia should be employed to avoid airway handling in patients with difficult airways, and adverse effects of general anesthesia in elderly patients with multiple comorbidities. Adequate pain management with multimodal analgesia is required for early mobilization and recovery of patients.

CHAPTER 33

Nonoperating Room Anesthesia (AS4.7)

Nikita Goel

Introduction

Diagnostic and therapeutic interventions outside the operating room (OR) have been happening for the past many decades. In the past, the patients encountered were simple, with almost no comorbidities and therefore did not require anesthesia. The increasing number of complex patients compounded by advanced procedures mandates the presence of and care by anesthetists to make procedures comfortable for the patients and improve patient outcomes.

The infrastructure, available human resources, along with their technical skills, are usually less familiar to anesthetists, unlike the OR.

"Administration of sedation/anesthesia to patients undergoing painful or uncomfortable procedures at off-site locations is referred to as nonoperating room anesthesia (NORA)."

Challenges Unique to NORA

Performing procedures outside of the OR creates a new set of challenges for anesthesiologists. The challenges are as follows:

- Patients scheduled for NORA suites are sometimes more complex and poorly optimized compared with the general OR population.
- NORA suites are designed to target the needs of the procedural operator, with less focus on the needs of anesthesiologists.
- The NORA suites are usually unfamiliar and crowded.

- Limited and inadequate access to patients.
- First-time visitors sometimes find it difficult to reach NORA suites due to their locations in deep trenches of the hospital.
- There is often limited access to resources such as space, monitors, anesthesia equipment, and medications.
- At times, anesthesia equipment is lacking in the NORA suites, and there may be delayed availability of additional help in case of need.
- The pressure to perform a rapid evaluation of patients with limited information and the urgent nature of the procedures may make anesthetic management challenging and risky.
- Anesthesiologists may be expected to recover patients in busy recovery suites without dedicated extended postoperative monitoring capabilities and with staff who may not routinely recover patients from general anesthetics.

All of these difficulties create a unique challenge that each anesthesiologist faces when delivering anesthetics in these locations. Some of the NORA sites include the following:

- Radiology.
  - ▶ Interventional.
  - ▶ MRI (all the equipment used in the MRI suite should be MRI-compatible. The types of equipment used in MRI are made up of aluminium).
  - ▶ CT scan.

- Gastroenterology endoscopies.
- Cardiac interventions:
  - ► Catheterization.
  - ► Interventional cardiology.
  - ► Transesophageal echocardiography.
- Lithotripsy.
- Electroconvulsive therapy sites.
- Obstetric labor and delivery.
- Ambulatory procedure rooms.

Role of Anesthesiologist in NORA

Anesthesiologists are supposed to execute their skills outside the OR settings in a timely fashion with accuracy. The functions of anesthesiologists include the following:

- Proper orientation to location and resources of the NORA suite.
- To understand the planned procedure and the requirements needed to perform it.
- A thorough screening of the patient and medical optimization for all disease states.
- To ensure the availability of additional help in case of crisis.
- To ensure the space, medications, equipment, dedicated staff, and monitors for postprocedure care.

Guidelines for Providing Care in NORA

According to the American Society of Anesthesiologists (ASA) statement of nonoperating room anesthetizing locations, minimum requirements for providing care include the following:

- The oxygen source should be reliable and last for the length of the procedure. At least

a full E cylinder should be available as a backup in case of failure of the main oxygen supply.

- A reliable source for suctioning.
- Scavenging system to vent out the waste anesthetic gases.
- The availability of a self-inflating resuscitator bag.
- Adequate anesthetic drugs, supplies, and equipment for the intended anesthetic care.
- Appropriate monitoring equipment that adheres to the ASA standards (refer to Chapter 6, *Monitoring in Anesthesia*).
- Sufficient electrical outlets that adhere to facility standards.
- Adequate illumination of the patient and equipment.
- Enough space to accommodate the necessary equipment and personnel.
- Immediate access to an emergency cart with a defibrillator, emergency drugs, and other equipment to provide cardiopulmonary resuscitation.
- Adequate anesthesia support staff.
- Availability of appropriate postoperative area with trained staff, monitoring equipment, and drugs for resuscitation.

Complications in NORA

- *Respiratory complications*: Hypoxemia as sequelae of respiratory depression, which is caused by an overdose of sedative/anesthetic drugs.
- *Hypothermia*: It is frequent in NORA suites due to the use of heavy air-conditioning devices. The children are more susceptible to hypothermia, and measures must be taken to ensure euthermia in this group of

patients. The common methods to prevents hypothermia are as follows:

▶ Use of warming blankets with surface heating.

▶ Padding the extremities with cotton.

▶ Covering the head with a cap.

▶ Heated fluids.

- *Aspiration*: The blunting of airway reflexes due to sedatives/anesthetics puts the patient at risk of aspiration. Adequate fasting for the type of food should be ensured before taking patients for the procedures.

- *Hypovolemia*: The volume-depleted patients exhibit an exaggerated response to vasodilation and cardiac depressant action of anesthetic drugs. Thus, maintaining appropriate hydration and a slow injection of drugs may prevent adverse events.

- *Postoperative nausea and vomiting*: Postoperative nausea and vomiting (PONV) is a recognizable and preventable cause of unplanned hospital admission.

Conclusion

Providing anesthesia outside the operating room is challenging due to inadequate infrastructure, unfamiliar surroundings, poor assistance from untrained staff, and the nonavailability of expert anesthetists in case of crisis. Less time for preoperative assessment and nonavailability of adequate infrastructure in the recovery area further compound challenges. A proper preoperative assessment and designing an appropriate plan with available resources can make things smoother and complication free.

CHAPTER 34

Anesthesia at Remote Locations (AS4.7)

Nikita Goel

Introduction

Human beings, being the most intelligent animal on this planet, keep on exploring the surroundings. Their habitat is not only limited to suitable physiological environments but also high mountains. The delivery of anesthesia care in such locations is challenging because of various factors like:

- Difficulty in reaching the location.
- The barometric pressure and temperature are different from that at sea level.
- The calibrated anesthesia equipment may not function optimally at locations other than sea levels.

The anesthetic challenges at high altitudes and those in hyperbaric chambers are overviewed in this chapter.

Anesthesia at High Altitude

More than 140 million members of the human race have permanent settlement at altitudes greater than 2,500 m, and many of them may require medical care. Anesthesia practitioners must understand the unique challenges at high altitude. The noteworthy physiological changes are as follows:

- The partial pressure of oxygen at high altitudes decreases with a decrease in atmospheric pressure.
- Increased 2,3-diphosphoglycerate in red blood cells shifts the oxygen dissociation curve to the right, leading to increased oxygen delivery and unloading in tissues.
- Respiratory alkalosis (secondary to hyperventilation) shifts the oxygen dissociation curve to the left. This increases oxygen's affinity to red blood cells and favors uptake through the alveolar circulation.

The mixed venous blood of a person at high altitude has the same PO_2 because of the following compensatory mechanisms:

- Hyperventilation (primary mechanism), which may increase alveolar oxygen tension by 25 to 30%.
- Lowered tissue metabolism due to decreased availability of oxygen.
- Adjustment of oxygen transport characterized by:

  a. Increase in pulmonary oxygen diffusion capacity by three- to fourfold.

  b. Increase in pulmonary capillary blood flow.

  c. Increase in lung volume and surface area of the alveolar membrane.

  d. Increase in blood supply to the upper lobes of the lung.

- Hypothermia: It leads to platelet dysfunction, cold injuries, and cardiac arrest in the worst scenario.
- Immune suppression: It results in ineffective healing and increased risk of infection.

Physiologic adaptations to high altitudes start around 2 to 3 weeks, and it may take months to complete. The decrease in the partial pressure of oxygen stimulates the kidney to produce more erythropoietin, which leads to a rise in hemoglobin (15 to 22 g/dL). The hematocrit increases from 45 to 65% as plasma volume drops by 10 to 20%, secondary to intravascular fluid shifts into the interstitial compartment.

Hypoxia leads to an increase in sympathetic output, which contributes to the rise in cardiac output, mostly due to the rise in heart rate. Stroke volume decreases due to a decrease in preload. Systemic blood pressure rises as a result of peripheral vasoconstriction.

Altitude Illness

The short-term and long-term stay at high altitude exposes the individuals to lower oxygen tension. This exposure can lead to a multiple forms of sickness, affecting the mainly respiratory and central nervous system. The common high altitude illnesses are:

a.   High-altitude pulmonary edema (HAPE)

It is noncardiogenic pulmonary edema seen at high altitudes in the setting of an elevation in pulmonary artery pressures. The underlying mechanisms are:

- Decreased barometric pressure and partial pressure of O_2, leading to pulmonary vasoconstriction and elevated pulmonary artery pressure (PAP).

- Patchy pulmonary vasoconstriction with some parts of the lungs receiving over perfusion cause fluid leakage, plus elevated PAP and increased blood viscosity, leading to capillary endothelial damage and fluid leakage.

- Fibrin thrombin formation in the lungs due to an increase in plasma fibrinogen levels.

- Increased production of oxygen-free radicals, causing oxidation of alveolar intracellular lipids and mitochondrial cell membranes.

Clinical Features

1. Common symptoms are dyspnea at rest, decreased exercise performance; chest congestion, and cough (frothy pink sputum).

2. Signs of HAPE include lung crackles, tachycardia, tachypnea, and cyanosis.

Treatment

- Urgent descent to a lower altitude.

- Management of pulmonary edema with supplemental oxygen, diuretics, calcium channel blocker (i.e., nifedipine), morphine, and noninvasive/invasive positive pressure ventilation.

- Hyperbaric oxygen therapy.

- Steroids.

- Phosphodiesterase inhibitor (tadalafil).

It is important to monitor respiratory rate and effort along with volume status, especially in the setting of treatment with opioids and diuretics.

b.   Acute motion sickness (AMS)

This condition is seen with the rapid ascent to high altitudes and thought to occur secondary to a hypoxia-induced subclinical cerebral edema. It is self-limiting and resolves within a week.

AMS presents as a throbbing generalized bilateral headache accompanied by anorexia, nausea, dizziness, fatigue, or insomnia.

Treatment

- Supplemental oxygen.

- Analgesics, antiemetics.

- Steroids.

- Acetazolamide.

Descent to a lower altitude is recommended as long as possible.

c.   High-altitude cerebral edema (HACE)

HACE is a severe form of AMS and is considered a medical emergency with a high risk of mortality. It results in a vasogenic and cytotoxic cerebral edema secondary to hypoxia. Symptoms are similar to AMS, in addition to gait ataxia, mental status alterations, hemiparesis, or coma.

The treatment requires urgent descent to normal altitudes. Medical management includes:

- Supplemental oxygen.

- Steroids, acetazolamide.

- Diuretics (e.g., furosemide).
- High carbohydrate diet.
- Hyperbaric chamber.

Anesthetic Considerations

- Because of the reduced ambient PO_2 at high altitudes, the risk of perioperative hypoxia is likely to be magnified.
- High altitude may exacerbate the respiratory-depressant effects of benzodiazepines and opioids.
- Hypothermia, if not addressed, may potentiate the effect of induction agents and muscle relaxants due to a decrease in drug metabolism. Ketamine may be the drug of choice due to its analgesic effects and respiratory preservation.
- There is an increased risk of perioperative bleeding due to high-venous pressure, vasodilation, and increased capillary density.
- Tobacco smoking increases carboxyhemoglobin levels, further impairing oxygen delivery.
- Alcohol, caffeine, and diuretics should be used with caution, as they increase diuresis and can aggravate dehydration.
- Nitrous oxide loses potency at high altitudes. It also limits inspired oxygen concentration and may further increase pulmonary artery pressures. Therefore, nitrous oxide is not recommended during delivery of anesthetics at high altitudes.
- There is a high incidence of dural puncture headache after spinal anesthesia, with the contributing factors being chronically increased cerebrospinal fluid (CSF) pressure and dehydration.

Delivery of Inhaled Anesthetics at High Altitude

- The potency of anesthetic gases is proportional to their partial pressure. Therefore,

the inhaled anesthetics have lower potency at high altitudes.

- Except for the Tec 6 Plus desflurane vaporizer (GE Healthcare), all other vaporizers do not need to be dialed up in order to adjust and compensate for the drop in atmospheric pressure at high altitudes.

Tec 6 Vaporizer

The Tec 6 vaporizer will deliver the dialed volume percentage at higher altitudes, but as soon as desflurane is exposed to the ambient pressure at high altitude, its partial pressure will decrease. Therefore, the Tec 6 vaporizer has to be dialed up to deliver the same partial pressure of desflurane at higher altitudes.

Perioperative Supplemental Oxygen

The hypoxic environment at high altitude induces hypoxia-mediated hyperventilation that increases alveolar oxygen tension. The blunting of hypoxic ventilatory drive by anesthetic drugs may precipitate hypoxia. The use of opioids may further worsen hypoxia by causing respiratory depression. Therefore, oxygen supplementation is a must, especially with opioid use.

Anesthesia in a Hyperbaric Chamber

Exposure to oxygen tension at 2 to 3 atmospheric pressure (hyperbaric oxygen) causes an increase in arterial and tissue partial pressure of oxygen but no effect on arterial pH or partial pressure of carbon dioxide. The increased arterial oxygen tension can result in:

- Vasoconstriction.
- Antibacterial action, particularly against anaerobic bacteria.
- Inhibition of endothelial neutrophil adhesion in injured tissue.

The Challenges Inside a Hyperbaric Chamber

The hyperbaric chamber poses unique challenges for the working personnel. The important ones are:

- The ambient temperature rises in proportion to the rate of pressurization inside the hyperbaric chamber.

- High atmospheric pressure is believed to cause more inflammation, although the evidence for it is meagre.

- The limited space inside the hyperbaric chamber makes the ergonomics difficult for the equipment and working staff.

- The noise of the compression pump interferes with one's ability to monitor heart and respiration by stethoscopic methods.

Anesthetic Considerations

- The exposure of medical personnel to inhaled anesthetics at high-ambient pressure inside the chamber may have deleterious pharmacologic effects.

- The use of nitrous oxide at high-ambient pressure saturates the tissue; the bubble formation can occur during the decompression phase.

- The hyperbaric nitrous oxide can dilute alveolar oxygen during the decompression phase, posing the patient at risk of hypoxia.

- The rotameter flow meters calibrated at 1 ATA will indicate false high values at increased ambient pressure because of the increased gas density.

- Intravenous anesthetics behave similarly and are unlikely to be affected within the usual clinical range of ambient pressure.

- The regional anesthesia is safe as well as effective in a hyperbaric environment and avoids the need for mechanical ventilation.

- Extreme care should be taken to ensure sterile technique because of the propensity for enhanced bacterial growth in the warm, humidified environment of a hyperbaric chamber.

Conclusion

Providing anesthesia at locations other than sea level requires knowledge of physiological changes at altitude and inside hyperbaric conditions. The risk of perioperative hypoxemia is magnified at high altitude due to low ambient PaO_2, while the increased solubility of gases inside hyperbaric chambers exposes the OT personnel to the deleterious effects of inhaled anesthetics and nitrous oxide.

CHAPTER 35

Anesthesia for Daycare Surgeries

Ajit Kumar and Kritika Saini

Introduction

Anesthesia has made surgery feasible by providing a relaxed, sedated, pain-free patient. However, surgeries and anesthesia have their complications. Managing the postoperative period is as important as managing the surgery itself. But with the advent of daycare surgeries (DCS), the overall burden of postoperative management and prolonged hospitalization has reduced. This has been made possible due to the emergence of minimally invasive surgeries and newer advances in techniques of anesthesia and analgesia.

History

- 1903: Surgeon James Nicoll Glasgow, operated 9000 children almost on daycare basis.
- 1912: Ralph Waters, USA, who, in his "The Down Town Anaesthesia Clinic," anesthetized various cases of minor outpatient surgery.
- 1960: First hospital-based ambulatory unit was developed.
- 1984: Foundation of the Society for Ambulatory Anaesthesia (SAMBA).

Terminology

Commonly used terms and abbreviations have been described in **Table 35.1**.

Advantages

DCS offer various advantages in terms of cost-effectiveness, reduced absenteeism from work, early ambulation, etc. (**Table 35.2**).

Patient Selection Criteria

The success of daycare procedures is broadly based on careful selection not only of the patient but also the surgical procedure. Overall safety and postoperative care of the patient is also an important issue that should be kept in mind. Thus, broadly speaking, patient selection is divided into three major domains—surgical, social, and medical.

Surgical Criteria

The advent of advanced minimally invasive surgical procedures has widened the boundaries of ambulatory anesthesia and DCS to a great extent. Surgeries not involving the breach of thoracic/abdominal cavities (except minimally

Table 35.1 Internationally agreed terminology, abbreviations, and definitions as proposed by the International Association for Ambulatory Surgery (World Health Organization 2007)

Terminology	Synonyms and definitions
Day surgery	• Ambulatory surgery, same-day surgery, day only
Extended recovery	• 23 h, overnight stay, single night • Treatments requiring an overnight stay before discharge
Short stay	• Treatments requiring 24–72 h in hospital before discharge
Office-based surgery	• An operation or procedure carried out in a medical surgery/office or practitioner's professional premises, which provide appropriately designed and equipped service room(s) for its safe performance

Table 35.2 Advantages of DCS

Patient benefits	Hospital benefits
• Less risk of hospital-acquired infections	• The lesser burden on hospital staff with optimal utilization of human resources
• Decreased risk of postoperative thromboembolic events	
• Minimally invasive surgeries and regional anesthesia techniques decrease the need for postoperative analgesia	• Avoids unnecessary occupation of hospital beds
• Less absenteeism from work	
• Lesser separation anxiety among children	• Organized scheduling of cases with minimal cancellation
• The benefit of early return to a familiar environment	
• Lesser burden on family members and caretaker	• Economically worthwhile

Abbreviation: DCS, daycare surgery.

invasive) or not followed by the risk of postoperative hemorrhage can be performed on a daycare basis. *Also, the procedure should not require postoperative intravenous fluid therapy or analgesics.* Examples of some surgical procedures that can be performed and not limited to have been mentioned in **Table 35.3.**

Social Criteria

A patient should be scheduled for a daycare procedure only after ensuring a safe home environment, a responsible caregiver, convenient transportation, and communication access (e.g., telephone) in case the need arises. All instructions should be discussed verbally and in a written format by both the anesthesiologist as well as the surgeon.

Medical Criteria

Selection criteria should be done, keeping in mind the overall "medical fitness" of the patient. Thorough and well-documented history should be taken. Preanesthetic checkup is, therefore, of paramount importance in making the decision.

Preanesthetic Checkup for Daycare Surgeries

The idea behind preanesthetic evaluation is to screen the patient for any comorbidities and assess the impact of the patient's fitness on the surgical outcome and perioperative management. Preoperative evaluation prevents needless delays and cancellations. This evaluation should be done based on structured format and can vary from one institution to another. But the following points must be specifically kept in mind while evaluating the patient for DCS:

1. Age: Despite having higher incidences of comorbidities, DCS in carefully selected geriatric patients offer all the advantages, as discussed above (**Table 35.2**). Also, there is reduced cognitive impairment and minimal separation from the home environment. Therefore, there is no upper limit of age, *but age > 80 years is considered to be associated with higher perioperative risk.*

2. American Society of Anesthesiologists (ASA) status: Performed with ASA status 1 or 2 to ensure early ambulation and discharge.

3. Comorbidities: Associated comorbidities and their preoperative evaluation are discussed below in this chapter.

Hypertension: Hypertension has a direct relation with increased perioperative adverse cardiac events, for example, myocardial ischemia. However, in the absence of associated end-organ

Table 35.3 Commonly performed surgeries on a daycare basis

Orthopedic surgery	• Diagnostic and therapeutic arthroscopic procedures • Anterior cruciate ligament repair • Carpal and tarsal tunnel release • Minimally invasive hip replacement
Otolaryngorhinology	• Adenotonsillectomy • Grommet insertion • Myringotomy • Tympanoplasty • Endoscopic sinus surgeries
General surgery	• Laparoscopic cholecystectomy • Ventral hernia repair • Gastric fundoplication perianal fistula repair • Pilonidal sinus excision
Gynecology	• Diagnostic laparoscopy and hysteroscopy • Laparoscopic tubal ligation • Endometrial ablation
Neurosurgery	• Vertebroplasty • Lumbar microdiscectomy • Stereotactic brain biopsy • Cranioplasty
Ophthalmic surgery	• Cataract surgery • Squint repair • Trabeculectomy • Occuloplasty
Dental surgery	• Tooth extraction • Apicectomies
Pediatric surgery	• Circumcision • Inguinal hernia repair • Orchiopexy • Hydrocele resection
Urology	• Vasectomies • Pyeloplasty
Vascular surgery	• Varicose vein surgery

damage, it is advised not to defer surgeries if blood pressure < 180/110 mm Hg.

Ischemic heart disease: *History of myocardial infarction within 6 months, angina at rest, or with minimal physical activity, all pose as contraindications to elective surgical procedures.* Detailed evaluation along with the assessment of high-risk factors like coexisting diabetes, peripheral vascular disease, poor exercise tolerance (<4 metabolic equivalents or METs) should be done before coming to the decision of whether or not to proceed with the procedure. β-*blocker therapy should be continued throughout the procedure.*

Asthma/chronic obstructive pulmonary disease (COPD): Asthmatic patients with good exercise tolerance, no recent history of asthma exacerbation/hospitalization, or systemic steroid intake can be posted for ambulatory anesthesia and DCS. Similarly, for COPD, asymptomatic patients without a recent history of smoking (>6–8 weeks) can be considered. *However, avoidance of airway manipulation and preference to local/regional anesthesia are always warranted in these patients.*

Acute upper respiratory tract infection: Afebrile patients with no features of lower respiratory tract involvement can be considered for regional anesthesia as day cases. It is best to avoid any tracheal manipulation, but if this cannot be avoided and the patient is febrile, then it is better to defer the case.

Obstructive sleep apnea (OSA): It is associated with a very high risk of perioperative adverse events like difficulty in airway handling, fall in oxygen saturation, airway obstruction, hypertension, and cardiac dysrhythmias. *Opioids should better be avoided, or dose should be limited.* These patients can be considered for DCS, provided the patient tolerates continuous positive airway pressure devices (CPAP) and is efficient in practicing this at home postdischarge.

Diabetes mellitus: Diabetic patients pose no contraindication to DCS unless they have associated comorbidities like autonomic dysfunction, cardiovascular or renal impairment (which can independently cause multiple complications). *It is advised to schedule these patients as the first case.* Patients should be clearly instructed to omit the morning dose of oral hypoglycemic agents or insulin. Their nil per oral time should be minimized postsurgery.

Renal and hepatic diseases: Patients with severe hepatic disease, a renal disease requiring dialysis, are not candidates for daycare procedures. However, minor procedures like dialysis fistula access can be performed under local/regional anesthesia on a daycare basis.

Fasting Guidelines for Daycare Surgeries

The standard guidelines of fasting, as proposed by ASA, are also followed for various daycare procedures (**Table 35.4**).

Technique of Anesthesia (AS4.6)

For the success of DCS, ideal anesthetic agents/techniques should offer the following qualities:

1. Quick recovery.
2. Should not be associated with emergence delirium.
3. Minimal postanesthesia sedation.

Table 35.4 Fasting guidelines

Ingested material	Minimum fasting period (h)
Clear fluids	2
Breast milk	4
Infant formula feed	6
Non-human milk	6
Light meal	6
Fatty meal, meat	8

4. No risk of respiratory depression.
5. Good postoperative pain relief.
6. No postoperative nausea/vomiting.

Just like any surgery, the DCS can be performed either in regional anesthesia or general anesthesia. The various techniques of regional anesthesia offer the advantage of minimal effect on the consciousness and awakening, with the added advantage of good analgesia. But with the advent of newer anesthetic agents that offer quicker offset of action and minimal side effects, even general and monitored anesthesia care have emerged as safe techniques.

Spinal Anesthesia

Central neuraxial blockade using short-acting local anesthetic agents (hyperbaric prilocaine 2% and 2-chloroprocaine) offers excellent anesthesia and analgesia for various orthopedic, gynecologic, urologic, and other surgical procedures. The patient can be discharged once the motor and sensory effects wear off. *Postdural puncture headache, a troublesome side effect of spinal anesthesia, has reduced since the introduction of smaller gauge and pencil-tipped needles.*

Regional Anesthesia: Peripheral Nerve Blocks

Various peripheral nerve blockade techniques are increasingly becoming popular nowadays, because they not only avoid the complications of intravenous and inhalational anesthetic agents but also provide excellent analgesia, especially when administered with adjuvants. Studies on adjuvants like alpha-2 agonists, opioids, and steroids like dexamethasone have shown how these can prolong the duration of postoperative analgesia. Furthermore, ultrasonography has minimized the complications along with increasing the chances of successful nerve blocks.

Other regional techniques that can be used include intravenous regional anesthesia, intra-articular blocks, and field blocks.

General Anesthesia

Agents like thiopentone, midazolam, and ketamine are not suitable for ambulatory anesthesia because of their prolonged action. Etomidate, on the other hand, has numerous side effects like increased risk of postoperative nausea and vomiting (PONV) and myoclonus. *Thus, among currently available agents, propofol seems to be most appropriate for DCS.*

Total Intravenous Anesthesia

Agents like propofol, dexmedetomidine, and remifentanil, which provide the benefit of minimal emergence and quicker recovery have laid the foundations of total intravenous anesthesia (TIVA), thus avoiding various side effects associated with inhalational agent usage. TIVA, therefore, offers the following advantages:

1. Quicker recovery and minimal emergence reactions.

2. Reduced incidence of PONV.

3. Minimizing operating room pollution.

4. Avoiding complications like malignant hyperthermia.

TIVA, however, lacks the muscle relaxation offered by inhalation agents. It also requires more intensive monitoring with devices like bispectral index (BIS) to have an accurate assessment of the depth of anesthesia. Also, there are a few disadvantages associated with propofol induction such as pain on injection, hypotension, and transient apnea.

Inhalational Anesthesia

Newer inhalational agents like sevoflurane and desflurane with a lower blood–gas partition (0.69 and 0.42, respectively) and blood–brain coefficients have the superiority of rapid reversal.

Sevoflurane being sweet-smelling also offers the benefit of rapid induction. It has bronchodilation properties and, therefore, can be safely used in patients with bronchial asthma.

Sevoflurane use is, however, associated with emergence delirium. This can be minimized by combining agents like dexmedetomidine.

Desflurane, on the other hand, causes bronchial irritation and is therefore not used for induction.

But it can be used as a maintenance agent with the fastest recovery time.

However, in the author's opinion, no single agent, be it intravenous or inhalational, offers ideal anesthesia, and hence induction using intravenous followed by maintenance can be used to combine the benefits from both. Also, other agents like nitrous oxide, muscle relaxants, and opioids can be used.

Nitrous Oxide

Although associated with increased risk of PONV, N_2O still holds its role in DCS because it deepens the plane of anesthesia and reduces the risk of awareness; it is cost-effective, minimizes inhalational agent requirements, and hastens recovery.

Muscle Relaxants

Short to intermediate-acting muscle relaxants can be used in surgeries that require good relaxation. The risks associated with muscle relaxants are serious, including residual paralysis and postoperative respiratory compromise. All these can prolong the postoperative stay. Therefore, minimal doses of muscle relaxants, along with neuromuscular monitoring, can be used to achieve optimal relaxation.

Opioids

Fentanyl administration minimizes postsurgical pain as well as pain associated with propofol injection. But it increases the risk of PONV and respiratory depression and can prolong overall recovery time. Remifentanil is ultra-short acting and is a part of TIVA, but it is also associated with the risk of PONV.

Analgesia

Pain during the perioperative period is associated with various complications such as the following:

1. Deferred recovery and ambulation.

2. Adverse respiratory effects (risk of basal atelectasis).

3. Tachycardia, increased myocardial oxygen demand, and ischemia.

4. Delayed ambulation or physical inactivity which, in turn, increases the risk of deep vein thrombosis.

5. Increased risk of PONV.

Adequate pain relief measures are thus of paramount importance in DCS because a patient in severe pain cannot be discharged. Various methods to provide good pain relief perioperatively are as follows:

1. Patient education (regarding the procedure).

2. Preemptive analgesia (i.e., analgesia commenced before surgical incision and included intra and postoperative periods as well).

3. Multimodal analgesia (optimized use of different classes of analgesics).

4. Use of regional anesthesia (nerve blocks and central neuraxial blocks).

5. Time to time pain assessment (using comprehensible pain scores like visual analog scale, numeric rating scale for adults, or FACES pain scale for children).

The commonly used analgesics are summarized in **Table 35.5**.

Postoperative Nausea and Vomiting

As highlighted in previous sections, PONV is not only associated with various anesthetic agents but also with different surgical procedures (e.g., breast, eye, ENT surgeries, etc.). PONV can postpone patient discharge. Therefore, antiemetic

Table 35.5 Some commonly used analgesics

Drug	Dose (IV)	Side effects	Caution in
Paracetamol	15 mg/kg	• Usually well-tolerated	• Hepatic diseases
NSAIDs Diclofenac Ketorolac	1–2 mg/g 0.5 mg/kg	• Peptic ulcers • Increased risk of perioperative bleeding • Bronchospasm • Exacerbation of asthma, renal insufficiency	• Hepatic diseases • Renal diseases
Opioids Tramadol Fentanyl Morphine	1–2 mg/kg 1–2 µg/kg 0.1–0.2 mg/kg	• Sedation • Respiratory depression • Nausea, vomiting • Chest wall rigidity • Urinary retention • Biliary spasm	• Hepatic diseases • Renal diseases
Alpha-2 agonists			
Dexmedetomidine	1 µg/kg loading dose over 10 min followed by 0.2–0.7 µg/kg/h	• Bradycardia • Hypotension	• Av block • Bradycardia • Hypotension
Clonidine	0.5–1.0 µg/kg		

Abbreviation: NSAID, nonsteroidal anti-inflammatory drug.

Table 35.6 Drugs for PONV prophylaxis

Drug	Action	Dose	Side effects
Droperidol	D2 antagonist	0.625–1.25 mg (IV)	• Extrapyramidal • Sedation • Gastrointestinal irritation • QT_C prolongation
Metoclopramide	D2 antagonist	10 mg (IV)	• Extrapyramidal • Sedation • Abdominal cramping
Ondansetron Granisetron Dolasetron Tropisetron	5-HT_3 antagonist	4 mg (IV) 0.35–1 mg (IV) 12.5 mg (IV) 5 mg (IV)	• Hypersensitivity • Dizziness • Headache
Dexamethasone	Steroid	4–8 mg (IV)	• Heartburn • Muscle weakness • Impaired wound healing • Increased blood sugar levels
Propofol	Serotonin antagonism	10–20 mg (IV) bolus, can be repeated after 15–20 mins	• Pain on injection site

Abbreviation: PONV, postoperative nausea and vomiting.

prophylaxis is a must. **Table 35.6** represents various drugs for PONV prophylaxis.

The scoring system designed by Apfel et al (**Table 35.7**) has a very simple structure and predicts PONV risk in adults undergoing surgeries under inhalational anesthesia. If at least two predictors are positive, there is almost 40% risk of PONV, and hence prophylaxis should be considered.

Postoperative Consideration and Discharge

Recovery is usually divided into three stages: early, intermediate, and late recovery stage.

Early stage—begins with the awakening of the patient along with recovery of protective reflexes.

Intermediate stage—starts form the transfer to postanesthesia care unit (PACU) until discharge of the patient.

Late stage—is the final physiological as well as psychological recovery of the patient from the surgical procedure performed.

Table 35.7 Apfel scoring system

Risk factors	Score
Female gender	1 point
Nonsmoker	1 point
History of the previous PONV	1 point
Postoperative use of opioids	1 point
Maximum score	4 points
Number of points	**Risk of PONV**
0	10%
1	20%
2	40%
3	60%
4	80%

Abbreviation: PONV, postoperative nausea and vomiting.

Various complications that should be well taken care of before discharging a DCS patient are bradycardia, hypotension, hemorrhage, emergence phenomenon, postdural puncture headache (PDPH), transient neurological symptoms, pain, respiratory depression, urinary retention, shivering, and PONV.

Scoring systems help in better monitoring and assessment of ambulatory surgery patients and help in safe discharge. Some commonly used scoring systems have been listed in **Box 35.1**.

Amongst these, the modified Aldrete score (**Table 35.8**) is more commonly used for monitoring, whereas PADSS (**Table 35.9**) is used primarily to assess discharge after anesthesia and surgery.

To summarize, the discharge of DCS patients should be well-planned, and the elimination of all the possible anesthesia/surgery-associated complications should be ensured. Along with the above-mentioned score, the following are a few important points that must be taken care of before discharging the patient:

1. Fully conscious and orientation to time, place and person.

2. Well-documented and stable vitals, exclusion of orthostatic hypotension.

3. Recovery from neuraxial anesthesia with the return of sensory (perianal area—S4/5) and motor functions (plantar flexion of the foot to preoperative level and adequate great toe proprioception).

4. Ensuring the presence of caregiver to escort the patient and provide necessary care postdischarge.

5. All the discharge instructions should be discussed with the patient and caregiver by both the anesthesiologist and the surgeon.

Box 35.1 Scoring system for monitoring and assessment of daycare patients

- Postanesthetic discharge scoring system (PADSS)
- Modified Aldrete score
- Clinical recovery score
- Stewart recovery score

Table 35.8 Modified Aldrete score

Variable	Score
Respiration	2 = able to take deep breath and cough 1 = dyspnea/shallow breathing 0 = apnea
O_2 saturation	2 = maintains > 92% on room air 1 = need oxygen supplementation to maintain saturation > 90% 0 = saturation less than 90% even with oxygen supplementation
Consciousness	2 = fully wake 1 = arousable on calling 0 = not responding
Circulation	2 = BP ± 20% of preanesthetic level 1 = BP ± 20–49% of preanesthetic level 0 = BP ± 50% of preanesthetic level
Activity	2 = able to move four extremities 1 = able to move two extremities 0 = unable to move any extremity

The total score is 10. Score ≥ 9 can be discharged

Table 35.9 Postanesthetic discharge scoring system

Variables	Score
Vital signs	
• Within 20% of the preoperative value	2
• Within 20–40% of the preoperative value	1
• >40% of the preoperative value	0
Ambulation and mental status	
• Oriented with a steady gait	2
• Oriented or has a steady gait	1
• Neither	0
Pain or nausea/vomiting	
• Minimal	2
• Moderate	1
• Severe	0
Surgical bleeding	
• Minimal	2
• Moderate	1
• Severe	0
Intake and output	
• Has had per oral fluids and voided	2
• Has had per oral fluids or voided	1
• Neither	0

Conclusion

DCS help reduce the burden on operating theaters, where patients require more complex surgeries with postoperative stay and care. Choosing a suitable patient, using short anesthetic agents, ensuring adequate pain management, and discharging the patient (with timely help in case of emergency) are the cornerstones of daycare surgical procedure.

CHAPTER 36

Pain and Anesthesia

Praveen Talawar and Vijaybabu Adabala

Introduction

Pain is an unpleasant experience with very high interindividual variations in terms of its perception. It is often a common reason to visit a physician. The management and taking care of a patient is not only challenging but also adds to increased healthcare costs, poor quality of life (QOL), and lost days of work. The proper assessment and treatment of pain with appropriate medical and surgical interventions alleviate patient's suffering and improves the QOL.

Pain and Pain Physiology (AS8.1)

The International Association for the Study of Pain (IASP) defines pain as "an unpleasant sensory and emotional experience associated with or resembling that associated with, actual or potential tissue damage."

The IASP emphasizes the complex nature of pain with its physical, emotional, and psychological components. The perception and interpretation of pain involve the transmission of painful stimuli from receptors to the cerebral cortex. The processing and transmission of pain can be understood through the following mechanisms:

- Transduction: It is the conversion of painful stimuli into electrical energy. The electrical energy induces an action potential when it reaches a threshold value, and the resultant impulse is carried toward the central nervous system through nerve fibers.
- Transmission: The sharp localized pain is carried by myelinated A-fibers, while the poorly localized, burning, and persistent pain is carried by unmyelinated C fibers. The pain impulse is transmitted from the periphery through the spinal cord, brain stem, and thalamus to the cortex.

- Perception: The somatosensory cortex identifies the location and intensity of pain, and the perception may manifest as arousal and attention, somatic as well as autonomic reflexes, endocrine responses, and emotional changes.

- Modulation: Modulation of pain involves changing or inhibiting pain impulses in the descending tract. The modulation can occur both at peripheral as well as central level. The neurotransmitters in pain modulation are:

  ▶ Excitatory neurotransmitters, for example, calcitonin gene-related peptide (CGRP), glutamate, aspartate, and adenosine triphosphate (ATP).

  ▶ Inhibitory neurotransmitters, for example, acetylcholine (Ach), glycine, gamma-aminobutyric acid (GABA), and enkephalins.

Assessment of Pain (AS8.2)

The assessment of pain is quite challenging because of high interindividual variation for the same painful stimulus. However, the common methods of pain assessment include a number of the pain rating scales and questionnaire (**Table 36.1**).

Acute Pain Management

Acute pain occurs because of noxious stimulation due to injury or a disease process or an abnormal

Table 36.1 Methods of pain assessment

Single-dimension scale	
• VAS	• It is a horizontal line with 0 end (no pain) and 10 end (worst imaginable pain). The patient is asked to point his pain on this line, and the actual score is measured with a measuring scale
• NRS	• It is similar to VAS, but the horizontal line is divided into 10 equal parts. The patient is asked to mark his/her pain on it
Multidimensional scale	
• McGill pain questionnaire	• It contains 20 sets of descriptive words. It determines pain intensity and also assesses cognitive components of pain
Pediatric scales	
• Neonates, infants, and toddlers	• Pain assessment is mainly observational. Pain, fear, anxiety, and distress are difficult to be distinguished. Examples are CRIES, FLACC, and comfort methods
• Toddlers and school-going children	Self-reported pain scale: • Wong–Baker (>3 years) • VAS (>5 years) Observational scale: • FLACC (2 months–7 years) • CHEOPS (1–7 years)

Abbreviations: CHEOPS, Children's Hospital of Eastern Ontario Pain Scale; CRIES, crying, requires SpO_2 > 95%, increased vital signs, expression, sleeplessness; FLACC, face, leg, activity, cry, consolability; NRS, numeric rating scale; VAS, visual analog scale.

function of muscle or viscera. Acute pain can occur after trauma, in the postoperative period, and in association with acute medical illnesses. The strategies for pain control include pharmacological and nonpharmacological options.

Pharmacological (AS8.3)

The goal is to maximize the positive effects and limit the side effects. The guiding principle is that balanced analgesia provides optimal pain relief. Multimodal analgesia is the preferred method of treating pain. It minimizes the adverse effects of using synergistic agents. The pharmacological methods include:

- Nonsteroidal anti-inflammatory drugs (NSAIDs): These are important components of multimodal analgesia and reduce the dose of opioids.

- Acetaminophen: Acetaminophen along with NSAIDs decrease the requirement of opioids.

- Opioids: These are the mainstay for the management of postoperative pain. Opioids can be given through intravenous (IV), intramuscular (IM), and epidural routes.

Nonpharmacological

Keeping in mind the biopsychosocial model of pain, nonpharmacological measures are employed. Psychological support is an integral part of acute trauma management as well as the rehabilitation phase. Other techniques like transcutaneous electrical nerve stimulation (TENS), hypnosis, relaxation techniques, biofeedback, and acupuncture are also useful. Regional blocks play a pivotal role in the alleviation of pain in this ultrasound era. The common regional techniques are:

- Thoracic paravertebral block: For thoracic, breast, and upper abdominal surgeries.

- Transversus abdominis plane block: For abdominal surgeries like cesarean and hernia repair.

- Lumbar plexus block: For knee and hip surgeries.

- Femoral nerve block: For hip fractures and surgeries on the hip.

- Brachial plexus block: For upper limb surgeries.

Chronic Pain Management

The chronic pain conditions have complex pathophysiology, with a varying incidence of 25 to 30%. The common clinical conditions associated with chronic pain are:

a. Low backache: The low backache is commonly encountered in clinical practice. It has a prevalence of 13.8 and an incidence of 31% in the general population. The proper evaluation in consultation with orthopedics is often warranted to rule out surgical causes of low backache. Red flag signs must be ruled out, which include:

    - Loss of control of the bowel or bladder.

    - Weakness or numbness in a leg or arm.

    - Foot drop, disturbed gait.

    - High fever.

    - Saddle anesthesia (numbness of the anus, perineum, or genitals).

    Low back pain can be:

    - Acute < 5 to 7 weeks.

    - Subacute > 7 weeks to 12 weeks.

    - Chronic > 12 weeks.

    Treatment is initiated once the pain generator is identified after the examination. The medical management supplemented by physiotherapy is employed as standard care. The interventions may be required in case of failure of medical management. The commonly used interventions are:

    - Epidural steroids.

    - Facet joint injection with steroids.

- Percutaneous discectomy for a prolapsed disc.

- Sacroiliac joint injection for sacroiliitis.

- Vertebroplasty for vertebral prolapse.

b. Neuropathic pain: Neuropathic pain can occur due to the dysfunction of peripheral as well as the central nervous system. The pathophysiology includes ectopic discharges, cross-excitation of nerves, collateral sprouting, and cerebral reorganization. The most common neuropathic pain conditions are:

    - Trigeminal neuralgia.

    - Postherpetic neuralgia.

    - Complex regional pain syndrome (CRPS).

    In neuropathic pain, there is increased activity and decreased inhibition in the somatosensory system. Pharmacotherapy is based on modulation of these phenomena by reducing the spontaneous activity and transmitter release and enhancing the inhibitory mechanisms. Pharmacotherapy is the most important treatment modality (**Table 36.2**). Complete pain relief is exceptional; hence, some pain relief is a realistic goal, which needs to be explained to the patient. The practical goals are:

    - Functional improvement and better QOL.

    - Better mood and sleep.

    - Relief of anxiety.

c. Cancer pain: Cancer pain syndromes can be divided into acute and chronic. Acute ones are usually a direct consequence of invasive diagnostic or therapeutic procedures, but they can less commonly be related to cancer itself. Chronic ones are more likely to be caused by the neoplastic process or antineoplastic therapy.

Table 36.2 Pharmacotherapy for neuropathic pain

Drug	Mechanism of action
Tricyclic antidepressants	Serotonin and noradrenaline reuptake inhibition, sodium channel blocking, NMDA antagonism
SNRIs	Serotonin and noradrenaline reuptake inhibition
Carbamazepine, oxcarbazepine	Sodium channel blockers
Topical lidocaine	Sodium channel blockers
Gabapentin, pregabalin ("gabapentinoids")	Regulation of voltage-dependent calcium channels in the central nervous system
Tramadol	Serotonin and noradrenaline reuptake inhibition, mu-opioid agonism
Opioids	mu-opioid agonism
Topical capsaicin	TRPV1-receptor agonism

Abbreviations: NMDA, N-methyl-D-aspartate; SNRI, serotonin-norepinephrine reuptake inhibitor; TRPV1, transient receptor potential cation channel subfamily V member 1.

The local expansion and metastases to distant organs result in the increasing severity of cancer pain. Treatment should be in an integrated fashion and the approach includes:

- Primary antitumor therapies.
- Analgesic modalities.
- Psychological and rehabilitative interventions.

The WHO ladder recommends nonopioid analgesics as possible options at all steps. Opioids are the mainstay of analgesic therapy and are stratified based on their ability to control pain. The dosing of opioids should be titrated based on the desired pain control and associated side effects. The cancer patients often report breakthrough pain in the background of optimized pain control for which immediate-release opioids are helpful.

d. Myofascial pain syndrome (MPS): MPS is characterized by local and referred pain and perceived as deep and aching in the presence of myofascial trigger points. It is distributed equally between men and women, with an overall prevalence of 40 to 70%. Myofascial pain (MP) causes a significant reduction in QOL and is a major cause of time lost from work. The treatment goals are:

- Correction of perpetuating factors.
- Trigger point inactivation: Either invasive or noninvasive methods.
- Prevention of recurrence.

The treatment methods are physiotherapy, transcutaneous electrical nerve stimulation, acupuncture, topical cooling of muscle, and trigger point injection with local anesthetics.

e. Fibromyalgia: Definition: "A common rheumatological syndrome characterized by chronic, diffuse musculoskeletal pain, and tenderness with a number of associated symptoms, among which sleep disturbances, fatigue, and affective dysfunction are particularly frequent."

The diagnostic criteria for fibromyalgia are:

- Widespread pain index (WPI) score > 7 and symptom severity (SS) scale score > 5 or WPI score of 3 to 6 and SS scale score > 9.

- Symptoms present at a similar level for at least 3 months.

- No disorder present that would otherwise explain the pain.

The treatment modalities are:

- Pharmacological: Tricyclic compounds, serotonin-norepinephrine reuptake inhibitors (SNRIs), and anticonvulsants.

- Nonpharmacological: Education, aerobic exercise, and cognitive-behavioral therapy.

Nerve Blocks in Pain Management

1. **Stellate ganglion block**

   a. Indications:

      - Complex regional pain syndrome (type 1 and 2).

      - Herpes zoster over face and neck.

      - Refractory anginal pain and phantom limb pain.

      - Raynaud's phenomenon, obliterative vascular disease.

      - Scleroderma.

   b. Contraindications:

      - Recent myocardial infarction.

      - Coagulopathy.

      - Glaucoma.

      - Pre-existing contralateral phrenic nerve palsy (may precipitate respiratory distress).

   c. Techniques:

      - Landmark technique: Chassaignac's tubercle is the identification mark.

      - Fluoroscopy assisted: The spread of radio-opaque dye is visualized in AP and lateral views.

      - Ultrasound-guided: The endpoint for injection is the ultrasound image, demonstrating the tip of the needle and penetrating the prevertebral fascia in the longus colli.

   d. Signs of successful stellate ganglion block: Successful block produces:

      - An ipsilateral Horner's syndrome (ptosis, miosis, and anhydrosis).

      - Flushing of the face.

      - The rise in temperature of the arm by at least one degree.

   e. Side effects:

      - Nerve injury (brachial plexus, recurrent laryngeal nerve, phrenic nerve).

      - Perforation of trachea/esophagus.

      - Inadvertent vascular or intrathecal injection, pneumothorax.

2. **Trigeminal nerve block:** Trigeminal nerve comprises ophthalmic, maxillary, and mandibular nerves.

   a. Indication:

      - Trigeminal neuralgia.

   b. Technique:

      - The block can be given at Gasserian ganglion or one of the branches (maxillary/mandibular), depending on the site of the lesion. The block can be performed either blindly or with the assistance of ultrasound/fluoroscopy.

   c. Complications:

      - Temporary blindness (due to optic nerve involvement).

      - Injury to the pharynx (during mandibular nerve block).

3. **Intercostal nerve (ICN) block**

   a. Indications:

      - Rib fractures.

- Chest and upper abdominal surgery such as thoracotomy, thoracostomy, mastectomy, gastrostomy, and cholecystectomy.

- Postmastectomy pain (T2) and postthoracotomy pain.

- Herpes zoster.

- Cancer pain.

b. Technique:

- The ICN is blocked by injecting local anesthetic in the plane between internal intercostal and innermost intercostal muscle in the midaxillary line. In adults, the most popular site for ICN block is at the angle of the rib (6–8 cm from the spinous processes).

c. Complications:

- Pneumothorax: Incidence—0.07%.

- Systemic toxicity.

- The blood level of local anesthetics is highest after an ICN block.

4. **Celiac plexus block:** Coeliac "plexus" is the largest plexus of the sympathetic nervous system that innervates the upper abdominal organs.

a. Indications:

- Gastric malignancy.

- Pancreatic malignancy.

b. Techniques: Fluoroscopic-guided approaches include:

- Posterior (retrocrural) approach: This approach targets celiac plexus through retrocrural space, which is located posterior-cephalad to the diaphragm.

- Anterior approach: The needle is put anterior to the crus of the diaphragm.

- Transaortic approach: The needle is placed immediately anterior to the aorta and advanced gradually with intermittent aspiration till aorta is entered, as evinced by the appearance of blood.

- Transcrural approach: The needle pierces the crus of diaphragm to finish anterior and caudad to the diaphragm in the same plane as aorta, anterior to it.

- Transintervertebral disc approach: This technique has been recently suggested, wherein the needle passes through the intervertebral disc.

- Recently, ultrasound-guided technique was introduced, which has advantages over fluoro-guided approaches like less time consuming, real-time image, avoidance of vascular structures and other organs, etc.

c. Complications:

- Hypotension.

5. **Lumbar sympathetic chain block:** The lumbar sympathetic chain is located in the prevertebral fascia, which lies on the anterolateral aspects of the vertebral bodies. The psoas muscle separates the lumbar sympathetic chain from the lumbar somatic nerves. A single injection of local anesthetic at the level of L2 will usually provide a complete block of postganglionic sympathetic efferents to the lower extremity because the lowest preganglionic sympathetic outflow to the chain is at the level of L2.

a. Indications:

- Vascular insufficiency.

- CRPS types 1 and 2.

- Neuropathic lower limb pain.
- Cancer pain.
- Cancer-related rectal tenesmus.
- Intractable back pain.

6. **Superior hypogastric block:** Superior hypogastric plexus is formed from pelvic sympathetic fibers of the aortic plexus and L2 and L3 splanchnic nerves. These afferent and efferent fibers innervate the pelvic viscera, including the uterus, bladder, vagina, and prostate. The plexus is located between the upper third of the first sacral vertebral body and the lower third of the fifth lumbar vertebral body, at the sacral promontory, in the retroperitoneal space.

   a. Indications:

      - Cancer and noncancer pelvic pain.

7. **Ganglion impar block:** Ganglion impar represents the termination of the para-vertebral sympathetic chains, converging at the sacrococcygeal level. It can be blocked fluoro-guided or ultrasound-guided.

   a. Indications:

      - Perineal pain.
      - Coccydynia.

Pain Management in Palliative Care (AS8.4)

Palliative care aims to reduce the severity of disease symptoms rather than provide a cure. The goal is to prevent and relieve suffering and improve people's quality of life facing serious, complex illnesses. The goals of pain management in palliative care include:

- Relief from suffering.
- Treatment of pain.
- Treatment of other distressing symptoms.
- Psychological and spiritual care.

- Daily living support system.
- Support system for the patient's family.

The basic principles of palliative care are as follows:

- Patients are often undertreated and hence require a competent pain assessment.
- A multidisciplinary approach is crucial to assess and provide optimal relief of pain and suffering.
- The collaborative involvement of patients, families, and care providers is needed to achieve the best result.
- A small proportion of patients do require a specialist referral, and these include:
  ▶ Neuropathic pain.
  ▶ Opioid intolerant pain.
  ▶ Unacceptable side effects of analgesics.
  ▶ A morbid fear of analgesics.
  ▶ Requests for euthanasia because of pain.
- Patients should be comfortable and pain-free with a minimum number of drugs needed.
- Reevaluate the patient regularly because the patient's need changes as the illness progresses.
- Always anticipate side effects, and always prescribe regular aperients and antiemetics.

The prescription of palliative care is incomplete without the "World Health Organization (WHO) pain ladder" (**Table 36.3** and **Fig. 36.1**).

Coanalgesics are drugs that, when used concurrently with analgesics, may contribute significantly to pain relief. A few examples of coanalgesics are listed in **Table 36.4**.

Pain Management in Terminally Ill Patients (AS8.5)

Pain management near the end of life is a professional, moral, and ethical obligation. Most patients equate the pain at the end of life

Table 36.3 The WHO pain ladder

Step	Severity of pain (score on VAS = 0–10)	Drugs
1	Mild (0–3)	Nonopioid analgesics plus coanalgesics
2	Moderate (4–6)	Weak opioids plus step 1 analgesics
3	Severe (7–10)	Strong opioids plus step 2 analgesics

Abbreviations: VAS, visual analogue scale; WHO, World Health Organization.

Table 36.4 Examples of coanalgesics

Coanalgesic type	Examples
NSAIDs	Ibuprofen, naproxen, diclofenac, ketorolac
Steroids	Dexamethasone
Antidepressants	Amitryptyline
Anticonvulsants	Carbamazepine, sodium valproate, clonazepam, gabapentin
Psychotropics	Diazepam, levomepromazine
NMDA receptor antagonists	Ketamine

Abbreviations: NMDA, N-methyl-D-aspartate; NSAIDs, nonsteroidal anti-inflammatory drugs.

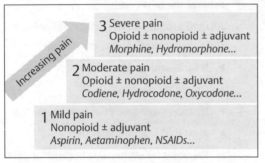

Fig. 36.1 The World Health Organization (WHO) pain ladder. NSAIDs, nonsteroidal anti-inflammatory drugs.

to consequences of illnesses like HIV, cancer, and degenerative diseases. However, the pain is not due to the underlying disease rather the consequences of underlying pathology. The care setting, availability of resources, and expertise substantially influence pain management. The principles of pain management in terminally ill patients are as follows:

- A thorough pain assessment using appropriate tools.
- Cognition often gets impaired near the end of life. Therefore, tools like pain assessment in advanced dementia (PAINAD), behavioral pain scale (BPS), and critical care pain observation tool (CPOT) are helpful.
- Pharmacotherapy remains the mainstay of treatment as guided by the WHO pain ladder.

- Opioids are the principal class of analgesics in terminally ill patients because of their potency, concomitant sedative and anxiolytic properties, and ability to be administered through multiple routes.
- Nonsteroidal anti-inflammatory drugs (NSAIDs) are usually not suitable in these patients because of their adverse effect profile.
- The oral, sublingual, and buccal route is appropriate in patients who can swallow. As the disease progresses, a switch to transdermal, rectal, vaginal, or neuraxial infusion may be needed.
- Neuraxial infusion of opioids will provide adequate analgesia in patients with refractory pain or intolerable side effects, owing to the systemic route.
- Patients with intolerable pain related to advanced cancer may require denervation of the affected area with alcohol, phenol, or glycerol.
- Finally, the patient not responding to pharmacologic as well as the interventional approach may require palliative sedation.

Conclusion

Pain is the most unpleasant experience for an individual. Assessment of pain with appropriate pain scale and managing it with various pharmacological and nonpharmacological techniques is important to avoid long-term complications, ensure early rehabilitation, and improve the quality of life. The WHO pain ladder is a simple guide to choose an appropriate medication, based on the severity of pain.

Section VI
Miscellaneous

CHAPTER 37

Gases Used in Anesthesia: Road to Mountain

Ranjitha Nethaji and Puneet Khanna

Introduction

The gases used in anesthesia practice deserve special attention. The existence of life without oxygen is known to all. Oxygen is the most frequently used gas by anesthetists in perioperative as well as critical care settings. In addition, nitrous oxide (N_2O), medical air, Entonox, carbon dioxide, and heliox are other gases of importance. The gases in anesthesia can be categorized as follows:

- Nonliquefied compressed gas: A nonliquefied compressed gas does not liquefy at ordinary ambient temperatures regardless of the pressure applied. Examples include *oxygen, air, nitrogen, and helium.*

- Liquefied compressed gas: Liquefied compressed gas is one that becomes liquid to a large extent in containers at ambient temperature and pressures from 25 to 1500 psig. Examples include *nitrous oxide and carbon dioxide.*

Oxygen

Joseph Priestley first synthesized oxygen. It is colorless and odorless with a boiling point of −183°C and a critical temperature of −118°C. The critical temperature of oxygen above the room temperature makes its existence as a gas at normal ambient temperature. The importance of it lies in the fact that reading on the pressure gauge correlates with the volume of oxygen remaining inside the cylinder.

Manufacture

Manufacturing of oxygen is a two-step process. First, atmospheric air is liquefied. Second, liquid air is separated into its components by fractional distillation. The commercial production of a large volume of oxygen also involves the fractional distillation of air.

Oxygen concentrators are portable devices that produce oxygen by absorption of nitrogen on zeolites. These are suitable for use in homes, hospitals, and remote locations.

Storage

- Medical oxygen is stored in oxygen cylinders at 2000 psi.
- Also stored as liquid oxygen in vacuum-insulated evaporator (VIE).

Heliox

Heliox comprises a variable proportion of oxygen and helium. The percentage of oxygen may vary from 21 to 50%. *Heliox is useful in patients with upper airway obstruction.* Theoretically, patients with airway obstruction offer more resistance to flow of gases, resulting in turbulent flow inside the airways. The low density (0.1669) of helium provides the advantage of low resistance to flow when breathed in as heliox. The decreased resistance lowers the work of breathing significantly.

Storage

Heliox is stored in black color cylinders with brown and white shoulders at the pressure of 2000 psi.

Xenon

Xenon is a rare gas, contributing no more than 0.0875 ppm of the atmosphere. *It is manufactured by fractional distillation of air.* Xenon has a good safety and efficacy profile, but its cost is the major barrier to its widespread clinical use.

The estimated minimum alveolar concentration (MAC) of xenon is 63%. Xenon has the lowest blood–gas partition coefficient (0.115) of all known inhaled anesthetics, making induction and emergence from anesthesia rapid. Other advantages are neuroprotection, less cardiovascular depression, and profound analgesia.

Carbon Dioxide

Carbon dioxide is the most commonly used as an insufflation gas during laparoscopy. It was used as a respiratory stimulant in the 1930s during the respiratory arrest. Other uses in the past were:

- To hasten recovery at the emergence.
- To open the glottis during blind intubation.
- Treatment of postdural puncture headache.

Manufacture

It is produced as a byproduct during the hydrogenation of ammonium.

Storage

It is stored in gray cylinders at the pressure of 750 psi.

Medical Air

Medical air is provided by the following three methods:

- Compressed air.
- Synthetic air.
- Cylinder manifolds.

Compressed medical air is formed by drawing ambient air into the compressor. There are a series of filters that remove the impurities before the compressed air enters the pipeline system.

Synthetic air is prepared by blending liquid nitrogen with liquid oxygen in the gaseous state.

Its advantage is that no power supply is required and there are no contamination problems.

Medical air seems to be the most suitable substitute for N_2O, as a mixture of oxygen with medical air can be universally used as a carrier gas. There are absolutely no contraindications for a combination of nitrogen with oxygen; it can be used in every patient and in every surgical condition.

Air is also used, at a higher pressure, to power a variety of surgical tools and other devices such as tourniquets pneumatic drills and saws.

Nitrous Oxide

Joseph Priestly first isolated N_2O in 1772, and subsequently, Humphery Davy recognized the analgesic property of N_2O and coined the term "laughing gas." Horace Wells, in 1845, used N_2O for pain-free dental extraction.

Manufacture

It is produced by heating ammonium nitrate at 250°C.

Storage

It is stored as a compressed liquefied gas at 760 psi.

Physical and Anesthetic Properties

- It is a colorless gas with a slightly sweet odor.
- It is 1.5 times heavier than air and 35 times more soluble than nitrogen.
- It has a critical temperature (36.5°C) above the room temperature, so it is stored as a liquid in pressurized cylinders.
- It is a good analgesic but has low-anesthetic potency because of its high MAC of 105. It means a larger quantity of N_2O is required to produce the effect. However, under anesthesia, a minimum of 30% oxygen

has to be provided to patients. Hence, only 70% N_2O can be provided and has to be supplemented with other inhalational anesthetics.

Advantages

- Its mild sympathetic effect counteracts the cardiovascular depression by other anesthetics.
- Its low solubility makes it highly controllable, resulting in rapid induction and recovery.
- The high-lipid solubility of N_2O results in its rapid transfer across the alveoli. The rapid transfer of nitrous from alveoli leads to increased uptake of volatile anesthetics. This is termed as "second-gas effect."
- Providing a higher concentration of N_2O or volatile anesthetic agents also increases the concentration of the inhaled anesthetic agent, which is referred to as the "*concentration effect*."

Disadvantages

There are several concerns about adverse effects and postoperative complications related to the use of N_2O. The noteworthy ones are as follows:

- *Diffusion hypoxia* is a well-known phenomenon that may occur during recovery from anesthesia. At the end of anesthesia, there is a rapid transfer of N_2O from the blood to alveoli. It leads to dilution of oxygen inside the alveoli and also impairment of the oxygen transfer across the alveoli to blood. These phenomena lead to hypoxia that can be offset by maintaining adequate minute ventilation and supplementing oxygen.
- Due to its tendency to vigorously diffuse into all air-filled spaces, N_2O is contraindicated in cases of the following:

- ▶ Pneumothorax.
- ▶ Bowel obstruction.
- ▶ Middle ear surgery.
- ▶ Pneumocephalus.
- ▶ In all cases with increased risk of air embolism.
- ▶ Ophthalmic surgeries with internal gas tamponade.

- Due to its vitamin B_{12} inactivating effect, depressing methionine and folate metabolism, it should not be used in the first trimester of pregnancy and in patients undergoing chemotherapy.
- Due to the increase of cerebral blood flow, the use of N_2O is a contraindication in cases with increased cranial pressure. N_2O should be avoided in all patients with a history of postoperative nausea and vomiting (PONV).

Entonox

It is the trade name for a compressed gas mixture containing 50% oxygen and 50% N_2O by volume. Entonox is stored in the cylinder (blue color body with blue and white shoulder) at a pressure of 1900 psig. It is mainly used for labor analgesia.

Conclusion

Anesthetic gases are an inseparable component of day-to-day perioperative care. Oxygen is required not only during the surgery but also in the postoperative period to prevent hypoxia. Nitrous oxide and air act as carrier gases during delivery of inhaled anesthetics, while Heliox and Entonox are used in upper airway obstruction and labor analgesia, respectively. Finally, the role of carbon dioxide in laparoscopic surgeries cannot be overlooked.

CHAPTER 38

Complications in Anesthesia

Abhishek Singh

Introduction

No domain in life is without risks, and complications do occur during patient care and treatment. In this regard, anesthesia is no more an exception. The complications can range from mild anaphylactoid reaction to death in the worst scenario. This chapter is an overview of complications that may arise during anesthetic care, and one should be aware of them. These are listed below:

- Mortality.
- Respiratory complications:
  ▸ Pulmonary aspiration.
  ▸ Pulmonary embolism.
  ▸ Hypoxia.
  ▸ Hypocapnia.
  ▸ Hypercapnia.
  ▸ Oxygen toxicity.
- Cardiovascular complications:
  ▸ Hypotension.
  ▸ Hypertension.
  ▸ Myocardial ischemia.
  ▸ Dysrhythmias.
  ▸ Cardiac arrest.
- Neurological complications:
  ▸ Postoperative cognitive dysfunction (POCD).
  ▸ Convulsion.
  ▸ Delayed recovery.
  ▸ Cranial nerve palsies.
  ▸ Awareness.
  ▸ Extrapyramidal side effects.
- ▸ Agitation, delirium, and emergence excitation.
  ▸ Peripheral neuropathies.
- Gastrointestinal complications:
  ▸ Postoperative nausea and vomiting (PONV).
- Renal complications.
- Hepatic complications:
  ▸ Postoperative jaundice.
  ▸ Postoperative hepatitis.
  ▸ Postoperative cholestasis.
- Positioning in anesthesia and their complication.
- Ocular complications.
- Temperature-related complications:
  ▸ Hypothermia and shivering.
  ▸ Hyperthermia.
  ▸ Malignant hyperthermia (MH).

Mortality

Evidence suggests that perioperative mortality due to anesthesia is between 1 in 13,000 and 1 in 15,000 cases, but the incidence of mortality exclusive due to anesthesia is rare. Certain patient and procedure-related factors add to increased mortality:

- Extremes of age (neonates, children less than 1 year, and elderly patients).
- Males.
- American Society of Anesthesiologists (ASA) III physical status or more.
- Emergency surgeries during general anesthesia.

- Cardiac surgery (followed by thoracic, vascular, abdominal, pediatric, and orthopedic surgeries).

The main causes of anesthesia-related mortality were airway management and cardiovascular events related to anesthesia and drug administration.

Respiratory Complications of Anesthesia

Pulmonary Aspiration

Aspiration is defined as the inhalation of oropharyngeal or gastric contents into the larynx and lower respiratory tract.

Mendelson's syndrome is defined as a chemical injury of the lung due to the entry of acidic gastric content.

Aspiration pneumonia is defined as the infectious process caused by the entry of oropharyngeal secretions or enteral content, colonized by pathogenic bacteria, into the lung.

Incidence

- 1 to 5 per 10,000 cases under general anesthesia.
- More frequent in emergency surgery than elective surgery.
- Three times more common in pregnancy.
- Extremes of age are at higher risk.

Protective Mechanism against Aspiration

The following structures help in preventing aspiration:

- *Upper esophageal sphincter (UES)*: It is formed by cricopharyngeous muscle, which is striated in nature. A conscious individual has a tone of around 25 to 38 cm of H_2O. Anesthetic agents except ketamine reduce the tone of the sphincter.
- *Lower esophageal sphincter (LES)*: It lies at the junction of the stomach and esophagus. The resting end-expiratory LES is approximately 8 to 20 cm of H_2O higher (barrier pressure) than resting end-expiratory intragastric pressure. *Since succinylcholine increases both the pressures, as a result, the barrier pressure is maintained.*
- *Gastroesophageal (GE) junction*: Diaphragmatic fibers act as pinchcock, thus preventing the regurgitation of content.
- *Protective laryngeal reflexes*: Protective reflexes like coughing, laryngospasm, etc., play important roles.

Risk Factors for Aspiration

The risk factors for pulmonary aspiration are summarized below:

- *Increased gastric volume*:
  - ► Recent meal.
  - ► Gastric insufflation.
  - ► Increased intra-abdominal pressure due to pregnancy or pneumoperitoneum.
  - ► Increased secretion of gastric acid.
- *Delayed gastric emptying*:
  - ► *High* protein or lipid diet.
  - ► *Gastric* outlet obstruction.
  - ► *Intestinal obstruction.*
  - ► Drugs like opioids and anticholinergics.
  - ► Obesity.
  - ► Diabetic gastropathy.
  - ► Peptic ulcer disease.
  - ► Condition of sympathetic nervous system stimulation like active labor, acute pain, or stress.
- *Decreased LES tone*:
  - ► Hiatus hernia.
  - ► Drugs like anticholinergics, opioids, and dopaminergic agonists.
  - ► Cricoid pressure.
  - ► Pregnancy.

- *Decreased UES tone*:
  - ▶ Procedural sedation.
  - ▶ General anesthesia.
  - ▶ Muscle relaxant.
- *Loss of protective airway reflexes*:
  - ▶ Advanced age.
  - ▶ Neurological diseases like multiple sclerosis, Guillain–Barre syndrome.
  - ▶ Neuromuscular disease like myasthenia gravis, myotonica dystrophica.
  - ▶ Altered consciousness due to sedative medication or coma.

Pathophysiological Manifestations

The aspiration of gastric content into the lungs can result in:

- Blocking of upper airway.
- Foreign body in the airway may lead to inflammation and granulomatous reaction.
- Mucosal irritation.
- Loss of surfactant may lead to alveolar collapse.
- Noncardiogenic pulmonary edema.
- Acute respiratory distress syndrome (ARDS).

Determinants of the Severity of Aspiration

The following factors affect the severity of aspiration:

- pH less than 2.5.
- The volume of aspirate: More than 0.4 mL/kg.
- Physical nature: Particulate and feculent matter causes severe pneumonitis.

Prevention Measures for Aspiration

The preventive measures against pulmonary aspiration are summarized below:

- *Adherence to ASA preoperative fasting guidelines.*

- ▶ *Adult*:
  - ○ 2 hours—water and clear fluids.
  - ○ 6 hours—light meal.
  - ○ 8 hours—heavy meal (fried/fatty food, meat).
- ▶ *Pediatric*:
  - ○ 2 hours—water and clear fluids.
  - ○ 4 hours—breast milk.
  - ○ 6 hour—infant formula, nonhuman milk, a light meal.
- ▶ *Diabetic*:
  - ○ 8 hours—semisolid food.
- ▶ *Pregnancy and labor*:
  - ○ Mothers are allowed to alleviate thirst during labor with sips of water or clear fluids.
  - ○ Intravenous (IV) hydration is preferred over oral intake in certain high-risk pregnancies with a difficult airway, difficult regional anesthesia, and high probability of cesarean section.
  - ○ Solid or semisolid foods are avoided once the mother is in active labor or has received opioid analgesics.
- *Pharmacoprophylaxis*:
  - ▶ *Regulation of gastric acid secretion*:
    - ○ *Neutralization of gastric acidity* by nonparticulate antacids: 30 mL of 0.3 M Na citrate.
    - ○ *Decrease acidity and volume of secretions*:
      - – H2-receptor antagonist—cimetidine, ranitidine, famotidine.
      - – Proton pump inhibitors—pantoprazole, omeprazole, rabeprazole.
    - ○ *Increase gastric emptying*: Metoclopramide, erythromycin.

- *Preoperative gastric emptying*:
  - ▶ Routine placement of the gastric tube is not recommended as it may impair the function of both LES and UES and does not guarantee an empty stomach.
- *Choosing the appropriate technique of anesthesia in full stomach patients*:
  - ▶ Regional technique is preferred.
  - ▶ Rapid sequence induction (RSI) if regional techniques are not feasible.
  - ▶ Awake intubation is reserved for difficult airway patients.

Rapid Sequence Induction

It is done to protect the airway from aspiration of gastric content. It minimizes the interval between loss of consciousness and endotracheal intubation. The RSI includes:

- Preoxygenation: Tidal volume breathing in 100% oxygen for 3 minutes or 4/8 vital capacity breaths in 30/60 seconds, respectively.
- Predetermined dose of induction agents (thiopentone sodium).
- Muscle relaxant: Scoline or rocuronium can be used.
- Cricoid pressure.
- Avoidance of positive pressure ventilation until the airway is secured with a cuffed endotracheal tube.

Modified Rapid Sequence Induction

Avoidance of positive pressure ventilation during conventional RSI precludes the ability of the clinician to check the airway and determine whether ventilation by the mask is possible. The failure to secure the airway during RSI may result in hypoxia, hypercarbia, and even death. Therefore, conventional RSI is modified. It consists of the following components:

- Preoxygenation.
- Induction of anesthesia.

- Application of cricoid pressure.
- Gentle positive pressure ventilation with pressure less than 20 cm of H_2O.
- Muscle relaxant.
- Securing of the airway with a cuffed endotracheal tube.

Sellick's Maneuver

Its main objective is to prevent aspiration by compressing the esophagus between the cricoid cartilage and body of C6 vertebra. The current recommendations regarding the amount of pressure are as follows:

- *Adults*: 1 to 20 N at the beginning of induction, which is gradually increased to 30 N as the patient loses consciousness.
- *Pediatrics*:
  - ▶ <1 year: 8 N
  - ▶ 1 to 4 years: 9 N
  - ▶ 4 to 8 years: 10 N
  - ▶ >10 years: 15 N

Adequacy of Pressure

The adequacy of Sellick's maneuver can be checked by the following:

- There will be blanching of more than half of the nail bed.
- Equivalent pressure will induce pain when applied to the bridge of the nose.

Limitations of Cricoid Pressure

The cricoid pressure is not without limitations, and the ones mentioned below are noteworthy:

- In an awake patient, it may induce vomiting due to reflex relaxation of LES.
- Coughing or retching may lead to rupture of the esophagus.
- It may worsen laryngoscopy view.
- Pressure > 40 N may distort airway anatomy, obstruct the airway, impair intubation, or mask ventilation.

- It may not occlude esophagus completely.
- It hinders successful placement of laryngeal mask airway (LMA).
- It may impede tracheal intubation through intubating LMA.
- Cricoid fracture has also been reported.

Precaution at Extubation and Postoperative Period

The following measures at the time of extubation can reduce the chances of aspiration to a great extent:

- Avoid extubation in the deeper plane of anesthesia in patients at risk of aspiration.
- Patients should be extubated only when conscious and obeying commands.
- Sim's position for recovery when the patient is drowsy and regurgitating or has upper airway bleeding.

Pulmonary Embolism

Pulmonary embolism (PE) is defined as a blockage of the pulmonary artery or one of its branches by a thrombus that had originated in the venous system or right side of the heart.

Clinical Manifestations

- Dyspnea is the most frequent symptom.
- Tachypnea is the most frequent sign.
- Chest pain is common and is usually sudden and pleuritic in origin and may mimic angina pectoris or myocardial infarction.
- Anxiety.
- Fever, tachycardia, apprehension, cough, diaphoresis, hemoptysis, and syncope.

Management

- **Emergency medical management:**
  - ▶ The immediate objective is to stabilize the cardiopulmonary system.

  - ▶ Oxygen is administered immediately to relieve hypoxemia, respiratory distress, and central cyanosis.
  - ▶ Vasopressors, inotropic agents, and anti-dysrhythmic agents may be indicated to support circulation.
  - ▶ Perfusion scan, hemodynamic monitoring, and serial arterial blood gas (ABG) analysis is needed to monitor the response to treatment.
  - ▶ The patient may need intubation and mechanical ventilation, depending upon the clinical picture and ABG result.
  - ▶ Small doses of IV morphine or sedative may be administered to relieve patient anxiety.
  - ▶ Elastic compression stocking or intermittent pneumatic leg compression devices may be used to reduce venous stasis.
- **Pharmacologic and surgical therapy:**
  - ▶ *Anticoagulation therapy*: Heparin and warfarin have traditionally been the primary method for managing acute deep venous thrombosis (DVT) and PE.
  - ▶ *Thrombolytic therapy (urokinase, streptokinase, alteplase, and reteplase)*: Thrombolytic therapy resolves the thrombi or emboli and restores the pulmonary circulation's normal hemodynamic functioning, thereby reducing pulmonary hypertension and improving perfusion, oxygenation, and cardiac output.
  - ▶ *Surgical management*: A surgical "embolectomy" is rarely performed but may be indicated if the patient has a massive PE or hemodynamic instability or if there are contraindications to thrombolytic therapy.

Prevention

For patients at risk of PE, the most effective approach for prevention is to prevent DVT by way of the following:

- Active leg exercises to avoid venous stasis.
- Early ambulation.
- Promoting the use of elastic compression stocking and sequential compression devices.

Hypoxia

Hypoxia is defined as the failure of oxygenation at the tissue level, while hypoxemia is defined as a condition where the arterial oxygen tension is below normal (normal PaO_2 = 80–100 mm Hg). The hypoxemia can be of the following types:

- *Hypoxemic hypoxia*: Insufficient oxygen is reaching the blood.
- *Stagnant or circulatory hypoxia*: Decreased blood flow to the tissues, leading to reduced oxygen delivery to the tissue.
- *Anemic hypoxia*: Due to the decreased oxygen-carrying capacity of the blood.
- *Histologic hypoxia*: Due to impaired utilization of oxygen by the tissues.

The hypoxemia can occur due to the causes listed in **Table 38.1**.

Treatment

- Treatment of the underlying cause.
- Ventilation with 100% oxygen.

Hypocapnia

Hypocapnia occurs when the level of carbon dioxide (CO_2) in the blood is less than 35 mm of Hg. Causes of hypocapnia are as follows:

- Increased elimination of CO_2:
  - ▶ Increased minute ventilation in patients on controlled ventilation.
  - ▶ Increased minute ventilation in spontaneously ventilating patients in response to the following:
    - ○ Pregnancy.
    - ○ Pain.
    - ○ Metabolic acidosis.
    - ○ Central nervous system (CNS) pathology like infection and tumor.
- Decreased dead space ventilation.
- Reduced pulmonary perfusion:
  - ▶ Hypovolemia.
  - ▶ Hypotension.
  - ▶ Cardiac arrest.
  - ▶ PE.
- Reduced CO_2 production:
  - ▶ Hypothermia.
  - ▶ Hypothyroidism.
  - ▶ Low metabolism.

Management

- Evaluate the oxygen status.
- Confirm hypocapnia by ABG.
- Decrease minute ventilation if hypocapnia is due to iatrogenic hyperventilation.
- Assess and maintain circulation.

Hypercapnia

Hypercapnia occurs when the level of CO_2 in the blood is more than 45 mm Hg. Causes of hypercapnia are as follows:

- *Hypoventilation*:
  - ▶ Reduced minute ventilation in patients on controlled ventilation.
  - ▶ Decreased minute ventilation in spontaneously ventilating patients due to drug-induced depression of the ventilatory response to CO_2. Common agents

Table 38.1 Causes of hypoxemia

Hypoventilation	A spontaneously breathing anesthetized patient may hypoventilate due to drug-induced respiratory depression, while in patient who is paralyzed and ventilated, hypoventilation may occur due to inadequate mechanical ventilation
Reduced functional residual capacity	Induction of general anesthesia causes a reduction in functional residual capacity by 15–20%, which is more pronounced in patients with preexisting lung disease and obesity
Atelectasis	It is a condition of alveolar collapse which may manifest as micro atelectasis, macro atelectasis, or lobar collapse. It leads to V/Q mismatch, right to left shunting of blood, and arterial hypoxemia
Diffusion defect	Even though the adequate oxygen is supplied to the alveoli, the defect at alveolar level may prevent its absorption into blood. This is due to: • Thickened alveolar membrane • Thickening of air–blood interface • Inflammation • Edema • Fibrosis or loss of alveolar surface area (sarcoidosis, emphysema)
Inhibition of HPV	It is a protective phenomenon to prevent hypoxemia. When PaO_2 decreases in a region of the lung, pulmonary vasoconstriction occurs in that particular region. It diverts the blood flow from the lung's hypoxic regions to better-ventilated regions, thus decreasing V/Q mismatch and preventing hypoxemia. Inhibition of HPV leads to the development of arterial hypoxemia
Poor oxygen delivery to tissues	It can occur due to: • Systemic hypoperfusion • Embolus • Sepsis • Local problems like a cold limb, Raynaud phenomenon, sickle cell disease, etc
Increased oxygen demand	It can occur in case of: • Fever • Malignant hyperpyrexia • Shivering • Sepsis

Abbreviation: HPV, hypoxic pulmonary vasoconstriction.

are opioids, benzodiazepines, sedative-hypnotics (propofol), and halogenated inhalational agents.

• *Increased dead space ventilation.*
• *Rebreathing*:
  ▶ Faulty breathing circuits.
  ▶ Inadequate fresh gas flow.
  ▶ Exhausted absorbent agents.
  ▶ Faulty expiratory check valves.
• *Increased CO_2 production*:
  ▶ Fever.
  ▶ Sepsis.
  ▶ Systemic absorption during laparoscopic procedures.
  ▶ Thyroid storm.
  ▶ MH.

Management

- Confirm hypercapnia by ABG.
- Treat the cause.

Oxygen Toxicity

Oxygen toxicity results from the harmful effects of breathing molecular oxygen at increased partial pressure. It is mostly associated with long-term oxygen therapy or hyperbaric oxygen therapy.

Risk Factors for Toxicity

- All the patients who are on high concentrations of supplemental oxygen for a long duration (100% oxygen for > 8–12 h).
- Infants and neonates getting 100% oxygen for > 2 to 3 hours.
- Mechanical ventilation with FiO_2 more than 50%.
- Premature babies.
- Exposure to chemicals that increase the risk for oxygen toxicity like chemotherapeutic agent bleomycin.
- Hyperbaric oxygen therapy.
- Underwater divers.

Mechanism of Toxicity

Partial reduction of oxygen by one or two electrons results in the formation of reactive oxygen species (ROS). Most commonly produced ROS are as follows:

- Superoxide anion.
- Hydroxyl radical.
- Hydrogen peroxide.
- Hypochlorous acid.

Oxygen radicals react with cell components and cause the following:

- Lipid peroxidation of membranes.
- Increased permeability and calcium influx, causing mitochondrial damage.
- Proteins are oxidized and degraded.
- DNA gets oxidized and ultimately breakdown.

Systemic Effects of Oxygen Toxicity

The systemic manifestations of oxygen toxicity are summarized below:

- *CNS effect*:
  - ▶ Initially, it manifests as visual changes (tunnel vision), followed by tinnitus, nausea, twitching (especially of the face).
  - ▶ Behavioral changes (irritability, anxiety, confusion, and dizziness).
  - ▶ Convulsions: Tonic-clonic type.
  - ▶ Unconsciousness.
- *Respiratory system effects*:
  - ▶ Dyspnea.
  - ▶ Absorption atelectasis.
  - ▶ ARDS.
  - ▶ Tracheobronchitis.
  - ▶ Bronchopulmonary dysplasia in neonates.
- *Ocular effects*:
  - ▶ Myopia.
  - ▶ Cataract.
  - ▶ Retinal detachments.
  - ▶ Retrolental fibroplasia/retinopathy of prematurity (ROP).

Prevention

- FiO_2 should be < 60% in patients on a mechanical ventilator.
- Monitoring of blood oxygen levels in premature infants receiving oxygen to balance hypoxia and ROP.
- Exogenous antioxidants, especially vitamins E and C, may be used prophylactically in high-risk infants.

- History of fever or seizure is a relative contraindication to hyperbaric oxygen treatment.

Cardiovascular Complication of Anesthesia

Hypotension

Perioperative hypotension is defined as mean arterial pressure values 25% below the patient's preoperative normal value. Many organ systems in our body autoregulate blood flow over a wide range of perfusion pressure, but hypotension beyond their autoregulation capacity may result in permanent ischemic damage.

Causes

Any change in systemic vascular resistance, stroke volume, and heart rate may produce hypotension (**Table 38.2**).

Prevention

Intraoperative hypotension is common in patients with existing hypertension taking angiotensin-converting enzyme (ACE) inhibitors or angiotensin II antagonists. Stopping ACE inhibitors or angiotensin II antagonists preoperatively for at least 10 hours is associated with a reduced risk of intraoperative hypotension.

Management

The first step in managing hypotension is identifying the cause. Preload should be optimized by giving a fluid bolus or by changing the position like Trendelenburg. High inhaled anesthetic concentration or rate of infusion anesthetic drug should be reduced. Inotropes like noradrenaline, adrenaline, ephedrine, and vasopressor like metaraminol and phenylephrine may be used for managing hypotension.

Hypertension

Intraoperative hypertension is defined as arterial pressure (systolic, mean, or diastolic) higher than 25% of preoperative values. Myocardial work is increased by increased afterload and left ventricular wall tension, increasing the risk of ischemia and infarction.

Table 38.2 Mechanism of hypotension

Fall in systemic vascular resistance	• Central neuraxial blockade • Drugs: Anesthetic agents, vasodilators • Sepsis • Hypersensitivity reaction
Decrease in heart rate	• Drugs: Beta-blockers, neostigmine • Vagal reflexes • Dysrhythmias

Decrease in stroke volume	• *Decreased preload*
	  ○ Hypovolemia: Hemorrhage, gastrointestinal fluid loss, poor resuscitation
	  ○ Positive pressure ventilation: High intrathoracic pressure
	  ○ Impaired cardiac filling: Pericardial effusion, aortocaval compression, pneumothorax, tamponade
	• *Increased afterload*
	  ○ Pulmonary embolism, aortic stenosis, left ventricular outflow tract obstruction
	• *Decreased contractility*
	  ○ Cardiac failure, myocardial ischemia, hypothermia, hypoxia, acidosis, ischemic heart disease, cardiomyopathy

Causes

- Presence of preexisting undiagnosed or poorly controlled hypertension.
- Sudden withdrawal of antihypertensive medication.
- Sympathetic nervous system activation due to hypercapnia, hypoxia, laryngoscopy, inadequate plane of anesthesia and analgesia.
- Drugs: Inotropes, vasopressors, ketamine.
- Intracranial hypertension (Cushing reflex).
- Other causes include MH, hyperthyroidism, carcinoid syndrome, pheochromocytoma.
- Postoperative period: Inadequate pain control, urinary retention, residual paralysis, anxiety, etc., act as causative factors for hypertension.
- Surgical procedure: More common in neuro, head and neck, vascular surgeries.

Treatment

Patients with preexisting hypertension should be treated first before elective surgery. Preoperative stoppage of antihypertensive medication should be avoided as this may result in rebound hypertension. Sedative premedication may be used to relieve anxiety and endogenous catecholamines. Antihypertensive agents like labetalol, esmolol, sodium nitroprusside, hydralazine, glyceryl trinitrate, and nifedipine may be used to control blood pressure.

Myocardial Ischemia

Perioperative cardiac ischemia and infarction are responsible for hospital mortality in up to 25% of the cases. In addition to this, a nonfatal perioperative myocardial ischemia (MI) is one of the risk factors for repeat MI or death within 6 months. In the majority of cases, these complications are preventable. Patients having a prior history of coronary artery disease are at a higher risk of developing this complication, but other factors like postoperative anemia, pain, and hypothermia can also contribute to this complication.

Causes

Nonoperative setting MI has different pathogenesis and clinical presentation than perioperative MI. Perioperative MI (PMI) can occur due to plaque rupture and subsequent thrombosis, and the imbalance between myocardial oxygen supply and demand. *Induction of anesthesia and extubation are the most vulnerable periods for developing PMI.* Emergence from anesthesia is associated with a rise in heart rate, sympathetic nervous activity (SNA), and blood pressure, increasing the risk of developing PMI.

Recognition

The typical clinical features of chest pain, ECG changes, and raised serum concentration of creatine kinase-MB (CK-MB) isoenzyme are generally absent in operation theater. As a result, the diagnosis of PMI needs high vigilance and an index of suspicion. *The presence of dysrhythmia, nonspecific ECG changes, and unexplained hypotension may be the only presenting feature during anesthesia.* Intraoperative continuous monitoring with five-lead ECG has a high sensitivity for detecting MI. Similarly, the echocardiographic finding of new regional wall motion abnormality gives early detection of ischemia. There are no standard diagnostic criteria for diagnosing PMI, and in the majority of cases, they are clinically silent. The change in the level of biochemical markers is difficult to interpret in the perioperative period. An appropriate cutoff level of cardiac troponins I and T for diagnosing clinically significant cardiac events are yet to be determined as noncardiac etiologies like kidney failure and PE may be associated with a rise in cardiac troponins.

Prevention and Management

Proper assessment and optimization of the cardiac condition are required for the prevention of PMI. Optimization may be achieved by drug therapy or cardiac revascularization procedure. The Lee revised cardiac index is used for stratifying patients who are at an increased risk of cardiac events. Evidence suggests that high-risk and intermediate-risk patients benefit from an additional investigation like stress echocardiography and myocardial viability studies and, if deemed necessary, by coronary revascularization procedure. *Currently, cardiac revascularization procedure before surgery is kept for patients with unstable or symptomatic heart disease.* Perioperative strategies like preventing hypothermic and sympathetic nervous system activation seem to be beneficial for preventing PMI. Definite treatment consists of identifying and treating reversible causes like hypoxia, hypothermia, and anemia. Other drugs like antiplatelet, thrombolytic, anticoagulants, aspirin, beta-blockers, statins, and ACE inhibitors have different efficacy and side effects in perioperative settings.

Dysrhythmias

Cardiac dysrhythmias occurring in 20 to 30% of noncardiac surgeries are among the major causes of morbidity and mortality in the perioperative setting.

Causes

During the perioperative period, most of the cardiac dysrhythmias occur in patients with preexisting cardiac disease who have undergone new insult. *Laparoscopic, cardiac, and thoracic surgeries are the most common surgeries prone to perioperative dysrhythmias* (**Table 38.3**).

Prevention and Management

All the reversible causes of dysthymias should be avoided in high-risk patients during the perioperative period. Perioperative beta-blockers and avoidance of overhydration are some of the other strategies. Unstable hemodynamics need synchronized cardioversion. Management of tachyarrhythmias consist of beta-blocker, amiodarone, calcium channel blocker, and digoxin, while for bradyarrhythmias or heart block, atropine, glycopyrrolate or temporary pacing may be needed.

Cardiac Arrest

The majority of cardiac arrests occur at the time of induction of anesthesia. The most common causes include difficulty in ventilation and intubation, side effects of anesthetic drugs used during the procedure, like severe hypotension caused by inhalational agents or bradycardia, asystole caused by Scoline, and sometimes anaphylaxis can cause cardiac arrest.

The management of cardiac arrest should follow advanced cardiac life support protocol.

Table 38.3 Causes of perioperative dysrhythmias

Drugs	Cardiac condition	Reversible causes	Rare causes
• Prolonged QT Antibiotics (fluroquinolone, macrolide) • Antipsychotic and antidepressant drugs class III antiarrhythmic agents (ondansetron, droperidol) • Sevoflurane • Local anesthetic toxicity • Digoxin toxicity • Inotropes	• Congenital heart disease • Long QT syndrome • Cardiomyopathy • Ischemic heart disease • Wolff–Parkinson–White syndrome	• Metabolic and electrolyte abnormalities • Hypoxia • Hypotension • Hypertension • Mechanical irritation: Central venous catheter insertion, chest drains • Hypothermia • Hypercarbia	• Subarachnoid hemorrhage • Pheochromocytoma • Malignant hyperthermia • Thyrotoxicosis • Carcinoid syndrome

Neurological Complications

Postoperative Cognitive Dysfunction

POCD is a condition in which a patient's memory and learning ability decline after undergoing surgery. POCD affects all age groups, but patients above 60 years of age are at a higher risk. Some common symptoms are as follows:

- Difficulty in recalling and remembering things.
- Difficulty or inability to finish the task that was done easily before surgery.
- Problem with intellectual performances.
- Problem with combining task or multitasking.
- Decreased psychomotor skills.
- Difficulty in comprehending language.
- Difficulty with merging with people in a social setting.

These symptoms vary among patients. Some patients may experience several aspects of this disorder, while others may only notice mild differences. The various patient and surgical factors that increase the risk of POCD are listed below.

Risk Factors

The various patient and surgical factors that increase the risk of POCD are listed below:

- *Surgical factors*:
  - *Type of surgery*: Orthopedic, vascular, and cardiac surgeries are associated with increased risk.
  - *Postoperative complications*: Respiratory and infective complications increase the risk.
  - Multiple surgeries in a short period.
- *Anesthesia related*:
  - General anesthesia poses higher risk than regional.
  - A longer duration of general anesthesia poses even more risk.
  - Intraoperative hypoxia, hypotension.
  - Poor analgesia.
- *Patient related*:
  - Age more than 60 years.
  - Preexisting cerebral, cardiac, or vascular disease.
  - Preexisting mental illness.
  - Sleep deprivation.
  - Low educational background.
  - History of alcohol abuse.

Diagnosis

It is diagnosed by a battery of tests called neurocognitive tests. These tests are conducted before surgery to get the baseline score and after the surgery to observe any changes.

Treatment

POCD can resolve by itself without any medication. In most patients, any cognitive impairment after surgery returns to baseline, that is, presurgery level within a few months of hospital discharge. However, in certain patients, it may last for several months. Currently, there is no approved medication for the treatment of POCD.

Convulsion

The causes of convulsion during the perioperative period are as follows:

- Hypoxia.
- Cerebrovascular disease.
- Drugs like methohexitone, etomidate, sevoflurane, and local anesthetic.

Treatment

- Care of airway, breathing, and circulation.
- Identifying and treating electrolyte disorders (mainly sodium).
- Anticonvulsant drugs.

Delayed Recovery

The causes of delayed recovery are as follows:

- Inadequate reversal of muscle paralysis.
- Drugs: An overdose of benzodiazepine, opioids, inhalational anesthetic agents, local anesthetic, etc.
- Acid-base imbalance.
- Electrolyte abnormalities.
- Altered hepatic and renal function, affecting the metabolism of drugs.
- Endocrine disorders like hypothyroidism.
- Metabolic: Hypoglycemia, hyperglycemia.
- Hypothermia.
- Central anticholinergic syndrome.
- Sepsis.
- Cerebrovascular event.
- Hypoxia.

Management

- Treatment of the cause and supportive therapy.

Cranial Nerve Palsies

- Combined unilateral palsy of cranial nerves X and XII is known as Tapia's syndrome. It is mainly caused by inflammation, carcinoma, injuries and, rarely, by airway manipulation during general anesthesia.
- Solitary hypoglossal nerve palsy (HNP) may occur as a rare complication of general anesthesia because of injury to the nerve during airway management.
- Abducens nerve palsy is one of the rare complications of spinal anesthesia.

Awareness

During anesthesia, awareness is defined as when a patient becomes conscious during a surgical procedure performed under general anesthesia and subsequently has a recall of these events. Its incidence ranges from 0.1 to 0.2%.

Risk Factors

- Women > men.
- Age < 60 years.
- Intravenous > inhalational.
- The long duration of surgery.
- Awareness history.

Causes

The causes of awareness are summarized below:

- *Light plane of anesthesia*:
  - Cardiac surgeries.
  - Cesarean section.
  - Surgery in trauma patients.
  - ASA physical status 4/5.
  - Premature discontinuation of anesthetic agents.
- *Increased anesthetic requirements*:
  - Chronic use of benzodiazepines or opioids.
  - Alcoholics.
  - Severely anxious patients.
  - Difficult intubation.
  - Previous awareness experience.
- *Improper equipment maintenance or anesthesiologist error*:
  - Failure to fill vaporizers.
  - Judgment errors related to drugs and volatile agents.
  - Disconnections and kinks in tubes from the ventilator.

Patient Perceptions of Awareness

The most common perceptions are as follows:

- Sounds and conversation—89 to 100%.
- The sensation of paralysis—85%.
- Anxiety and panic.
- Helplessness and powerlessness.
- Pain—39%.

Prevention

- *Preoperative evaluation*:
  - ▶ A detailed history and physical examination.
  - ▶ Identifying patients' risk factors for intraoperative awareness.
  - ▶ Informing high-risk patients regarding the possibility of intraoperative awareness.
- *Preinduction of general anesthesia*:
  - ▶ Prophylactic administration of benzodiazepines.
  - ▶ Checking the functioning of anesthesia delivery systems.
- *Intraoperative interventions*:
  - ▶ Cautionary use of the neuromuscular blocking agents.
  - ▶ Inhalational anesthetics must be monitored with end-tidal gas analyzers and the minimum alveolar concentration (MAC) of anesthetic agents should be maintained > 0.8.
  - ▶ Bispectral index (BIS) value should be 40 to 60.
- *Postoperative interventions*:
  - ▶ Postoperative interview to report awareness.
  - ▶ Providing postoperative counseling or psychological support.

Extrapyramidal Side Effect during Anesthesia

Metoclopramide, ondansetron, pregabalin, fentanyl, and droperidol have been associated with extrapyramidal side effect.

Agitation, Delirium, and Emergence Excitation

Pain and full bladder are the most common causes of agitation in the perioperative period. Emergence excitation is usually seen in children coming out of general anesthesia. It is usually a transient confusional state. Delirium in the perioperative period is usually due to the side effects of drugs like ketamine. *Treatment consists of benzodiazepines and the underlying cause.*

Peripheral Neuropathies

According to the recent ASA closed claim studies, *brachial plexus injury is the most common nerve injury in the postoperative period associated with general anesthesia*, followed by ulnar nerve injury. After spinal anesthesia, lumbosacral nerve roots are most commonly injured, followed by the spinal cord. The combined general and regional approach most commonly affects the spinal cord, followed by brachial plexus.

Gastrointestinal Complications

Postoperative Nausea and Vomiting

Patients rank PONV as one of the most unpleasant memories associated with their hospital stay. When severe, it can lead to increased length of hospital stay, increased bleeding, incisional hernias, and even life-threatening aspiration pneumonia. It is one of the most common problems in the ambulatory surgery patient population, occurring in an estimated 35% of all patients.

Risk Factors

The risk factors for PONV are listed below:

- *Patient-related risk factors*:
  - ▶ Gender: Female > male. Incidence of PONV increases during menstruation and decreases after menopause. After 70 years of age, both sexes are equally affected.
  - ▶ Age: PONV is rare in children less than 2 years of age. From more than 3 years to puberty, the risk is higher than adults.
  - ▶ Nonsmokers.

- ▶ Obese patients.
- ▶ Previous history of PONV/motion sickness.
- ▶ Early ambulation, early postoperative eating, and drinking.
- ▶ Anxiety.
- • *Surgery-related risk factors*:
  - ▶ Intra-abdominal.
  - ▶ Intracranial and middle ear surgery.
  - ▶ Squint surgery: The highest PONV risk surgery in children.
  - ▶ Gynecological surgeries.
  - ▶ Prolonged surgery.
  - ▶ Significant surgical pain.
- • *Anesthesia-related risk factors*:
  - ▶ Use of opioids.
  - ▶ Inhalational agents.
  - ▶ Nitrous oxide.
  - ▶ Prolonged anesthesia.
  - ▶ Spinal anesthesia (block above T5) and hypotension.
  - ▶ Intraoperative and preoperative dehydration.
  - ▶ Gastric distension.

The risk assessment for PONV can be done with Apfel's scoring system (**Table 38.4**).

Treatment

- • Serotonin antagonist: Ondansetron and granisetron remain important drugs for treatment and prophylaxis of PONV.

Table 38.4 Apfel's simplified score for adults

Risk factors	Points
Female gender	1
Nonsmoker	1
History of PONV	1
Postoperative opioids	1
Risk score	0 to 4

Abbreviation: PONV, postoperative nausea and vomiting.

- • Metoclopramide: First choice in situations associated with high risk of inspiration.
- • Dexamethasone: Evidence has suggested its efficacy similar to ondansetron.
- • Aprepitant: It is a neurokinin (NK-1) receptor antagonist associated with a 69% reduction in risk of PONV. However, its high cost limits its use.
- • Transdermal scopolamine effectively prevents PONV if applied the night before surgery (44%) or the coming morning (59%).
- • Droperidol is very effective in small doses (0.625–1.25 mg) to prevent and treat PONV. Unfortunately, its use has declined after its association with rare fatal arrhythmias. *The Food and Drug Administration (FDA) has given a black box warning. It is contraindicated in suspected QT prolongation patients.*

If a single agent's dose is ineffective, an additional dose of the same agent is unlikely to increase efficacy. In fact, it is likely to increase the risk of side effects. It is preferable to administer drugs that have not been used previously.

Renal Complications

Acute Kidney Injury

Perioperative acute kidney injury (AKI) is one of the major causes of morbidity and mortality. In perioperative AKI requiring renal replacement therapy (RRT), the mortality may reach up to 46%. They are associated with an increased risk of coagulopathy, sepsis, and prolonged mechanical ventilation.

Development of AKI, as defined by observed changes in serum creatinine (SCr) and/or urine output, is now known to be a significant cause of both morbidity and mortality, and when severe enough to require RRT, the observed mortality approaches 46%. Moreover, the development of AKI in the perioperative period is associated with increased risks of sepsis, coagulopathy, and prolonged mechanical ventilation.

Risk Factors

The risk factors for AKI during the perioperative period are highlighted in **Table 38.5**.

Reducing the Risk of Renal Complication

Some risk factors are fixed and offer little in terms of modifiable actions, particularly acutely. Nonmodifiable risk factors include age, the presence of chronic kidney disease (CKD), cardiovascular comorbidities, and obesity.

Management

The management of established AKI is supportive in nature, but different modalities can minimize perioperative renal complications. These are as follows:

- *During the preoperative period*:
  - ▸ Every effort should be made to minimize unnecessary fasting.

- ▸ Adequate hydration should be made maintained preoperatively.
- ▸ All drugs having nephrotoxic potential should be stopped preoperatively.
- ▸ ACE inhibitors and angiotensin receptor blockers are associated with intra-operative hypotension and reduction in glomerular perfusion pressure. Therefore, these drugs may be stopped before surgery and should be started postoperatively, depending upon the patient's status.
- ▸ Nonsteroidal anti-inflammatory drugs (NSAIDs) should be used with caution.

- *During the intraoperative period*:
  - ▸ All efforts should be made to avoid intraoperative hypotension as it is an independent risk factor for postoperative AKI.

Table 38.5 Risk factors for the development of perioperative AKI

Category	Risk factors	Comments
Demographics	• Age • Sex	• Age > 65 years and neonates • Male are at higher risk
Comorbidities	• Diabetes mellitus • Chronic kidney disease • Coronary artery disease • Hypertension • Heart failure • Chronic obstructive pulmonary disease • Obesity • Liver disease • Anemia	• May have preexisting diabetic nephropathy and CKD • The major risk for AKI • Increased risk of postoperative AKI • Metabolic syndrome increases the risk • Increased risk • Increased risk
Status of patient	• ASA score • ICU admission	• Higher score increases the risk • Increased risk
Pathology	• Acute illness • Sepsis • Multiorgan dysfunction • Trauma • Abdominal hypertension	• All factors associated with increased risk of AKI

Abbreviations: AKI, acute kidney injury; ASA, American Society of Anesthesiologists; CKD, chronic kidney disease; ICU, intensive care unit.

- ▸ Goal-directed fluid therapy may be used in patients at high risk of developing postoperative AKI.

- ▸ Vasopressors and inotropes should be used judiciously to avoid intraoperative hypotension.

- ▸ Common risk factors include the presence of vascular disease, CKD, hypertension, cardiac failure and diabetes, all of which are strongly associated with postoperative nonmodifiable risk factors.

- ▸ Every effort should be made to avoid the development of hypercapnia, hypoxia, and acidosis.

- ▸ There is limited evidence regarding the superiority of regional over general anesthesia with respect to renal protection.

- ▸ Halogenated volatile anesthetic agent methoxyflurane has been associated with nephrotoxicity through inorganic fluoride formation.

- • *During the postoperative period*:
  - ▸ Maintaining adequate hydration, renal perfusion, and avoiding nephrotoxic drugs.

  - ▸ Postoperative hemorrhage, sepsis, and cardiac dysfunction should be managed promptly.

  - ▸ Established AKI may require prompt RRT and aggressive management of metabolic acidosis, uremia, and hyperkalemia.

Hepatic Complications

Major surgeries may be associated with mild liver dysfunction, even in normal liver. It may be due to hepatic ischemia or due to the effect of anesthesia on the liver. Patients with liver disease, which is well controlled, usually tolerate the stress of surgery uneventfully. But few patients may experience certain complications. These are briefly explained further.

Postoperative Jaundice

Mixed hyperbilirubinemia of multifactorial origin is the most common cause of postoperative jaundice. It mainly results from increased production and decreased hepatic clearance of bilirubin. Major surgery or extensive trauma requiring multiple blood transfusions may result in postoperative jaundice. The presence of sepsis, hemolysis, and hematomas increases the bilirubin load along with hypoxemia, hepatic ischemia, and other poorly understood etiologies that can impair liver function, resulting in jaundice. Development of permanent hepatic damage is rare, and jaundice usually resolves slowly but completely.

Postoperative Hepatitis

Ischemic postoperative hepatitis is caused by poor liver perfusion in the perioperative period, which results from transient perioperative hypotension or hypoxia. Aminotransferase levels increase rapidly but come to normal within a few days.

Halothane-induced hepatitis usually develops within 2 weeks of exposure. It is marked by an acute increase in serum aminotransferase levels and the occurrence of jaundice within 2 weeks of surgery. It may be associated with fever and eosinophilia in up to 30% of the cases. The liver injury is usually self-limiting and resolves with 4 to 8 weeks.

Sometimes, postoperative hepatitis may result from transmission of hepatitis C during a blood transfusion.

Postoperative Cholestasis

Postoperative cholestasis may result from extrahepatic biliary obstruction occurring as a result of intra-abdominal complications or due to drugs given postoperatively. It may also result after a major surgery like abdominal or cardiovascular.

The exact pathogenesis is unknown, but the condition is self-limited and resolves slowly and spontaneously.

Positioning in Anesthesia and Their Complication

Patients require various forms of positioning during surgery to facilitate easy access to the surgical site. However, each position has its complications.

Lithotomy

- It is associated with a reduction in functional residual capacity and vital capacity by 20%, resulting in increased ventilation and perfusion mismatch.
- Nerve injuries associated with lithotomy position (most common being peroneal nerve).
- Compartment syndrome: One of the rare complications caused by inadequate tissue perfusion due to extreme tightening of the straps.
- Injury to fingers when lower section of bed is raised.
- Elevation of legs during positioning results in increased venous return, resulting in increased cardiac load.

Trendelenburg

- The Trendelenburg position is often used to increase venous return during hypotension, improve exposure during abdominal and laparoscopic surgery, and prevent air emboli and facilitate cannulation during central line placement.
- The Trendelenburg position has significant cardiovascular and respiratory consequences. Increased venous return is associated with the increased cardiac load. The cephalic movement of the abdominal viscera against the diaphragm decreases the functional residual capacity and pulmonary compliance.
- The stomach also lies above the glottis. Endotracheal intubation is often preferred to protect the airway from pulmonary aspiration, related to reflux, and to reduce atelectasis.
- Prolonged head-down position leads to swelling of the face, conjunctiva, larynx, and tongue, with an increased potential for postoperative upper airway obstruction.
- It is also associated with increased central venous, intracranial, and intraocular pressures.

Sitting Position

- Venous air emboli.
- Hypotension.
- Brainstem manipulations resulting in hemodynamic changes.
- Risk of airway obstruction.
- Pneumocephalus.
- Spinal cord ischemia and quadriplegia can occur due to extreme flexion of the neck.
- Brachial plexus injury.
- Femoral and obturator nerve injury due to angulation at the thigh.

Lateral/Prone Position

- Brachial plexus injury.
- Spinal cord ischemia.
- Radial and ulnar nerve injury.
- Breast injury.
- Genital organ injury.
- Compartment syndrome of the hand.
- Accidental extubation.
- Obstruction of the endotracheal tube with bloody secretions or sputum plugs.
- Facial and airway edema.
- Visual loss.

Ocular Complications

Exposure keratitis is a common complication of general anesthesia, which occurs if eyes remain open for a prolonged duration. It can be prevented by using artificial tears, eye ointment, and adequately covering the eyes with an eye pad.

Postoperative visual loss due to ischemic optic neuropathy and central retinal artery occlusion is one of the dreaded complications, which may result in blindness. It may result from prolonged hypotension, long surgery duration, large blood loss, large crystalloid use, anemia, hemodilution, increased intraocular pressure, and venous pressure from the prone position.

Temperature-Related Complications

Hypothermia and Shivering

Hypothermia is the most common temperature imbalance seen in anesthesia. The heat is lost to the atmosphere from the human body in four ways:

- Radiation.
- Conduction.
- Convection.
- Evaporation.

Low operation theater temperature leads to intraoperative hypothermia, mainly through radiant heat loss. Conductive heat loss occurs when the patient is placed on the cold operating room table, while laminar airflow contributes to heat loss through convection. In addition to the above mechanism, operative cleansing solutions aid in heat loss through evaporation.

Type of Anesthesia and Hypothermia

General Anesthesia

Autonomic temperature control is impaired by general anesthesia. Body heat redistribution occurs from the central compartment to the periphery via vasodilation after anesthesia induction, resulting in heat loss to the environment. The redistribution of heat is responsible for more than an 80% drop in core temperature. Along with redistribution, the patient's ventilation with cold and dry gas, cutaneous heat loss, and surgical skin preparation also contribute to intraoperative hypothermia.

Neuraxial Anesthesia

Autonomic temperature control is also impaired by neuraxial anesthesia. The redistributive heat loss during regional anesthesia is 50% of general anesthesia, but it still is the important cause of perioperative hypothermia. The blocked portion of the body under regional anesthesia is not able to shiver or vasoconstriction. As a result, a long case under neuraxial anesthesia may cause more heat loss than general anesthesia.

Implications of Perioperative Hypothermia

- *Blood loss*: Hypothermia-induced coagulation cascade and platelet dysfunction are the important causes of increased blood loss.

- *Surgical wound infection*: Intraoperative hypothermia has been linked with an increased risk of surgical site infection. Hypothermia-induced vasoconstriction results in reduced oxygen delivery to the surgical site, leading to collagen lattice and scar's poor strength. It also impairs chemotaxis, phagocytosis, and antibody production by white blood cells and the immune system.

- *Length of hospital stay and postanesthesia care unit (PACU) recovery time* is increased if patients suffer from perioperative hypothermia.

- *Drug metabolism*: Hypothermia impairs enzymes responsible for the metabolism of anesthetic drugs. The duration of action of morphine, midazolam, propofol, and many muscle relaxants like vecuronium, atracurium, and rocuronium is prolonged due to the pharmacokinetic effect of hypothermia.

- *Shivering*: Shivering is one of the protective mechanisms against hypothermia. Shivering is four times more dependent on core temperature than skin temperature. Oxygen consumption during shivering can increase up to 400%. As a result, oxygen should be given to the patient during shivering. Shivering can be controlled by pethidine as well as tramadol.

- *Cardiac events*: Patients suffering from perioperative hypothermia have an increased incidence of postoperative cardiac events, including angina, ischemia, infarction, and cardiac arrest.

Hypothermia Prevention and Treatment

- *Passive warming*: One of the simplest methods to reduce heat loss from the body is by raising ambient temperature. Heat loss can be prevented by insulating the patient with reflective or mass covering. Reflective covering prevents heat loss by reflecting the radiant heat back to the body. Surgical drapes and blankets are examples of mass covering, which prevents heat loss by halting airflow between the patient and coverings.

- *Active warming*: It consists of warming the body by forced-air warming systems, warming blanket, or mattress. Forced-air warming systems are safe, effective, easy to use, and relatively inexpensive. Warming blanket and mattress get heated when current is passed through the resistant polymer. They work on the principle of conduction and prevent heat loss by warming the surface, which will come in contact with the patient.

Hyperthermia

Causes of hyperthermia in anesthesia are as follows:

- Hypermetabolic states like pheochromocytoma, thyrotoxicosis, etc.
- Neuroleptic malignant syndrome.
- Drugs induced like pethidine, amphetamines, MAO inhibitors, tricyclic antidepressants, and atropine.
- Injury to the temperature-regulating center of the hypothalamus.
- MH.

Prevention and Treatment

- Identifying patients at risk.
- Decreasing ambient temperature.
- Use of cold IV fluids and cold sponging of the body surface.

Malignant Hyperthermia

MH is a life-threatening elevation in body temperature usually resulting from a hypermetabolic response to concurrent use of a depolarizing muscle relaxant and a potent, volatile inhalational general anesthetic.

Incidence and Epidemiology

- 1:1,00,000 administered anesthetics.
- Approximately half of the patients who develop acute MH have one or two uneventful exposures to triggering agents.
- It affects all ethnic groups.
- Cases are reported from all parts of the world.
- Males > females (2:1).
- Children < 19 years (45–52% of reported events).

Pathophysiology

- Genetic skeletal muscle receptor abnormality.

- Mutations encoding for abnormal ryanodine receptors (RYR1) or dihydropyridine (DHP) receptors.

- Triggering agents (volatile anesthetics) lead to the unregulated passage of calcium from the sarcoplasmic reticulum into the intracellular space, causing sustained muscle contraction.

- Hyperthermia occurs minutes to hours following the initial onset of symptoms.

- Clinical manifestations occur due to cellular hypermetabolism, leading to sustained muscular contraction and breakdown (rhabdomyolysis), anaerobic metabolism, acidosis, and sequelae.

Triggers

- Volatile anesthetic agent (e.g., halothane, isoflurane, sevoflurane, desflurane).

- MH has been reported following administration of succinylcholine in the absence of an inhalational agent (e.g., to facilitate endotracheal intubation).

- MH crisis may develop at first exposure to a triggering agent; however, the patient has had previous exposures before having a documented reaction.

Clinical Signs and Complications

The MH-related complications and the clinical signs are highlighted in **Table 38.6**.

Diagnosis

- Clinical evaluation.

- Testing for complications.

- Susceptibility testing for people at risk.

The appearance suspects the diagnosis of typical symptoms and signs within 10 minutes to, occasionally, several hours after inhalational anesthesia is begun. Early diagnosis can be facilitated by prompt recognition of jaw rigidity, tachypnea, tachycardia, and increased end-tidal CO_2.

Table 38.6 Clinical signs and complications of MH

Clinical signs	
Early	**Late**

• Hypercarbia
 • Sinus tachycardia
 • Masseter muscle rigidity
 • Generalized muscle rigidity
   ○ Most common initial sign of an MH crisis is an unexpected rise in end tidal CO_2 (ETCO > 60 mm Hg), which is difficult to decrease as minute ventilation is increased
   ○ MMR (in the presence of succinylcholine and volatile agents)
   ○ Generalized muscle rigidity in the presence of neuromuscular blockade is virtually pathognomonic for MH when other signs are present
	• Electrocardiogram changes due to hyperkalemia
	 • Ventricular ectopy/bigeminy
	 • Ventricular tachycardia/fibrillation
	 • Hyperthermia
	 • Myoglobinuria
	 • Excessive bleeding due to DIC

Complications	
• Hyperkalemia • Respiratory and metabolic acidosis • Rhabdomyolysis with CK elevation and myoglobinuria may occur • Coagulation abnormalities (particularly DIC). In older patients and patients with comorbidities, DIC may increase the risk of death	

Abbreviations: CK, creatine kinase; DIC, disseminated intravascular coagulation; MH, malignant hyperthermia; MMR, masseter muscle rigidity.

There are no immediately confirmatory tests, but patients should have testing for complications, including ECG, blood tests (complete blood count with platelets, electrolytes, blood urea nitrogen, creatinine, creatinine kinase, calcium, PT, PTT, fibrinogen, D-dimer), and urine testing for myoglobinuria.

Other diagnoses must be excluded and include the following:

- Perioperative sepsis (may cause hyperthermia but rarely as soon after induction).
- Inadequate anesthesia (can cause increased muscle tone and tachycardia but not elevated temperature).
- Thyroid storm and pheochromocytoma (rarely manifest immediately after anesthetic induction).

Susceptibility Testing

Recommended for people at risk based on:

- Family history of the disorder.
- Personal history of a severe or incompletely characterized previous adverse reaction to general anesthesia.

The caffeine halothane contracture test (CHCT) is the most accurate. It measures the response of a muscle tissue sample to caffeine and halothane. This test can be done only at certain referral centers and requires excision of about 2 g of muscle tissue. Genetic testing has limited sensitivity (about 30%) but is quite specific.

Treatment

MH has high mortality and may not respond to even early and aggressive therapy. The treatment includes the following:

- *Rapid cooling and supportive measures*: It is critical to cool patients as quickly and effectively as possible to prevent damage to the CNS and also to give patients supportive treatment to correct metabolic abnormalities. The outcome is best when treatment begins before muscular rigidity becomes generalized and before the development of rhabdomyolysis, severe hyperthermia, and disseminated intravascular coagulation (DIC).
- *Dantrolene* (a muscle relaxant) (2.5 mg/kg IV q 5 min as needed, up to a total dose of 10 mg/kg) should be given in addition to the usual physical cooling measures. In some patients, tracheal intubation, paralysis, and induced coma are required to control symptoms and provide support.
- Benzodiazepines given IV, often in high doses, can be used to control agitation.

Prevention

- Local or regional anesthesia is preferred to general anesthesia when possible.
- Potent inhalational anesthetics and depolarizing muscular relaxants should be avoided in patients who are susceptible.
- Nondepolarizing muscular blockers are the preferred anesthetic drugs. Preferred induction agents include barbiturates (e.g., thiopental), etomidate, and propofol.
- Dantrolene should be available at the bedside.

Conclusion

Complications during perioperative care are not uncommon. The complication may range from a mild drop in saturation to death. The risk of complications increases in patients with higher ASA grades, male gender, neonates, and emergency surgery. Meticulous preoperative assessment, optimization of comorbid illness, adequate preparation in operation theater, vigilant monitoring, and prompt action in case of complications are the cornerstones to prevent untoward adverse events.

CHAPTER 39

The Newer Concept in Anesthesiology: Artificial Intelligence

Ajit Kumar and Ravishankar Kumar

Introduction

Artificial intelligence has been defined as the study of algorithms which give machines the ability to reason and perform functions such as problem-solving, object and word recognition, inference of world states, and decision-making. In simple words, it is the human handshake with a machine.

Artificial intelligence in biosciences, including anesthesiology, critical care, and pain medicine, brings about a Brobdingnagian amount of excitement and expectation for the betterment of current treatment strategies.

Machine learning involving artificial intelligence helps develop algorithms that can assist devices in creating choices relating to the administration of anesthetic agents and thus determine numerous issues related to anesthetic management.

History of Artificial Intelligence

History of artificial intelligence dates back to 1950 when Mayo and Bickford used early machines for self-administration of volatile anesthetic agents via reading electroencephalograms (EEG) to monitor the depth of anesthesia. In this era, artificial intelligence created a phase of excitement among the various field of medicine. Then, came the phase of machine learning in the 1980s in which Servo anesthesia theory was additionally postulated, which is also the early integration of artificial intelligence into anesthesiology. Throughout the 1990s, target-controlled drug infusion (TCI) was brought into action, which used

artificial intelligence technology for its practical demand. Since 2010, it is the section of deep learning which is gaining importance in recent years. Recently, automatic drug delivery systems of anesthetic robots, the assistant operating system of anesthetic technology robots, and the automatic system of anesthesia evaluation and diagnosis robots have developed rapidly.

Working Principle of Artificial Intelligence

There are three approaches to machine learning, that is, supervised learning, unsupervised learning, and reinforcement learning.

- Supervised learning: It is the machine learning task of learning a function that maps an input to an output based on, for, example input-output pairs. In supervised learning, every example is a pair consisting of an associate degree input object (typically a vector) and the desired output value (also known as the supervisory signal). An example of a supervised learning study is to use electronic health records of patients to identify postinduction hypotension.

- Unsupervised learning: It is a sort of machine learning that looks for antecedently undetected patterns in a data set with no pre-existing labels and minimal human supervision. In contrast to supervised learning that typically uses human-labeled data, unsupervised learning, additionally far-famed as self-organization, allows for modeling of probability densities over inputs. An associate example of unsupervised learning is a study carried out by Bisgin et al who used this technique to obtain data from Food and Drug Administration (FDA) drug labels like specific adverse events to classify drugs consequently.

- Reinforcement learning: It refers to the method by which an algorithm is asked to aim at a particular task (e.g., deliver inhalational anesthesia to a patient) and to learn from its ensuant mistakes and successes. An associate degree example of reinforcement is to assess a patient's bispectral index (BIS) and mean arterial pressure (MAP) to manage the propofol infusion rates (in a simulated patient model).

Numerous techniques are utilized by the approaches mentioned above to machine learning. Typically used techniques are as follows:

- Fuzzy logic: 1965 was the year when Fuzzy theory was published. A device that uses "fuzzy logic" is programmed to resemble human judgment; in associate degree, accelerated means even in complicated situations. Classical or normal logic allows for correct mathematical value of say 1.0 and incorrect value as 0.0, while fuzzy logic mathematical value might dwell between 0.0 and 1.0, that is, the partial value. Thereafter, comparison could also be created between probable theory and the extent to that a sentence is correct. For example, the probable theory could be "a laparoscopic cholecystectomy procedure will be scheduled for tomorrow," while a true or real theory maybe "there is 90% chance of laparoscopic cholecystectomy procedure being scheduled tomorrow." Thus, this sort of technique is quite similar to that of human decision-making with discrete or inaccurate information.

- Classical machine learning: Here, characteristics are developed or chosen by the authority to help the algorithms explore the sophisticated data. The decision trees can be used to predict total patient-controlled analgesia (PCA) consumption from features such as patient demographics, vital signs, aspects of their medical history, surgery type, and PCA doses delivered with the promise of using such approaches to optimize PCA dosing regimens.

- Neural networks and deep learning: Neural networks are driven by human nervous systems, transmitting signals in clusters of biological or, say, computational units, that is, neurons. Here, one network constitutes associate degree input bundle of neurons which has characteristics of the information. It has one concealed layer of connection which carries out the numerical modification of the initial data. The third layer is the output which ultimately provides the result. As compared to classical machine learning, where characteristics are hand-designed, deep learning has an auto-learning character based on the data itself. In anesthesiology, examples of neural networks and deep learning are monitoring of depth of anesthesia and control of anesthesia delivery.

- Bayesian methods: This technique provides an account of the probability of an incident which is based on experience or data about factors that may influence that incident.

Applications of Artificial Intelligence

- Monitoring of depth of anesthesia: Utilizing BIS and EEG, artificial intelligence can help monitor the depth of anesthesia. In recent times, alternative characters like midlatency auditory-evoked potentials and heart rate variability have been used to determine the depth of anesthesia.

- Management of delivery of anesthetic agents: Artificial intelligence can help assist the control of the delivery of anesthetic agents like neuromuscular blocking agents, volatile anesthetic agents, or other related drugs. Based on various approaches of machine learning, a closed loop anesthesia delivery system can also be operated. A famous example of artificial intelligence integrated delivery of anesthetic agents is Sedasys system, that is, a computer-assisted personalized sedation device.

- Perioperative care or alternative risk prediction: Numerous techniques in machine learning, neural networks, and fuzzy logic have all been applied for the prediction of events like perioperative complications, duration of stay, awareness, etc. For instance, neural networks with the assistance of BIS can be used to predict the hypnotic impact of an induction agent bolus dosage like that of propofol.

- Ultrasound guidance: Ultrasound-based procedures can be assisted, and the most typically utilized technique of achieving ultrasound image classification is via neural network technique. The most common ultrasound-guided procedures are blocks for postoperative pain relief and placement of central venous cannulas.

- Pain management: In pain management, artificial intelligence can assist from opioids dose and analgesic response prediction to patient identification that will get benefitted from preoperative consultation. In recent times, it has helped in the manufacturing of various patient-controlled anesthesia devices. An example

of machine learning assistance was the development of a nociception level index using photoplethysmography and skin conductance waveforms. Another example is the development of various simulators and virtual reality-based devices for regional anesthesia and pain management.

- Operating room logistics: Artificial intelligence can even assist in operating room provisions such as planning operation theater time or pursuit movements and actions of anesthesiologists.

- Other uses: Other places where artificial intelligence techniques can be implied are intensive care units, imaging suits, virtual reality tools for training anesthesia residents, automated anesthesia carts, preoperative and postoperative suits, etc.

Famous examples of artificial intelligence in anesthesiology are as follows:

- McSleepy: World's first robot anesthesiologist.

- Sedasys: A computer-assisted personalized sedation system.

- Kepler intubating system: It consists of robotic arm, joystick, Pentax-AWS video-laryngoscope, and software control system.

Benefits of Artificial Intelligence

- Cost reduction.

- Time reduction.

- No interindividual difference.

Limitations of Artificial Intelligence

- Errors with a Brobdingnagian learning curve.

- Absent emotional intelligence.

- Moral and ethical implications.

- Downside determination restricted.

- Safety concerns.

Conclusion

Artificial intelligence can impact anesthesia's clinical application from perioperative support and critical care delivery to outpatient pain management. Thus, anesthesiologists ought to partner with other caregivers (e.g., surgeons, interventionists, intensivists, nurses) and patients to assist in the development of strategy for the best use of artificial intelligence.

CHAPTER 40

Cardiopulmonary Resuscitation

Ajay Singh and Michelle Sirin Lazzar

The goal of cardiopulmonary resuscitation (CPR) is to achieve the best possible outcome for individuals who are experiencing a life-threatening event.

History and Basics of CPR

The history of CPR traces back to the biblical ages. James Elan and Peter Safar reinforced and explained the importance of ventilation by mouth-to-mouth breathing. William B Kouwenhoven had introduced chest compressions, while defibrillation to break ventricular fibrillations was introduced by Claude Beck and Paul Zoll. The standards for CPR performance were generated at the National Research Council conference in 1966, when the modern era of CPR began.

Theories of CPR

The blood flow generated by chest compressions provided during CPR can be explained by two theories, which include:

- Thoracic pump theory.
- Cardiac pump theory.

Thoracic Pump Theory

The chest compressions cause a rise in the intrathoracic pressures more than that of extrathoracic regions, which cause the blood to flow. The direction of flow of blood toward the arterial tree is explained by the presence of venous valves, which prevent retrograde flow of blood at the thoracic inlet.

Cardiac Pump Theory

This theory states that blood flow is generated due to compression of the heart between the sternum and vertebral column.

Transesophageal echocardiography (TEE) during CPR in humans has helped in real-time visualization of changes in the heart and blood flow. During the chest's compression, blood is ejected from the ventricles into the aorta and pulmonary system while the tricuspid and mitral valves close. When the pressure on the chest is released, the pressure gradient allows the heart's venous flow. Any factors that affect the intrathoracic pressure like high-pressure mechanical ventilation, inadequate recoil of the chest also hinders adequate heart-filling and decreases chances of restoration of spontaneous circulation (ROSC). Providing adequate chest compressions is vital soon after a sudden cardiac arrest (SCA) because blood flow rather than oxygen content is the limiting factor for oxygen delivery to vital organs like the brain and heart. In most cases, this holds unless hypoxia is the cause of the arrest as in conditions like suffocation or drowning.

Basic Life Support (AS2.1)

Basic life support (BLS) includes some fundamental steps to be taken in case of any cardiac arrest, which are as follows:

- Recognition of SCA.
- Ensure scene safety.
- Activation of the emergency response team/call for help.
- Rapid initiation of high-quality CPR with chest compressions.
- Defibrillation using automated external defibrillator (AED).

The BLS interventions are all time-sensitive and designed to increase the probability of ROSC.

If the rescuer encounters an unresponsive individual, the steps to be followed include:

- Verify the safety of the scene for both the victim and the provider.
- Check the responsiveness of the victim by tapping the shoulder and shout, *"Are you OK?"*
- If the victim is unresponsive, call for help.
- Activate the emergency response team appropriate to your setting (if alone).

If another person is available, send the person to get the AED and emergency equipment and activate the emergency response team.

- If alone, get the AED and emergency equipment.

Assess for Breathing and Pulse

The victim's breathing and pulse should be assessed simultaneously to minimize delay, and this should not take more than 10 seconds.

To assess breathing:

- Look for chest rise and fall.
- If breathing, monitor victim until help arrives.
- If gasping or not breathing, it indicates cardiac arrest.

To assess pulse:

- In an adult, palpate the carotid.
- If no pulse can be felt within 10 seconds, initiate high-quality CPR with chest compressions.

To locate the carotid, locate the trachea using two or three fingers, and slide them to the groove between the trachea and muscles. If no pulse can be palpated within 10 seconds, chest compressions should be started. The assessment of breathing and pulse, followed by appropriate action, is tabulated below (**Table 40.1**).

Chest Compressions

- Rate: 100 to 120/min.
- Depth: At least 2 inches (5 cm).
- Push hard and push fast.
- Allow adequate chest recoil after each compression.
- Minimize interruptions in chest compression.

If two rescuers are available, then a compression is to ventilation ratio of 30:2 has to be maintained.

- The victim should preferably be placed on a firm surface in order to provide effective chest compressions. A soft surface does not allow adequate compression for blood pumping, and the compression provided will push the body into the soft surface.

Steps to Provide Good Quality Chest Compressions

- Position yourself by the victim's side.
- Make sure the victim is lying supine and on a firm surface. If the victim is in the prone position, positioning should be done

Table 40.1 Assessment of victim of cardiac arrest

Assessment	Next step
If breathing and pulse are normal	Monitor the victim until, emergency response team arrives
If normal pulse is present, but victim is not breathing normally	Provide rescue breathing and confirm that emergency response team has been activated
If victim has no pulse and is not breathing normally	Start high-quality CPR, with chest compressions

Abbreviation: CPR, cardiopulmonary resuscitation.

carefully, keeping the head, neck, and torso in a line.

- Positioning yourself: Heel of one hand rests in the center of the victim's chest on the lower half of the breastbone (sternum). Heel of the other hand rests on top of the first hand. Position yourself such that your shoulders are directly over your hands.

- Provide chest compressions at a rate of 100 to 120/min.

- Push at least 5 cm during each compression.

- Allow adequate chest recoil after each compression.

- Minimize interruptions.

Providing Breaths during CPR

The victim's airway has to be opened using two maneuvers:

- Head tilt-chin lift.
- Jaw thrust.

If a cervical spine injury is suspected, use ONLY jaw thrust maneuver to minimize neck spine movement.

Head Tilt–Chin Lift Maneuver

Place one hand on the victim's forehead and tilt the head backward, while the other hand is used to lift the victim's chin and bring it forward by placing fingers on the bony part of the lower jaw.

Jaw Thrust Maneuver

Place your hands on either side of the victim's head and your fingers under the lower jaw's angles. The jaw needs to be lifted with both hands and displaced anteriorly. The provider can rest the elbows on the surface on which the victim is lying.

The rate of infection from victim to health care provider is very low during CPR. However, all personal precautions should be taken because some cases of infectious transmission have been reported.

For providing mouth-to-mouth breaths, a pocket mask with a one-way valve can be used, which helps to divert the air exhaled by the victim away from the provider. Alternatively, bag and mask devices can be used.

Advanced Cardiovascular Life Support (AS2.2)

The BLS skills include performing effective chest compressions, use of the bag and mask for ventilation, and use of an AED and is usually provided by the emergency response team. However, health care workers (HCWs) and physicians require to provide more advanced assessment and management (**Flowchart 40.1**).

Primary Assessment

The unconscious patient's primary assessment is done after the BLS, while in conscious patients, the primary assessment is done right away. The primary assessment is done under the following heads:

- A—airway.
- B—breathing.

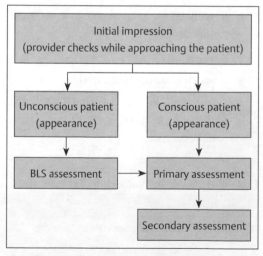

Flowchart 40.1 Systematic approach by the ACLS provider. Abbreviations: ACLS, advanced cardiovascular life support; BLS, basic life support.

- C—circulation.
- D—disability.
- E—exposure.

Airway

The assessment of airway and appropriate actions is summarized in **Table 40.2**.

Breathing

The assessment of breathing and appropriate actions is summarized in **Table 40.3**.

Circulation

The assessment of circulation and appropriate actions is summarized in **Table 40.4**.

Disability

- Check for neurologic function.
- Check for the pupillary response, level of consciousness, and responsiveness.
- Alert, voice, pain, unresponsive (AVPU).

Table 40.2 Airway assessment

Assessment	Actions to be taken
• Is the airway patent? • Is there an indication for an advanced airway to be placed? • Is the advanced airway placed properly? • Is the advanced airway securely placed and position reconfirmed?	• Airway patency is to be maintained in the unconscious by head tilt, chin lift, nasopharyngeal, or oropharyngeal airway placement • More advanced airways to be used if required • Confirm proper placement • Secure the advanced airway • Proper placement and position to be monitored continuously by waveform capnography

Table 40.3 Assessment of breathing

Assessment	Actions to be taken
• Is the ventilation and oxygenation being provided adequate? • Is the oxyhemoglobin saturation and quantitative capnograph being monitored continuously?	• Oxygen supplementation to be provided as required, to maintain a saturation of 94% or greater • For patients of cardiac arrest, 100% oxygen to be administered • Excessive ventilation to be avoided • Adequacy of oxygenation and ventilation should be monitored using quantitative capnography and pulse oximetry

Table 40.4 Assessment of circulation

Assessment	Actions to be taken
• Assess the adequacy of chest compressions • Assess the cardiac rhythm • Is there a requirement of defibrillation or cardioversion? • IV/IO access has been established and secured? • Is ROSC present? • Is there a need to administer medication for maintenance of pulse and blood pressure?	• CPR quality can be monitored by intra-arterial pressure and end-tidal CO_2 monitoring • Provide defibrillation/cardioversion as necessary • Obtain IV/IO access • Intravenous fluids to be administered if needed • Drugs are required to maintain rhythm and blood pressure to be administered as needed • Glucose and temperature to be monitored

Abbreviations: CPR, cardiopulmonary resuscitation; IO, intraosseous; IV, intravenous; ROSC, return of spontaneous circulation.

Exposure

All clothing is removed and looked for obvious injuries, burns, bleeding, or any other signs of trauma.

Secondary Assessment

This involves a focused history and search for the cause of cardiac arrest. A focused history is recommended by the American Heart Association (AHA) using the mnemonic SAMPLE.

S—signs and symptoms.

A—allergies.

M—medications (including the last dose taken).

P—past medical history.

L—last meal consumed.

E—events.

The most common causes of cardiac arrest should be kept in mind while managing cardiac arrest (**Table 40.5**).

When the patient shows ROSC, post cardiac arrest care should be initiated.

The cardiac arrest algorithm consists of two limbs: The management of a shockable rhythm, while the other is regarding the nonshockable rhythm, including asystole and pulseless electrical activity (PEA).

Following 2 minutes of uninterrupted CPR, a rhythm check should be done, which should not exceed 10 seconds. Other noteworthy points are as follows:

- In the case of no electrical activity, epinephrine bolus is given, and chest compressions should be resumed.

- If electrical activity is present, then the pulse should be palpated.
- If palpable, then post cardiac arrest care is initiated.
- If no pulse is palpable or there is a doubt regarding the pulse palpability, then the chest compressions should be resumed without exceeding an interruption of 10 seconds (**Flowchart 40.2**).

Post Cardiac Arrest Care

Post cardiac arrest care has known to reduce the early mortality caused by hemodynamic instability, and later morbidity and mortality caused by multiorgan dysfunction and brain injury. The further management required to ensure the success of post cardiac arrest care includes:

- Optimization of oxygenation and ventilation.
- Optimization of hemodynamics.
- Initiation of targeted temperature management.
- Immediate coronary reperfusion by percutaneous coronary intervention (PCI).
- Immediate neurologic care.

The treatment of the cause of the cardiac arrest should be initiated, and if unknown, then investigations required to identify the precipitating cause of arrest should be advised. A comprehensive, multidisciplinary system of care should be implemented for the care of post cardiac arrest patients.

Table 40.5 Common causes of cardiac arrest

Hs	Ts
Hypovolemia	Tension pneumothorax
Hypoxia	Tamponade
Hydrogen ions (acidosis)	Toxins
Hypo/hyperkalemia	Thrombosis (pulmonary)
Hypothermia	Thrombosis (coronary)

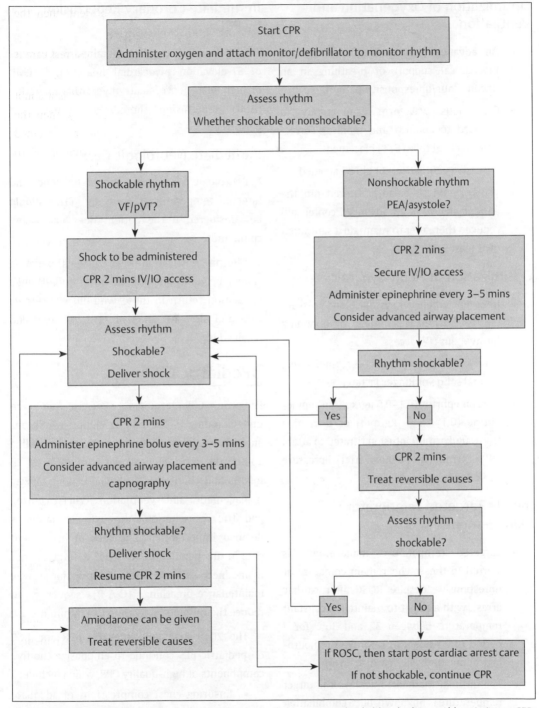

Flowchart 40.2 Algorithm for management of shockable or nonshockable rhythms. Abbreviations: CPR, cardiopulmonary resuscitation; IO, intraosseous; IV, intravascular; PEA, pulseless electrical activity; ROSC, return of spontaneous circulation; VF/PVT, ventricular fibrillation/pulseless ventricular tachycardia.

Optimization of Oxygenation and Ventilation

- An advanced airway can be placed for mechanical support of breathing in an unconscious/unresponsive patient.

- Continuous waveform capnography to be used to confirm and monitor correct endotracheal tube (ETT) placement.

- Excessive ventilation should be avoided.

- 100% oxygen can be administered until the patient arrives in an advanced center and reduced thereafter to maintain a saturation of at least 94%.

Optimization of Hemodynamics

- Intervene whenever systolic blood pressure (SBP) < 90 mm Hg, initially by obtaining intravenous (IV) access.

- Fluid bolus—1 to 2 L to be administered, normal saline or Ringer lactate.

- Norepinephrine (0.1–0.5 µg/kg/min)/epinephrine (0.1–0.5 µg/kg/min) or dopamine (5–10 µg/kg/min) infusion titrated to attain SBP > 90 mm Hg or a mean arterial pressure of > 65 mm Hg.

Initiate Targeted Temperature Management

- Targeted temperature management is started in those who remain comatose or unresponsive despite ROSC after cardiac arrest, with a target to maintain a constant temperature between 32 and 36°C for a period of 24 hours to improve the neurological outcome after cardiac arrest.

- The optimal method to achieve the target temperature is unknown, but a combination of various techniques like the rapid infusion of ice-cold, isotonic, nonglucose containing liquid (30 mL/kg), surface cooling devices, or simple surface techniques like ice bags are used commonly.

Immediate Coronary Reperfusion by PCI

Twelve-lead ECG should be obtained, and in cases of ST-elevation myocardial infarction (STEMI) or high suspicion of acute myocardial infarction (AMI), reperfusion should be planned and performed.

Immediate Neurologic Care

A neurologic assessment should be done, and targeted temperature monitoring (TTM) should be considered if the patient does not follow commands.

The prognostication of neurological outcome should be done after 72 hours of spontaneous circulation return in those who did not receive TTM and after 72 hours of TTM in those who received it.

Pediatric CPR

Pediatric CPR requires expertise and an understanding of the unique clinical conditions and their therapeutic considerations. Unlike adults, the most common of cardiac arrest in infants and children is asphyxia, making airway management and ventilation crucial during pediatric resuscitation. Although ventilation is deemed important, due to lack of insufficient data in this population, the 2015 AHA guidelines maintained the chest compression-airway maintenance-breathing (C-A-B) sequence to reduce the no-blood flow time to a minimum.

The 2015 AHA guidelines for CPR and ECC on pediatric BLS continue to emphasize the five components of high-quality CPR, which include:

- Ensuring chest compressions of adequate rate.

- Ensuring chest compressions of adequate depth.

- Allowing full chest recoil between compressions.

- Minimizing interruptions in chest compressions.
- Avoiding excessive ventilation.

Recommendations

Rate: 100 to 120/min.

Location: In infants, two fingers are used, placed below the inframammary line on the sternum.

In children, the lower half of the sternum (avoiding the xiphoid process) with one or two hands.

Depth of compression: One-third of the antero-posterior diameter of the chest (approximately 1.5 inches [4 cm] in infants to 2 inches [5 cm] in children).

The guidelines also recommend the usage of feedback devices to ensure adequate rate and depth.

A manual defibrillator is preferable in infants when a health care provider identifies a shockable rhythm. An AED with pediatric attenuator and pediatric pads can be used in children up to 8 years, with pads placed in an anteroposterior position.

In pediatric cardiac arrest, initial defibrillation energy of 2 J/kg is used and may be increased to 4 J/kg in the second shock. Increased energy levels may be subsequently considered but should not exceed 10 J/kg. If a pediatric defibrillator is not available, then an adult AED can be used without hesitation.

For pediatric patients, management of different life-threatening arrhythmias, PEA arrest/asystole, or ventricular fibrillation (VF)/ventricular tachy-cardia (VT) arrest is similar to adults, except for the dosage (defibrillation/medication) for children is weight-based. Actual body weight is recommended to calculate initial resuscitation drug doses. Vascular access can be challenging in critically ill children; therefore, intraosseous (IO) access is recommended in difficult IV access cases.

To Ensure Administration of Quality CPR

- Push hard (up to one-third of AP diameter of the chest).
- Push fast (100–120/min).
- Allow complete chest recoil.
- Minimize interruptions between chest compressions.
- Avoid excessive ventilation.
- Rotate compressor every 2 minutes or sooner in case of fatigue.
- If no advanced airway, a 15:2 ratio of compression: ventilation is to be followed.
- If an advanced airway is placed, the position to be confirmed by waveform capnography and continuous monitoring can be done. One breath to be administered every 6 seconds (10 breaths/min) along with chest compressions.

Drug Dosage (IO/IV)

- *Adrenaline/epinephrine*: 0.01 mg/kg (1 in 10,000) concentration to be repeated every 3 to 5 minutes.

  If IO/IV access is not available, then 0.1 mg/kg dose can be administered via endotracheal route.

- *Amiodarone*: 5 mg/kg bolus, can be repeated twice for refractory VF or pulseless VT.

- *Lignocaine*: 1 mg/kg loading dose, followed by 20 to 50 µg/kg/min infusion (bolus to be repeated if infusion started after 15 mins of initial bolus).

Reversible Causes of Cardiac Arrest in Children

- Hypovolemia.
- Hypoxia.
- Hydrogen ion (acidosis).
- Hypoglycemia.

- Hypo/hyperkalemia.
- Hypothermia.
- Tension pneumothorax.
- Tamponade (cardiac).
- Toxins.
- Thrombosis (pulmonary).
- Thrombosis (cardiac).

Some relevant differences between adult and pediatric CPR are highlighted in **Table 40.6**.

CPR in Pregnancy

Cardiac arrest in pregnancy is rare (1:30,000). The most common causes include:

- Bleeding.
- Eclampsia.
- Amniotic fluid embolism.
- Drug toxicities.
- Anaphylaxis.
- Peripartum cardiomyopathy.

Table 40.6 Comparison of adult and pediatric CPR

Component	Adults and adolescents	Children (age 1 year to puberty)	Infants (age less than 1 year and excluding newborn)
Scene safety	Make sure the environment is safe for rescuers and victim		
Recognition of cardiac arrest	• Check responsive/unresponsive • Breathing or apnea • Pulse: Palpable/unpalpable		

Activation of emergency response system	• If alone, leave victim and activate emergency response team
	• Else, send the other person to activate response team and start CPR immediately
		• *Witnessed collapse*: Same steps as adults
		• *Unwitnessed collapse*:
		  ○ Give 2 min CPR
		  ○ Leave the victim to activate emergency response system, return and restart CPR	

Compression ventilation ratio (without advanced airway)	• 1 or 2 rescuers • 30:2	• 1 rescuer • 30:2 • 2 or more rescuers • 15:2	
Compression ventilation ratio (with advanced airway)	• Continuous chest compressions at 100–120/min • One breath to be given every 6 s		
Compression rate	100–120/min		
Compression depth	At least 2 inches (5 cm)	At least one-third of AP diameter of chest, about 2 inches (5 cm)	At least one-third of AP diameter, 1.5 inches (4 cm)
Hand placement	2 hands on the lower half of the sternum	2 or 1 hand on lower half of the sternum	*Single rescuer*: 2 fingers in the centre of the chest, just below the nipple line 2 rescuers: 2 thumbs encircling the chest, just below the nipple line
Chest recoil	Full recoil of the chest to be allowed after each compression		
Minimizing interruptions	Interruptions should be limited to less than 10 s		

Several modifications are implemented during the CPR of a pregnant individual:

- The wedge is placed to give left lateral tilt.
- Hands are placed higher on the sternum for chest compressions.
- Intubation is preferred early.
- The preparation for the perimortem cesarean section should be initiated and performed with 4 minutes of arrest. It is beneficial for both the baby (helps save the baby) and the mother (relieves aortocaval compression).

Complications of CPR

Chest compressions can result in a fracture of the ribs and sternum.

Artificial respiration using a bag and mask ventilation can cause gastric insufflation, leading to vomiting, aspiration, and airway compromise.

Drugs in CPR

Fluid Administration

Fluid administration should be titrated along with vasoactive agents to optimize heart rate, blood pressure, cardiac output, and systemic perfusion to maintain a mean arterial pressure of at least 65 mm Hg. In hypovolemia cases, normal saline or Ringer lactate is used to restore the volume status, and D_5 saline is avoided.

Epinephrine

Indications

- Cardiac arrest: VF, pulseless VT, asystole, PEA.
- Symptomatic bradycardia: Can be considered as an alternative to dopamine infusion.
- Severe hypotension: Can be used when pacing and atropine fail, when hypotension

accompanies bradycardia, or with phosphodiesterase inhibitor.

- Anaphylaxis, severe allergic reactions.

Dose

- 1 mg (10 mL of 1:10,000 dilution) administered every 3 to 5 minutes, followed by 20 mL saline flush and limb elevation for 10 to 20 seconds after administration.
- Higher doses: Up to 0.2 mg/kg are used in special conditions like beta-blocker or calcium channel blocker overdose.
- Continuous infusion: 0.1 to 0.5 µg/kg/min, titrated to response.
- Endotracheal route: 2 to 2.5 mg diluted in 10-mL saline.
- Profound bradycardia or hypotension: 2 to 10 µg/min infusion, titrated to response.

Antiarrhythmic Agents Used

Amiodarone: VF or pulseless VT unresponsive to shock.

Dose: 300 mg IV/IO push for the first dose, and if VF and pulseless VT persists, then the second dose 150 mg IV or IO can be administered 3 to 5 minutes after the first dose.

Lignocaine: Alternative antiarrhythmic with no proven efficacy in cardiac arrest; however, it is used when amiodarone is not available.

Dose: 1 to 1.5 mg/kg IV or IO and repeated every 5 to 10 minutes up to a maximum dose of 3 mg/kg (endotracheal administration— 2–4 mg/kg).

Magnesium sulphate: To prevent or terminate torsades de pointes in patients who have a prolonged QT interval.

Dose: 1 to 2 g IV or IO diluted in normal saline or D5 over 5 to 20 minutes.

To treat pulseless VT, immediate high-energy shock is preferred, while magnesium is used as an adjunctive to prevent recurrent or persistent VT associated with torsades de pointes.

Other Drugs Used in ACLS and in Post Cardiac Arrest Cases

- *Adenosine*: First drug for most forms of narrow complex supraventricular tachycardia (SVT).

  Dose: 6 mg rapid IV bolus followed by 20 mL of saline flush and extremity elevation if given via cannula in the limb. The second dose of 12 mg can be given in 1 to 2 minutes.

  To be given under proper monitoring, with full facility for resuscitation made available.

- *Atropine sulphate*: First drug for symptomatic bradycardia and also used in organophosphate poisoning.

  Dose: 0.5 mg IV every 3 to 5 minutes up to a maximum of 0.04 mg/kg (total 3 mg). In organophosphate poisoning, larger doses may be required.

- *Dopamine*: (IV infusion) second-line drug for symptomatic bradycardia after atropine. Also administered in hypotension with signs and symptoms of shock (SBP ≤ 70–100 mm Hg).

  Dose: 2 to 20 µg/kg/min infusion, titrated to response.

Hypovolemia should be corrected with IV fluids before dopamine is started.

CPR in COVID-19 Pandemic

The AHA has made certain recommendations in order to balance the immediate needs of the patient without compromising their safety. HCWs are at the highest risk of contracting this disease, further compounded by the worldwide shortage of personal protective equipment (PPE). BLS and advanced cardiac life support (ACLS) involve many aerosol-generating procedures, including chest compressions, intubation, positive pressure ventilation, suctioning, etc. The aerosols generated can remain suspended and be inhaled by those nearby, which is of particular importance because resuscitation usually involves multiple HCWs who work nearby. The recommendations made by the AHA are about three main specific steps:

- Reduction of exposure of the HCW.
- Prioritization of ventilation and oxygenation strategies which carry a lower risk of aerosolization.
- Considering the appropriateness of the resuscitation.

Reduction of Exposure of the HCW

Important points to consider here are as follows:

- Don PPE before entering the room/scene.
- Limit the number of personnel in the area.
- The COVID-19 status should be communicated to any new providers to minimize errors.
- Mechanical compression devices should be considered if available and if the individual meets the device's height and weight criteria.

Prioritization of Ventilation and Oxygenation Strategies which Carry a Lower Risk of Aerosolization

This includes the following:

- The high-efficiency particulate air (HEPA) filter should be used for all ventilation if available.
- Intubation with a cuffed tube should be done early and put on a mechanical ventilator.
- The first attempt to intubate should be the best attempt with all conditions made favorable.
- Chest compressions to be paused while intubating.
- Video laryngoscope should be used when available.

- Prior to intubation, a bag and mask device with a tight seal and HEPA filter may be used (T-piece in neonates).
- Supraglottic airway device may be considered if intubation is delayed.
- Circuit disconnections should be reduced to a minimum.
- Passive oxygenation using a nonrebreathing mask may be considered for adults for a short duration instead of a bag and mask device.

Considering the Appropriateness of the Resuscitation

This includes due consideration of the following:

- The goals of care for the patient should be addressed.
- Policies that guide the determination should be adopted while taking into account the risk factors for survival.

In case of arrest in an intubated patient:

- The patient should be left on a mechanical ventilator with a HEPA filter, and a closed-circuit should be maintained.
- Ventilator to be adjusted to allow asynchronous ventilation.

- FiO_2 should be increased to 1.0.
- The tidal volume of 4 to 6 mL/kg targeted.
- Trigger to be turned "off" to prevent the auto-trigger from chest compressions.
- Respiratory rate to be adjusted to 10 beats per minute (BPM) for adults and 30 BPM for neonates.

Flowchart 40.3 highlights the management algorithm in case of arrest of a patient in the prone position.

The 2020 Update

The updates of the 2020 guidelines of CPR by the AHA are tabulated in **Table 40.7**.

Adult Resuscitation

Flowcharts 40.4 and **40.5** detail the chain of survival for adult in-hospital cardiac arrest (IHCA) and out of hospital cardiac arrest (OHCA), respectively.

Pediatric Resuscitation

The CPR updates of 2020 in the pediatric population are highlighted in **Table 40.8**. **Flowcharts 40.6** and **40.7** detail the chain of survival for pediatric IHCA and OHCA, respectively.

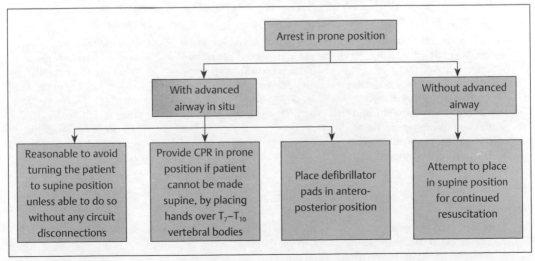

Flowchart 40.3 Management algorithm in case of arrest of a patient in the prone position.

Table 40.7 Updates of 2020 CPR by AHA

(a) Early initiation of CPR by lay rescuers		
Older version (2010)	**Update (2020)**	**Evidence**
• Previously, it was recommended that a lay rescuer not check for a pulse and assume an arrest if the person collapses or is unresponsive, while health care providers should not spend more than 10 s to palpate a pulse • Chest compressions to be started if no definite pulse felt	• Laypersons should initiate chest compressions for any presumed cardiac arrest, as the risk of harm to the patient is low	• The risk of harm to any individual receiving chest compressions even if not in cardiac arrest is low, when compared to those where lay rescues found it difficult to determine the pulse leading to a delay in initiating CPR

Early administration of epinephrine

Unchanged/reaffirmed	**Unchanged/reaffirmed**	**Update (2020)**
• Nonshockable rhythm: Administer epinephrine as soon as possible	• Shockable rhythm: Epinephrine can be administered after a failure of initial defibrillation attempts	• For nonshockable rhythms, an association was found between the early administration of epinephrine and ROSC, although improved survival rate was not confirmed • CPR and defibrillation attempts are to be made earlier and epinephrine administered following failed attempts of CPR and defibrillation for shockable rhythms

Real-time audio-visual feedback

Unchanged/reaffirmed (2020)	**Evidence**
• Audio-visual feedback devices may be used during CPR to optimize the resuscitation	• RCT done had reported a 25% increase in survival rates of IHCA with devices providing feedback on the quality of chest compressions

(b) Physiological monitoring of CPR		
Older version (2015)	**Update (2020)**	**Evidence**
• It was not recommended but reasonable to use physiologic parameters like quantitative waveform capnography, arterial relaxation diastolic pressure, arterial pressure monitoring, and central venous oxygen saturation to guide when feasible to monitor guide CPR quality, vasopressor therapy, and ROSC	• It is considered reasonable to use parameters like invasive blood pressure monitoring or end-tidal carbon dioxide when feasible in order to monitor and optimize the quality of CPR	• The usage of these monitoring strategies is supported by data that shows a higher possibility of ROSC when an $EtCO_2$ of at least 10 or ideally 20 mm Hg or greater was targeted. Ideal targets have not been identified yet

DSD: Not supported

New (2020)	**Evidence**
• There is no recommendation on the usefulness of double sequential defibrillation for refractory VF/VT	• Based on the evidence by current studies and case reports, the benefit of DSD or DCD is not known

(Continued)

Table 40.7 (*Continued*)

IV access preferred over IO

Older version (2010)	New (2020)/ update (2020)	Evidence
• CPR providers may consider establishing IO access if IV access is not readily available	• New: Providers may first attempt to establish IO access for drug administration in arrest situations • Update: IO access may be considered if there is no success in establishing IV access	• Administration of drugs via the IV route was associated with better outcomes. Thus, IV access is preferred, while IO may be considered if IV access could not be secured

(c) Cardiac arrest in pregnancy

New (2020)	Reason
• Prioritization of oxygenation and airway management is recommended during resuscitation of a pregnant individual because this group is more prone to hypoxia • Fetal monitoring is not recommended during the resuscitation of the pregnant individual as it may interfere with the process • Targeted temperature management is recommended in those who are comatose in the postarrest recovery phase • Fetal monitoring is recommended during the targeted temperature management of the mother due to potential complications like bradycardia	• Airway, ventilation, and oxygenation are important in pregnancy because of multiple risk factors that can cause hypoxia, including increased metabolism, decreased FRC, and the potential risk of fetal brain damage during the event • Evaluating the fetal heart during maternal CPR may cause distraction from the actual process

Abbreviations: AHA, American Heart Association; CPR, cardiopulmonary resuscitation; DCD, donation after circulatory death; DSD, double-sequence defibrillation; EtCO$_2$, end-tidal CO$_2$; FRC, functional residual capacity; IHCA, in-hospital cardiac arrest; IO, intraosseous; IV, intravenous; RCT, randomized controlled trial; ROSC, return of spontaneous circulation; VF, ventricular fibrillation; VT, ventricular tachycardia.

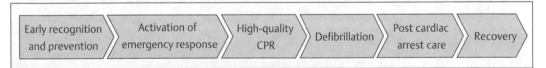

Flowchart 40.4 Algorithm depicting chain of survival for adult IHCA. Abbreviation: IHCA, in-hospital cardiac arrest.

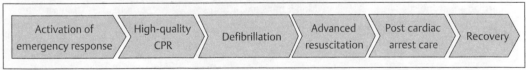

Flowchart 40.5 Algorithm depicting chain of survival for adult OHCA. Abbreviation: OHCA, out of hospital cardiac arrest.

Note: Prior guidelines had no recommendations regarding the choice of vasopressor or corticosteroids in septic shock, but later studies have proved that epinephrine is superior to dopamine as the initial vasoactive medication and that norepinephrine may also be used. Also, the benefit was found by corticosteroid administration in some pediatric cases with refractory septic shock.

Table 40.8 2020 CPR updates in pediatric population

Changes in assisted ventilation rate: Rescue breathing		
Older (2010)	**Update (2020)**	**Evidence**
• Palpable pulse 60/min or greater with inadequate breathing: Rescue breaths at 12–20/min	• Palpable pulse 60/min or greater with inadequate breathing: Rescue breaths at 20–30/min	–

Changes to assisted ventilation rate during CPR with advanced airway		
Older (2010)	**Update (2020)**	**Evidence**
• One breath every 10 s, i.e., 10/min	• One breath every 2–3 s, i.e., 20–30/min	• Higher ventilation rates are associated with higher rates of ROSC and survival

Cuffed ETTs		
Older (2010)	**Update (2020)**	**Evidence**
• Both cuffed and uncuffed tubes were accepted; however, a cuffed tube may be preferred with proper precautions in certain conditions	• The cuffed tube is recommended over the uncuffed tube, with proper consideration to size, position, and cuff pressures	• Studies support the safety associated with cuffed tubes and a decreased need to reintubate

Cricoid pressure during intubation		
Older (2010)	**Update (2020)**	**Evidence**
• Routine application for the prevention of aspiration during endotracheal intubation in children was supported by insufficient evidence	• Cricoid pressure is not recommended as a routine practice	• Cricoid pressure decreases the rate of intubation success and also does not reduce the risk of aspiration

Early administration of epinephrine		
Older (2015)	**Update (2020)**	**Evidence**
• Epinephrine could be administered in pediatric cardiac arrest (no specific recommendation on time)	• Epinephrine preferably to be administered early, within 5 mins of starting chest compressions	• Children who were administered epinephrine early (within 5 mins) were more likely to survive to discharge than those who were administered later. For every minute delay, a significant decrease in ROSC, survival at 24 h, survival to discharge, and survival with favorable neurological outcome was found

(Continued)

Table 40.8 (*Continued*)

Invasive blood pressure monitoring to assess CPR quality

Older (2015)	Update (2020)	Evidence
• For those who have an invasive monitoring line in situ, it is preferable to use blood pressure as a guide to CPR quality	• For those who have an invasive monitoring line in situ, it is preferable to use the diastolic blood pressure to assess CPR quality	• Higher survival rates with favorable neurological outcomes were found when diastolic pressure was at least 25 mm Hg in infants and 30 mm Hg in children during CPR

Detecting and treating seizures after ROSC

Older (2015)	Update (2020)	Evidence
• EEG (electroencephalography) should be done for the diagnosis of seizures • EEG monitoring should be done frequently or continuously in comatose after ROSC • Anticonvulsant medications used in status epilepticus may be considered in case of seizures after ROSC	• When available, continuous EEG monitoring is recommended in post cardiac arrest with persistent encephalopathy • Clinical seizures post cardiac arrest should be treated • Nonconvulsive status postarrest may be treated with expert consultation	• A nonconvulsive epileptic activity cannot be detected without EEG monitoring, thus recommended to be done continuously in all postarrest with persistent encephalopathy • Both clinical and nonconvulsive status epilepticus is associated with poor outcome. Thus, it may be beneficial to administer treatment of status epilepticus in both cases

Evaluation and support for cardiac arrest survivors

Update (2020)	Evidence
• Pediatric cardiac arrest survivors should be evaluated for rehabilitation services • Pediatric cardiac arrest survivors can be referred for ongoing neurologic evaluation for at least a year after the arrest	• Recovery from cardiac arrest continues long after the initial hospitalization. Survivors require support for months to years after their arrest. Supporting these patients is important for the best possible long-term outcome

Septic shock: Fluid boluses

Older (2015)	Updated (2020)
• Initial administration of a 20 mL/kg bolus was considered reasonable in conditions like severe sepsis, severe malaria, and dengue	• In septic shock, a total fluid bolus of 10–20 mL/kg may be administered in aliquots, with the frequent assessment

Septic shock: Choice of vasopressor

Update (2020)	Update (2020)
• In infants and children with fluid refractory septic shock, either epinephrine or norepinephrine infusion could be used as the initial vasoactive medication	• In infants and children with fluid refractory septic shock, dopamine may be considered if epinephrine and norepinephrine are not available

(*Continued*)

Table 40.8 (*Continued*)

Septic shock: Corticosteroid medication	
• Stress dose of corticosteroid may be considered in infants and pediatric age group in septic shock unresponsive to fluid bolus and requiring vasoactive support	• In those administered high fluid volumes rapidly, increased morbidity was observed secondary to fluid overload and may require mechanical ventilation. Thus, it was recommended to administer fluid in aliquots with frequent assessments

Hemorrhagic shock	
Update (2020)	**Evidence**
• In infants and children with hemorrhagic shock following trauma, blood products should be preferably administered instead of crystalloids when available for resuscitation	• Prior versions did not differentiate hemorrhagic shock from other hypovolemic shocks. Data support a balance resuscitation using packed red blood cells, fresh frozen plasma, and platelets

Abbreviations: CPR, cardiopulmonary resuscitation; ETT, endotracheal tube; ROSC, return of spontaneous circulation.

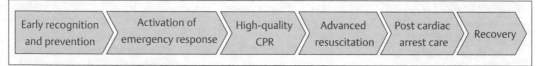

Flowchart 40.6 Algorithm depicting the chain of survival for pediatric IHCA. Abbreviation: IHCA, in-hospital cardiac arrest.

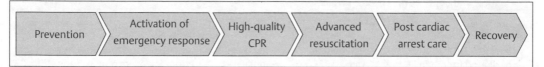

Flowchart 40.7 Algorithm depicting the chain of survival for pediatric OHCA. Abbreviation: OHCA, out of hospital cardiac arrest.

Neonatal Life Support

Following listed are some of the key points that need to be considered while providing neonatal life support:

- Most newborns do not require cord clamping or resuscitation attempts immediately. These can be evaluated during skin contact with their mothers.

- Skin-to-skin contact helps promote bonding with mother, breastfeeding, and normothermia. It is also to emphasize the importance of preventing hypothermia in neonatal resuscitation.

- Ventilation is of priority (in comparison to chest compression) in newborns.

- Heart rate is the single most important indicator of effective resuscitations in this age group.

- Pulse oximetry may be used as a guide during resuscitation.

- Endotracheal suctioning in all newborns with meconium-stained amniotic fluid should not be a routine practice. Suctioning is recommended only when there is airway obstruction during positive pressure ventilation.

- Chest compressions are started only if the heart rate does not rise in response to adequate ventilation measures (which includes endotracheal intubation).

- Heart rate response to resuscitation should be monitored using ECG.

- Vascular access: The order should be: umbilical vein preferred > IV access > IO access (may be considered when IV not feasible).

- Epinephrine may be administered if there is poor response to chest compressions.

- If the infant shows no response to epinephrine and has a history or examination finding suggestive of blood loss, volume expansion should be considered.

- Despite all these resuscitative efforts, if there is no heart rate response in 20 minutes, discuss redirection of care with team and family.

Recommendations for Some Special Conditions

Opioid overdose: **Flowchart 40.8** depicts the management algorithm for lay responders in case of opioid overdose.

Flowchart 40.9 depicts the management algorithm for emergency health care providers in case of opioid overdose.

Myocarditis

Important recommendations are as follows:

- In children with acute myocarditis who demonstrate arrhythmias, heart block, ST-segment changes, and low cardiac output, transfer to ICU and monitoring is recommended because they have a high risk of cardiac arrest.

- In children with myocarditis or cardiomyopathy and refractory low cardiac output state, the use of mechanical circulatory support or extracorporeal membrane

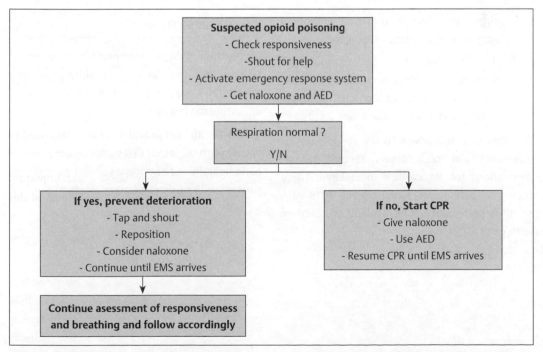

Flowchart 40.8 Lay responders' algorithm for opioid overdose. Abbreviations: AED, automated external defibrillator; CPR, cardiopulmonary resuscitation; EMS, emergency medical service.

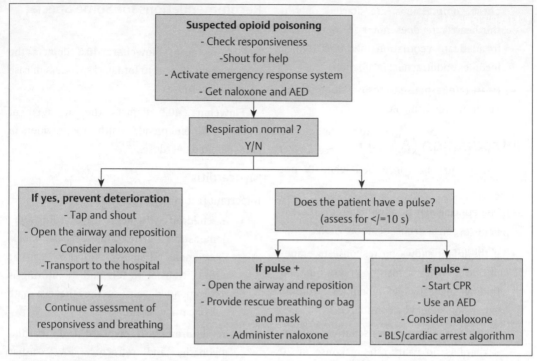

Flowchart 40.9 Emergency health care providers in opioid overdose. Abbreviations: AED, automated external defibrillator; BLS, basic life support; CPR, cardiopulmonary resuscitation.

oxygenation may help provide end-organ support and prevent cardiac arrest.

- Due to high challenges to successful resuscitation in children with myocarditis, early initiation of extracorporeal CPR may be beneficial once cardiac arrest occurs.

Previous pediatric advanced life support (PALS) guidelines did not contain specific recommendations for myocarditis in children. These recommendations are based on the 2018 AHA scientific statement on CPR in infants and children with cardiac disease.

Conclusion

To conclude, CPR is an important management skill to save lives in case of cardiorespiratory arrest which happen to occur inside the hospital or outside the hospital.

The health care providers of all strata need to update with the recent CPR guidelines and require periodic training to improve survival outcomes of patients with cardiorespiratory arrest.

CHAPTER 41

Anesthesiology: Ethics, Career, Medication, and Medical Errors

Ranjitha Nethaji, Tazeen Khan, and Puneet Khanna

Introduction (AS1.1)

The medical profession has long subscribed to a body of ethical statements developed primarily for the patient's benefit. As a member of this profession, a physician must recognize the responsibility to patients, first and foremost, and society as well as other health professionals and self. This chapter examines the ethical bases of the practices of medicine and the implications for anesthesiologists.

Guidelines for the Ethical Practice of Anesthesiology (AS1.3)

The Medical Council Act, 1956 incorporates ethics and regulations to govern the registered medical graduates in India. Therefore, qualified physicians must abide by regulations under the Indian Medical Council Act, especially Professional, Etiquette & Ethics Regulations, 2002, and subsequent amendments. The American Society of Anesthesiologists (ASA) has published a set of guidelines for anesthesiology's ethical practice which was amended in 2020. The Indian Society of Anesthesiologists (ISA) has also emphasized the importance of ethics in anesthesia practice. Some basic principles within the medical ethics are discussed below.

Basic Principles of Medical Ethics (AS1.3)

- **Nonmaleficence**: The doctrine of "do no harm" to patients.
- **Autonomy:** Ability to choose without controlling interferences by others.
- **Justice:** Fair when providing their services to patients.
- **Beneficence**: The doctrine of "do good" for the patient in every situation.

Informed Written Consent

Obtaining consent by the treating physician for a given procedure from an individual in a sound mind is not just enough. It is the basic right of individuals to know the alternative treatments, steps, risks, and outcomes associated with the procedure they undergo. A good rapport and communication is an essential key to informed written consent.

Preoperative Testing

Performing diagnostic tests on an individual is not without an ethical dimension. The intention of performing tests is to help the patient (beneficence) or use it to minimize other risks (nonmaleficence). However, medical tests may also carry implications for patients' autonomy, privacy, and even social justice.

Intraoperative Period

The anesthesiologist is responsible for patient positioning, and hence, we must be aware of various positions and their associated complications. The "captain of the ship" doctrine, which held the surgeon responsible for every aspect of the patient's perioperative care, is no longer a valid notion when an anesthesiologist is present. The surgeon and anesthesiologist as a team are ultimately answerable to the patient rather than to each other.

Postoperative Period

An anesthetist's responsibility does not end with completing the surgery; it extends to the postoperative period and follow-up of the patient until his discharge. Proper assessment and pain management have to be the area of focus.

Prospects of Anesthesiology as a Career (AS1.2, AS1.4)

An anesthesiologist is a well-trained specialist who works as a perioperative physician, makes anesthesia-related decisions, and is responsible for the patient's safety and well-being inside the operation theater. Providing anesthesia involves putting the patient in a state of controlled unconsciousness for amnesia, providing pain relief, and monitoring critical life functions as they are affected throughout the surgical, obstetrical, and other medical procedures.

Choosing a specialty as a career choice is made either during medical school or during the internship. Several factors affect this choice: intrinsic (personal attributes) or extrinsic (local/medical/environmental effects). Among them, exposure to a subspecialty in the undergraduate/postgraduate curriculum may significantly affect the trainee's career preferences.

Anesthesiology in the current era has evolved into a vast specialty not just limited to the operating room, with its subspecialties ranging from perioperative patient care, trauma care, obstetric and pediatric care to pain management and palliative care.

Various studies conducted to assess the awareness of anesthesiology's scope as a career and subspecialty options stated that most students joining anesthesia training were unaware of it. Hence, the need to increase awareness both at the undergraduate and postgraduate levels is imperative. This has a vital implication in national workforce planning and future recruitment strategies for specialist doctors in our health care system. The various career opportunities in anesthesia are described below:

Career Path and Subspecialties

- Cardiac anesthesiology.
- Neuroanesthesia.
- Obstetric anesthesia.
- Pediatric anesthesia.
- Pain medicine.
- Critical care medicine.
- Research careers in anesthesiology.

Cardiac Anesthesiology

A cardiac surgical patient's unique characteristics eventually led to cardiac anesthesiology's development as a subspecialty. A cardiac anesthesiologist is a perioperative physician trained to manage cardiac patients undergoing various cardiothoracic surgeries and repair of congenital heart defects, heart transplantations, and implantation of mechanical assist devices. They also have expertise in vascular surgeries and serve as attending physicians in cardiothoracic intensive care units.

Neuroanesthesia

The brain, which is the most important organ system and the principal target of anesthetic action, is still the least understood and most difficult to monitor. The development of neuroanesthesia as a subspecialty happened with the advances in understanding the intricacies of neurophysiology, pharmacology, and the pathophysiologic processes that underlie the nervous system's response to injury and ischemia. This enabled better management of neurosurgical patients in the perioperative period, with the implementation of neuroprotective and neuromonitoring techniques, resulting in better postoperative outcomes.

Obstetric Anesthesiology

It aims at the anesthetic care of women during pregnancy. Obstetric anesthesiologists have expertise in maternal and neonatal physiology as well as regional anesthesia. They provide anesthesia for in vitro fertilization, cerclage placements, nonobstetric surgery for parturient, postpartum procedures, and, of course, anesthesia for labor and cesarean deliveries.

With the increasing use of anesthesia for obstetric procedures, combined with advances in understanding the physiological and pharmacological difference between a pregnant and nonpregnant patient, the incidence of perioperative mortality and morbidity reduced and provided better patient satisfaction.

Pediatric Anesthesiology

This subspecialty of anesthesia focuses on the care of children and sometimes young adults. Children are not just small adults but differ in multiple aspects, anatomically, physiologically, and pharmacodynamically; thus, pediatric anesthesiology is necessary. Children born with congenital heart defects, congenital disabilities, or metabolic disorders require a special set of skills and knowledge that a pediatric anesthetist possesses. Neonates and children with severe or chronic illness pose a challenge when managing children with perfect bodies.

Pain Medicine

It is the subspecialty of anesthesiology that focuses on diagnosing and managing patients with acute, chronic, and cancer-related pain. This specialty differs drastically from the practice of anesthesiology in the operating room; a pain physician works in the outpatient clinic and involves long-term care of patients with chronic illness. This specialty suits individuals who enjoy anesthesia's technical aspects, particularly regional anesthesia, patient–physician interactions, and the challenges of diagnostic evaluation.

Acute pain specialists have expertise and skills in performing regional anesthesia and have chosen to extend these techniques into postoperative settings.

Comprehensive diagnostic evaluation, medical management, and applying neural blockage to the patient with pain are among the skills needed for a pain specialist. Many specialists have also gained minor surgical skills to independently perform implantation of devices in order to control chronic pain, such as spinal cord stimulators and spinal drug delivery systems.

Critical Care Medicine

Intensivist or critical care physicians consist of diverse clinicians, mainly anesthetists and specialists from internal medicine and pulmonary medicine as well as pediatricians. These individuals need to be well-versed in managing critically ill patients with multiple comorbidities, mechanical ventilation, invasive monitoring, and airway management. They need to be prompt in diagnosing and managing most medical conditions and handling emergencies related to airway and cardiopulmonary stability.

Research Careers in Anesthesiology

Research endeavors range from molecular biology to observational patient studies and clinical trials. The mainstay of focus has been the pharmacology of drugs used in the perioperative period, its impact on physiology, and management and assessment of various pathogenic mechanisms related to various conditions.

To sum up, anesthesiology is a diverse practice of acute care medicine that was originally developed to alleviate pain but has been involved in specialty that aims to make the perioperative period safe and comfortable for both the patient and the treating physician.

Common Medical and Medication Errors in Anesthesiology (AS10.4)

The crucial role of medicines and medical interventions in the prevention and treatment of various medical conditions is well appreciated. However, errors related to drug administration or intervention could have undesirable effects and be life-threatening. Medication errors are common in the health care system and reported to be the seventh most common cause of death worldwide, thus an area of huge concern and caution.

Definitions

- **Medical errors**: The failure of a planned action to be completed as intended or the use of a wrong plan to achieve an aim.
- **Medication error:** Any error in the medication process, whether there are any adverse consequences or not.
- **Adverse drug event (ADE)**: Any injury related to the use of a drug. Not all ADEs are caused by medical errors and vice versa.

Critical events occur most commonly during the middle of anesthesia, followed by during induction and at the beginning of the procedure. Administration of a single dose of a drug to a patient requires multiple steps: prescription, transcription, preparation, dispersion, and administration.

Most errors occur during the administration stage (53%), followed by prescription (17%), preparation (14%), and transcription (11%).

Risk Factors for Errors during Anesthesia

- Inadequate experience.
- Inadequate familiarity with equipment/device.
- Poor communication with team.

- Haste.
- Inattention.
- Fatigue.
- Failure to perform a normal check.
- Lack of enough supervision.
- Mental or physical factors.

Drugs Involved in Medication Errors

- Induction agents—thiopentone sodium, ketamine, depolarizing and nondepolarizing muscle relaxants.
- Narcotics and sedatives.
- Local anesthetics.

Medication errors occur either due to misidentification, wrong labeling, syringe swap, inattention, or haste.

Steps to Prevent Medical/Medication Errors

- Labels of all ampoules and syringes to be checked twice before drawing or being used.
- Legibility and contents of labels on ampoules and syringes should be optimized as per standardization.
- Standardized anesthetic cart and trays and consider usage and placement patterns.
- Separation of a look like drugs should be done.
- Errors during administration should be reported.
- Avoid the use of dangerous abbreviations and dose expressions.
- Enhance communication mechanism.
- Consistent documentation and complete operative medication history to be noted before administration of any drug.
- Drugs to drawn up and labeled by the anesthesia providers.

- Color coding by class of drugs should be according to an agreed national/international standard.
- Coding of syringes to position or size should be done.

Simple vigilance, standardization of protocols, and attentiveness at all times is the key to avoid the occurrence of medication errors. As the famous Chinese proverb goes, "the error of one moment becomes the sorrow of whole life," one needs to very careful with drug administration and medical interventions.

Conclusion

Anesthesia is a rapidly growing specialty in the field of medicine with budding subspecialties. Increasing legal claims against doctors across the globe mandate practicing anesthesia with imbibition of ethical aspects to ensure the safety of patient as well as the anesthesia provider. Like other specialties, medication errors do occur in daily anesthesia practice. Choosing the right drug, proper labeling, and communicating through a closed loop is a must to prevent medication errors.

CHAPTER 42

Postanesthesia Care Unit

Tazeen Khan and Puneet Khanna

Introduction (AS6.1)

Emergency critical care has become a growing area of concern in the present century, with particular concern for postoperative morbidity and mortality among high-risk patients; with the advent of the postanesthesia care unit (PACU), the quality of patient care along with postoperative morbidity has significantly improved.

The National Confidential Enquiry into patient outcome and death reported that a system was needed to be devised for patients with a high risk of perioperative complications, including postoperative care, hence emphasizing the need for PACU.

PACU or recovery room is specifically structured and staffed to monitor and manage patients recovering from the effects of anesthesia and surgery, thereby serving as a bridge from one-to-one monitoring in the operation theater (OT) to less focused monitoring in the ward.

Structure

Recovery room/PACU is usually built close to the OT complex and has a specified number of beds, depending upon the number of OTs and OT turnover. The facility should be open to allow each recovery bay to be observed at all times. The beds are to be spaced out to allow unobstructed access to trolleys, X-ray equipment, and resuscitation carts. The basic structure consists of the following:

- Beds (Fowlers's cot with side rails).
- Multipara monitors.
- Oxygen port and various devices for oxygen therapy.
- Suction port.
- Crash cart (with all emergency drugs and equipment).

Crash Cart (AS6.2)

It is a term used to describe a self-contained mobile unit that virtually contains all of the materials, drugs, and devices necessary to perform a code. It is placed in an easily accessible location and can be moved on wheels when needed. It is a tall, five-drawer cart, with each drawer having a separate set of contents with a list attached to it.

External Contents

This is placed on top of the crash cart and has the following:

- Biphasic defibrillator with paddles/pads.
- Ambu bag with a face mask of different sizes.
- Oxygen tube connector.

Internal Contents

It is divided and placed in five different drawers, depending on the use and requirement.

a. First drawer:

The first drawer comprises four rows with specific constituents (**Table 42.1**).

b. Second drawer:

The second drawer has also four rows with specific contents (**Table 42.2**).

c. Third drawer:

The third drawer is reserved mainly for materials to establish peripheral intravenous (PIV) access and contains some other miscellaneous items. The drawer contains:

Table 42.1 First drawer contents

Row	Contents
First	Medications used in a cardiac arrest (epinephrine, amiodarone, sodium bicarbonate, and calcium)
Second	RSI medications needed for intubation and medications for bradycardia
Third	Medications predominantly used in tachyarrhythmias
Fourth	Medications needed for hypotensive emergencies and patients with low CO. Hydrocortisone is included for its use in refractory hypotension and suspected adrenal crisis

Abbreviations: CO, cardiac output; RSI, rapid sequence induction.

Table 42.2 Second drawer contents

Row	Contents
First	Medications for hypertensive emergencies and decreased mental status due to hypoglycemia and opioid overdose
Second	IV and inhaled medications for acute exacerbations of respiratory diseases (asthma, chronic obstructive pulmonary disease, and upper airway edema) and medications for allergic reactions
Third	Antiepileptics, diuretics
Fourth	Thiamine

Abbreviation: IV, intravenous.

- Angiocatheters (14, 16, 18, 20, 22, 24 G) for emergent decompression of tension pneumothorax.

- For PIV access, contents include needles (16, 18, 21, 25 G), alcohol wipes, syringes (1, 3, 5, 10, 20, 30 mL).

- Long spinal needles (peds: 20, 22 G; adults: 18 G) for emergency pericardiocentesis, scalpel blades (10, 11, 15).

- Sutures (nylon 2.0, 3.0, 4.0; prolene 2.0), radial and femoral arterial line catheters (peds: 22, 24 G; adults: 20 G).

- Nasal packs and balloons (unilateral and bilateral) for severe nose bleeding and a magnet to reset malfunctioning pacemakers/defibrillators.

d. Fourth drawer:

The fourth drawer is designed to store respiratory equipment and supplies for both adults and pediatric patients. The front half of the drawer can be divided into two detachable compartments (pediatric and adult), one of which can be removed and placed at the head of the bed during resuscitation, depending on the patient's age group. The back half will contain the rest of the supplies: compact surgical airway set (cricothyroidotomy), batteries and light bulbs for the laryngoscope, tape, endotracheal tube holders, CO_2 detector, and xylocaine spray.

e. Fifth drawer:

The fifth drawer is reserved for larger instruments and supplies needed for special procedures. The contents of this drawer include central venous catheters (3–7 Fr/single and triple lumen); intraosseous kit; cut-down tray; umbilical catheterization set (3.5 and 5 F); chest tubes (sizes 10–42); thoracostomy kit; thoracotomy kit; suture set; delivery set; trauma tourniquets; pericardiocentesis kit; sterile stapler; and burr hole manual drill kit.

The crash cart needs to be checked and restocked regularly to detect any equipment malfunction or removal and replacement of expired drugs.

Staffing Requirements

- It is staffed by specially trained nurses, trained specifically toward postoperative care, and who can recognize common postoperative complications and manage them.
- It also requires an adequate number of ancillary staff such as operating room technicians, ward boys, and support staff.
- There should be an anesthetist or a professional with suitably qualified airway skills who is available for patients in the PACU within 3 minutes in case of an airway emergency.
- A physician is responsible for the discharge of patients from the recovery room.

Admission to PACU (AS6.1)

The patient is shifted from the OT to the recovery room/PACU, accompanied by the anesthesiologist who has complete knowledge about the patient's condition and any intraoperative events. The patient would be continuously evaluated and treated during transport with monitoring and support appropriate to the patient's condition.

Upon arrival to PACU, the patient shall be reevaluated, and a verbal report is given to the PACU nurse in charge, given by the anesthesiologist, and the status documented on arrival.

Management of patients in PACU mainly has two components:

- Monitoring.
- Resuscitation (early detection and management of complications).

Monitoring (AS6.1)

On admission to recovery/PACU, patients are closely monitored till they are stable enough to be shifted to their respective wards.

The main parameters monitored are as follows:

- Mental status.
- Hemodynamics (heart rate [HR] and blood pressure [BP]).
- Respiration (oxygenation and ventilation).
- Temperature.
- Pain.

Mental Status

Alertness and responsiveness need to be periodically monitored. Normally, a response to stimulation occurs within 60 to 90 minutes, even in cases of prolonged surgery and anesthesia. If the patient is still not alert/responsive or there is deterioration in the awareness, then the underlying cause needs to be evaluated and managed.

Hemodynamics

Maintaining hemodynamic stability forms an integral part of postanesthesia care:

- HR and BP being the two main parameters that are to be routinely monitored.
- ECG is mandatory for HR monitoring. It also enables early diagnosis and management of dysrhythmias, for example, bradycardia, tachycardia, or arrhythmias.
- BP can be monitored by either a noninvasive blood pressure (NIBP) monitoring at a minimum interval of every 15 minutes or an invasive blood pressure (IBP) monitoring if an arterial line is in situ.

Monitoring and maintaining stable hemodynamics during the immediate postoperative period is crucial in preventing major postoperative complications while the patient is recovering from anesthesia and the surgery's physiological effects.

Respiratory Monitoring

It involves the assessment of:

- Airway patency.
- Oxygen saturation (SpO_2).
- Respiratory rate (RR).
- Special attention should be given to the type of breathing and breathing patterns in the immediate postoperative period, for example, normal tidal respiration/rapid and shallow/slow and deep.

Pulse oximetry is an efficient way of assessing oxygenation, and capnography is used to assess the ventilation aspect. Patients maintaining a saturation < 94% postanesthesia mostly require oxygen therapy either through a face mask/nasal prongs or various continuous positive airway pressure (CPAP) devices.

Early detection of an airway collapse, altered breathing pattern, sudden desaturation, and prompt intervention can prevent life-threatening complications.

Temperature Monitoring

The patient's temperature must be periodically monitored, and signs and symptoms suggestive of hypo/hyperthermia, such as shivering or sweating, are to be looked out for.

Pain

Patients' pains score should be periodically assessed during their stay in the recovery, and appropriate interventions are to be made when and where required.

Other Factors to be Monitored

- Postoperative nausea and vomiting (PONV).
- Hydration status.
- Urine output (UO)—minimum of 0.5 mL/kg/h.
- Drainage and bleeding.

Complications and Its Management (AS6.3)

Upper Airway Obstruction

It is one of the most common complications in a postoperative recovery room.

Cause

It occurs due to loss of parapharyngeal muscle tone in a sedated patient under the persistent effect of anesthetics, neuromuscular blockers, or opioids.

Presentation

Snoring, paradoxical breathing pattern, and desaturation.

Management

Relieved by opening the airway with "jaw thrust maneuver" or "CPAP "(5–15 cm of H_2O) applied via a face mask. Placement of a nasopharyngeal airway or laryngeal mask airway may also be required in a few patients.

Systemic Hypertension

Common in patients with a history of essential hypertension during the immediate postoperative period.

Precipitating factors:

- Missed morning dose of antihypertensives.
- Pain.
- Nausea vomiting.
- Hypoventilation and hypercapnia.
- Hypoxia.
- Emergence excitement.
- Urinary retention.

It is managed by treating the underlying cause along with the use of antihypertensives in some cases.

Systemic Hypotension

It is the most common complication in the immediate postoperative period.

Causes

- Hypovolemic (decreased preload):

  Etiology:

  ▶ Ongoing third space loss.

  ▶ Bleeding.

  ▶ Inadequate intraoperative fluid replacement.

  ▶ Loss of sympathetic nervous system tone as a result of neuraxial blockage.

- Distributive (decreased afterload):

  Etiology—iatrogenic sympathectomy, allergic reactions, sepsis.

- Cardiogenic (intrinsic pump failure):

  Etiology—myocardial infarction, cardio-myopathy, cardiac arrhythmias, and tamponade.

  Presentation—tachycardia, hypotension, tachypnea, mottled skin, altered mentation, and nausea vomiting.

  Management:

  ▶ Judicious fluid therapy and transfusion if necessary in the forms of fluid bolus in addition to the maintenance fluid.

  ▶ Use of sympathomimetic drugs, for example, ephedrine (5–25 mg) or ino-tropes, for example, noradrenaline (0.1–0.5 µg/kg/min), use of antiarrhythmics.

  ▶ Treatment of the underlying cause.

Hypothermia and Shivering

Hypothermia is defined as the core temperature of < 36 °C. It occurs after both general or neuraxial anesthesia. Shivering leads to increased oxygen consumption, thereby increasing HR and cardiac output (CO), leading to myocardial ischemia in a few patients.

Cause

Secondary to heat loss during surgery by radiation, convection, evaporation, and conduction.

Management

Use of forced air warmers, warm fluids, and drugs such opioids, clonidine, and ketamine. Meperidine 12.5 to 25 mg IV is most commonly used to prevent shivering in adults.

Postoperative Nausea and Vomiting

The risk factors are:

- Inhalational anesthesia.
- Female gender.
- Nonsmoker.
- Prior history of PONV or motion sickness.
- Need for postoperative opioids.

PONV leads to a delay in discharge from PACU, prolongs hospital stay, increases the risk of aspiration, and causes significant postoperative discomfort.

Prevention and Treatment

Commonly used drugs are:

- Ondansetron 4 mg IV 30 minutes before completion of surgery.
- Dexamethasone 4 mg IV after induction of anesthesia.
- Metoclopramide 10 mg IV.
- Promethazine 12.5 to 25 mg IV.

Postoperative Pain

Acute postoperative pains remain a major problem in the immediate postoperative period and have multiple undesirable outcomes. Assessment is usually made using the visual analog scale (VAS), numerical rating scale (NRS), or verbal rating scale (VRS).

Management

Use of IV opioids (fentanyl/morphine) in the form of small boluses, as a continuous infusion, or as a patient control analgesia (PCA) is the most common modality.

Nonopioid analgesics such as nonsteroidal anti-inflammatory drugs (NSAIDs) (IV ketorolac 0.5mg/kg), gabapentin, small doses of ketamine, and dexmedetomidine have been found to relieve postoperative pain and opioid consumption.

Other techniques involve epidural analgesia, perineural blocks, and infiltrative techniques using local anesthetics as the mainstay for pain relief.

Discharge Criteria

It may vary from one setup to another, but the general principles are universally acceptable. The general principles before discharge are as follows:

- A fixed duration of stay in PACU is not necessary.
- Must be observed till they are fully alert with a clear mental status.
- No risk of ventilatory depression.
- Stable hemodynamics.
- No complaints of pain.
- Able to move lower limbs/flex knee post neuraxial block.

Multiple scoring systems are used for discharge from PACU, with the most common being the Modified Aldrete score and postanesthesia discharge scoring system (PADSS). The details of these scoring systems are mentioned in Chapter 35 (*Anesthesia for Daycare Surgeries*).

Conclusion

The postanesthesia care unit acts as a bridge between OT and ward. Immediately after the surgery, patients are at risk of desaturation, hypotension, and upper airway obstruction. Monitoring patients in PACU ensures stabilization of patients before they can be sent back to wards or home. Adequate infrastructure, availability of trained staff, and vigilant monitoring is required to have a stable patient without complications.

CHAPTER 43

Basics of Ventilator

Gourav Mittal and Puneet Khanna

Introduction

In the modern era, a sick patient's care cannot be imagined without a mechanical ventilator. With growing life expectancy and the burden of comorbid illness, more patients get admitted to the intensive care unit (ICU) and require ventilatory support in one or the other forms. The orientation and understanding of the ventilator are a must for all intensivists.

A mechanical ventilator is an automated machine that transforms the energy in a predetermined manner to augment or replace the patient's muscles in performing the work of breathing.

Components of a Ventilator

The functioning of a ventilator can be visualized in terms of the following components:

- Power source.
- Controls.
- Monitors.
- Safety features.

Power Source

It includes a gas supply system, batteries, and the power source for the mechanical ventilator.

Various Options for Power Supply

- Gas pressure to operate inspiratory flow and run valves and switches by supplying mechanical power.
- Gas pressure to drive inspiratory flow, and electrically powered valves and switches (most commonly used).

- Electrically powered turbines/compressors for inspiratory gas flow as well as to run valves/switches.

The generation of inspiratory flows can be achieved in various ways (**Table 43.1**).

Controls

The controls are meant for regulating the timing and characteristics of the delivered gas. The controls consist of various parts with specific functions.

a. Gas Blender

It controls the proportion of air and oxygen.

b. Gas Accumulator

It is the component of a ventilator that requires precise control of gas mixtures and cannot rely on proportioning valves to produce this level of precision, that is, where the gas flows are very low.

c. Inspiratory Flow Regulator

It is usually a solenoid valve which ensures that the respiratory circuit receives the prescribed gas flow.

d. Humidification Equipment

It is required for maintaining the humidity of the circuit. It can either be a device that heats and evaporates water into the supplied gas mixture (active humidifier) or a passive humidifier like a heat/moisture exchanger.

e. Circuit

It is a corrugated tubing with its characteristic compliance and resistance to airflow.

Table 43.1 Techniques of generation of inspiratory flows

Technique	Mechanism
Pneumatic	The gas supply from the gas pipeline or cylinder is used to generate required inspiratory flows • Achievable flow rate—200 L/min • Minimal battery power consumption • It requires a stable supply of pressurized gas, with a minimum flow and pressure of 120–150 L/min and 200 kPa, respectively
Turbine	A compressor generates pressurized gas flows • Achievable flow rates—240 L/min • Able to compensate for a large amount of leaks • It does not require a compressed air supply • Does need compressed oxygen supply (120 L/min)
Bellows	A flexible gas reservoir produces inspiratory flows • Can precisely control the composition of the gas mixture • Does not require 200 kPa supply (suitable for low-flow gas supply) • Has more moving parts and points and hence high chances of failure • Not suitable for NIV use because of inability to compensate for large leaks
Piston	The volume of the rigid chamber is mechanically manipulated to generate inspiratory flows • Controls the delivery of volume more accurately • More economical on gas use • Poor compensation for gas leak

Abbreviation: NIV, noninvasive ventilation.

f. Expiratory Pressure Regulator (PEEP Valve)

It controls and maintains positive airway pressure through a solenoid valve.

Monitors

Monitors are the eyes of the ventilator to assess gas delivery and the patient's respiratory system mechanics. It can provide information about the following parameters.

a. Gas Concentration

It is usually measured by either voltaic cells or spectrophotometers.

b. Flow

The modern ventilators systems use various techniques to measure flow (hot wire anemometry, variable orifice flow meters, and screen pneumotachograph).

c. Pressure

In modern ventilators, integrated silicon wafer pressure transducers are often used to monitor pressure.

d. Volume

This is not directly measured in modern ventilators. It is calculated from flow measurements (volume = flow × time).

Safety Features

Filters and alarms constitute integral safety features of a ventilator as described below:

a. Inspiratory Filters

It purifies the inspired gas by removing airborne particles and bacteria.

b. Expiratory Filters

Expiratory filters bleach out the great clouds of aerosolized pathogens and protect the ICU staff.

c. Alarms

Alarms safeguard against unintentional changes to the ventilator settings and weird misapplications of ventilation.

Setting up a Ventilator (AS7.4)

Before setting up a ventilator for invasive mechanical ventilation, we need some baseline information which includes:

- Ideal body weight:
  - ▸ Males = height (cm)–100.
  - ▸ Female = height (cm)–110.
- Comorbidities (e.g., obesity, asthma, chronic obstructive pulmonary disorder [COPD]).
- Baseline evidence of lung injury (e.g., acute lung injury, bronchospasm, alveolar overdistension, bronchopleural fistula).
- Expected time to being spontaneous ventilation.
- Baseline hemodynamics: Whether stable or not.
- Recent paralysis.
- Temperature.

After baseline information, we have to select various variables:

Choose mode

- If the patient is apneic or paralyzed, preferred modes are: volume control (VC)/pressure control (PC)/pressure-regulated volume control (PRVC).
- If spontaneous respiratory effort present: Synchronized intermittent mandatory ventilation (SIMV) + pressure-support ventilation (PSV).
- If spontaneous breathing with adequate efforts presents: Pressure support (PS)/volume support (VS)/continuous positive airway pressure (CPAP).

Set tidal volume

- 6 to 8 mL/kg of ideal body weight.

Respiratory rate (not for fully spontaneous modes)

- 10 to 15/min; rate needs to be set higher in case of metabolic acidosis.

Inspired oxygen fraction (FiO$_2$)

- 0.21 to 1.0 (depending upon the requirement of the patient in order to maintain SpO$_2$ > 92%.

Positive end-expiratory pressure (PEEP)

- Usually in the range of 0 to 20 cm H$_2$O. It has to be optimized, according to respiratory mechanics as well as hemodynamics.

Inspiratory to the expiratory ratio (I:E)

- <1:1 (prolonged expiratory time often needed for patients with obstructive airway disease like asthma, COPD).

Inspiratory flow rate

- 40–60 L/min (higher flow rate may be required in patients with obstructive airway disease like asthma, COPD).

Trigger

- When we allow the patient to breathe spontaneously, we need a trigger, which is a signal that the ventilator will sense and provide a flow of gases whenever required.
- Two types of trigger are usually used, that is, pressure and flow. However, flow trigger is most commonly used because it is often associated with less work of breathing.

Alarms

- Minute ventilation targets: Ensure adequate ventilation (minute ventilation [MV] = tidal volume [TV] × respiratory rate [RR]).

- Leak: To avoid significant loss of flow, which may lead to hypoventilation and respiratory acidosis.

- Peak airway pressure: To avoid trauma to patients' airway.

- FiO_2 alarm: To avoid inadvertently delivery of a hypoxic gas mixture.

Method of humidification

- Often decided based on the duration of mechanical ventilation, respiratory secretions, and availability. The options include a heat moisture exchanger (HME) and wet circuit humidifier.

Conclusion

A ventilator is an artificial respiratory support system. It is used to support patients' respiratory systems until they recover from illness, breathe normally, and meet their physiological needs. Thorough knowledge is required about the design and operational characteristics of a ventilator to use it efficiently and troubleshoot the alarms.

CHAPTER 44

Intensive Care Unit

Gourav Mittal and Puneet Khanna

Introduction

The intensive care unit (ICU) consists of advanced medical technologies like modern ventilators, advanced hemodynamic monitoring systems, and skilled, trained personnel to support organ systems in critically ill patients.

As per definition, "critical care is defined as the direct delivery by a physician (s) of medical care for a critically ill or critically injured patient. A critical illness or injury acutely impairs one or more vital organ systems, such that there is a high probability of imminent or life-threatening deterioration in the patient's condition."

Admission to ICU (AS7.2)

The admission to intensive care is guided by the institutional policy that usually considers local population subtype (trauma, burns, medical) and their limitations like ICU size and expertise. The optimal resource utilization plus improving outcomes should be considered while admitting someone to ICU. The important considerations are as follows:

- The specific patient needs like life-supportive therapies that can be only addressed in the ICU.
- Available clinical expertise.
- Diagnosis at the time of admission.
- Unoccupied beds in ICU.
- Objective health parameters at the time of referral.
- Potential that patient will benefit from interventions.
- Prognosis.

Patients requiring life-sustaining interventions, including cardiopulmonary resuscitation having a good prognosis, should be given priority over one with a significantly lower probability of recovery. The patients requiring mechanical ventilation or in sepsis should be admitted to ICU.

Patients should not be transferred to the general ward unless the ward is a high-dependency unit.

The following table is a summary of resource allocation and monitoring of patients receiving in-hospital care (**Table 44.1**).

ICU Functioning (AS7.1)

The functioning of ICU depends upon the organization model followed by a given ICU. A given ICU can be open, closed, or semiclosed type as described below:

- **Open ICU:** The specialty teams hold the admission right, and the intensivist acts as a consulting physician.
- **Closed ICU:** The intensivist decides on admitting a patient, and the specialty team helps the intensivist.
- **Hybrid/transitional/semiclosed ICU:** The intensivist and the specialty physician work in collaboration with equal distribution of decision-making power with regard to the patients.

The comparative summary of types of ICU is tabulated in **Table 44.2**.

"We do not have 'his or her' patients, we have 'our' patients, and if the home team feels that there may be aspects of our treatment that require explanation, we are only too happy to discuss this with them—civilly."

Table 44.1 Framework to guide the level of intensive monitoring and care

Level	Types of patients	Nurse-to-patient ratio	Intervention
ICU (level 3)	Critically ill requiring hourly as well invasive hemodynamic monitoring	1:1 to ≤ 1:2	Advanced hemodynamic support, invasive mechanical ventilation, renal replacement therapy, ECMO
Intermediate medical unit (level 2)	Unstable patients requiring nursing interventions, laboratory workup or 4 hourly monitoring	≤ 1:3	Noninvasive ventilation, IV drug administration, antiarrhythmic drugs
Telemetry (level 1)	Stable patients but requiring frequent monitoring	≤ 1:4	IV drugs
Ward (level 0)	Stable patient not requiring testing as well as monitoring lesser than 4 hourly	≤ 1:5	IV antibiotics, radiology, and laboratory workup

Abbreviations: ECMO, extracorporeal membrane oxygenation; ICU, intensive care unit; IV, intravenous.

Table 44.2 Types of ICU

Feature	Open	Closed	Hybrid	Advantage/disadvantage
The primary physician managing the case	Yes	No	Yes	More satisfaction to attendants
Intensivist	+/−	Always	Always	Presence leads to better resource utilization, better management
Physician conflict	Less likely	May be	More than closed	May lead to conflict on patient's treatment decision
Workforce	Less	More	Moderate	Shortage of trained intensivists
Efficiency	Less efficient	More efficient	More efficient	Evidence-based medicine leads to more efficiency of closed as well as hybrid ICU

Abbreviation: ICU, intensive care unit.

Explanation: The above quotation says that the intensivists and the treating physicians should treat each patient by a team approach and not by an individual approach. The treatment decisions and steps must be discussed and best one should be chosen in the part of patient's welfare.

Monitoring in ICU (AS7.5)

The patients admitted to the ICU are critically ill, have multiple organ dysfunction, and hence require vigilant monitoring of each organ function with the timely institution of intervention to improve patient's outcome.

According to the National Institute for Health and Care Excellence (NICE) guidelines, monitoring of heart rate, respiratory rate, blood pressure, and oxygen saturation is minimum in all intensive care patients. However, more advanced and invasive monitoring should be used for patients with a poor cardiorespiratory reserve and raised intracranial pressure.

The mnemonic "FAST HUGS BID" is simple to use and apply in critically ill patients and guides an intensivist not to miss any aspect of patient care during ICU stay.

- **F-Feeding** (to provide adequate calorie and protein).

- **A-Analgesia** (pain relief in surgical patients OR during the painful procedure).

- **S-Sedation** (to tolerate the discomfort of the endotracheal tube and other invasive lines/catheters).

- **T-Thromboprophylaxis** (use of mechanical or pharmacological means to prevent deep vein thrombosis).

- **H-Head elevation** (30-45 degree to prevent aspiration and ventilator-associated pneumonia).

- **U-Ulcer prophylaxis** (use of antacid/proton pump inhibitor or H2 blockers to prevent stress ulcer of the gastrointestinal tract).

- **G-Glycemic control** (tight control sugar helps to avoid infectious complications and improve survival, target <200 mg/dL).

- **S-Spontaneous breathing trial** (to check for readiness for liberation from mechanical ventilation).

- **B-Bowel care** (to ensure normal bowel movement with initial of early feeding and taking care of constipation).

- **I-Indwelling catheters** (removal of invasive lines and catheters when these are no more required to prevent infectious and thrombotic complications).

- **D-Deescalation of antibiotics** (stopping or switching of antibiotics to narrow-spectrum to decrease antibiotic resistance).

Discharge Criteria (AS7.2)

Once the patient recovers from acute illness, the decision needs to be taken to shift the patient out of ICU. Followings are the guiding principles while discharging a patient from ICU:

- Follow local ICU policy.

- Patient prognosis.

- Stability of organ systems.

- Ongoing active interventions.

- Avoid discharge from ICU at odd hours ("night shift" after 7 pm in institutions with 12-hour shifts).

- Discharge patients at high risk of mortality and readmission to a step-down unit or long-term acute care hospital instead of the regular ward. The patients with multiple comorbid illnesses, high severity of illness at the time of admission, and those requiring organ support come under the high-risk category.

Unconscious Patient (AS7.3)

Encountering a patient in an altered sensorium is not uncommon. Timely identification, evaluation, and institution of appropriate treatment are crucial in such a scenario. The altered state can range from clouding of consciousness to stupor or coma:

- Clouding of consciousness refers to a mild form of altered mental status in which the patient has inattention and reduced wakefulness.

- A confusional state is a more profound deficit that includes disorientation and difficulty following commands.

- Lethargy refers to the arousal of the patient by moderate stimuli and then drifting back to sleep.

- Stupor refers to the patient's arousal by repeated, vigorous stimuli, and when left undisturbed, the patient will immediately lapse back to the unresponsive state.

The causes of unconsciousness or altered sensorium are summarized in **Table 44.3**.

Table 44.3 Causes of altered sensorium

With focal signs	
Vascular causes	• Stroke • Critical vessel stenosis of some specific vessel • Intracranial hemorrhage
Infections	• Brain abscess • Meningoencephalitis
Neoplastic causes	• Space-occupying lesions
Traumatic causes	• Focal neurological injury due to head trauma • Increased intracranial pressure, giving rise to false localizing signs
Unconsciousness with no specific features	
Vascular causes	• Brainstem stroke with damage to the reticular activating system • Diffuse cerebral small vessel disease
Infections	• Septic encephalopathy
Drug-related causes	• Decreased clearance of sedatives, opioids
Intrinsic neurological cause	• Nonconvulsive status epilepticus • Raised ICP • ICU delirium
Traumatic causes	• Diffuse axonal injury
Endocrine and metabolic causes	• Hypoadrenalism • Hypothyroidism • Hepatic encephalopathy • Uremic encephalopathy • Wernicke's encephalopathy

Abbreviation: ICP, intracranial pressure; ICU, intensive care unit.

Examination of an Unconscious Patient

The examination of an unconscious patient starts with documentation of the consciousness level, which is guided by the Glasgow coma scale (GCS) score. Examination of pupils and respiratory patterns helps to identify the possible etiologies of altered sensorium.

Glasgow Coma Scale

It was originally designed to assess the consciousness level of patients with a head injury. However, it has widespread applicability in all groups of patients with altered sensorium. The component of GCS and their scores are described in **Table 44.4**.

Pupils

Pupil examination is pivotal in patients with altered sensorium. The types of pupils and their corresponding etiologies are summarized in **Table 44.5**.

Respiratory Pattern

The pattern of respiration is another important clinical tool to identify the cause of altered sensorium. The pattern of respiration and their etiologies are summarized in **Table 44.6**.

Table 44.4 The Glasgow coma scale

Response	Scale	Score
Eye-opening response	Spontaneous eye-opening	4
	Eye-opening to verbal command, shout	3
	Eye-opening to pain	2
	No eye-opening at all	1
Verbal response	Oriented	5
	Confused	4
	Inappropriate speech	3
	Incomprehensible sounds or speech	2
	No verbal response	1
Motor response	Obeys command	6
	Localizes pain	5
	Withdraws from pain	4
	Abnormal flexion, decorticate posture	3
	Extension response, decerebrate posture	2
	No motor response	1

Score = 3–15

Minor brain injury = 13–15 points, moderate brain injury = 9–12 points, mild brain injury = 3–8 points

Table 44.5 Pupil abnormality and the causes of altered sensorium

Unilateral miosis	Bilateral miosis	Unilateral mydriasis	Bilateral mydriasis
Horner's syndrome	Opioids	Uncal herniation	Hypoxic brain injury
Damaged sympathetic	Organophosphate poisoning	Midbrain lesion	Bilateral midbrain lesion
	Cholinergic		Sympathomimetic drugs
	Clonidine		Anticholinergic drugs
	Pontine lesion		
	Thalamic lesions		

Management

- Always follow airway, breathing, and circulation protocol:
  - ▶ Keep the airway patent (apply head tilt–chin lift and jaw-thrust maneuver wherever required).
  - ▶ Go for intubation if GCS is less than 8.
  - ▶ Assume cervical spine injury in all trauma patients and stabilize it.
  - ▶ Provide oxygen (through a nasal cannula, facemask, oxy mask, or nonrebreathing mask).
  - ▶ Secure an adequate intravenous (IV) access.
  - ▶ Infuse IV fluids to achieve optimal blood pressure.
- Give 50% glucose (50 mL).

Table 44.6 Respiratory pattern abnormality and the causes

Respiratory pattern	Metabolic pattern	PH, PaCO₂, HCO₃	Causes
Hyperventilation	Metabolic acidosis	PH < 7.35, $PaCO_2$ < 30 mm Hg, HCO_3 < 17 mmol/L	• Uremia • Diabetic ketoacidosis, lactic acidosis • Methanol • Salicylates
Hyperventilation	Respiratory alkalosis	PH > 7.45, $PaCO_2$ < 30 mm Hg, HCO_3 > 17 mmol/L	• Hepatic failure • Sepsis
Hypoventilation	Respiratory acidosis	PH < 7.35, $PaCO_2$ > 90 mm Hg, HCO_3 > 17 mmol/L	• Respiratory failure from the central or peripheral cause • Chest wall deformity
Hypoventilation	Metabolic alkalosis	PH > 7.45, $PaCO_2$ > 45 mm Hg, HCO_3 > 30 mmol/L	• Vomiting • Alkali ingestion

- Do give thiamine 100 mg IV to patients with a history of chronic alcoholism.
- Rule out metabolic, electrolyte abnormality, and infectious etiologies if a patient is present with seizures.
- Use phenytoin to treat definite seizures.
- Consider empiric treatments for the following conditions:
  ▶ Possible bacterial or viral meningitis:
    ○ Ceftriaxone and vancomycin.
    ○ Acyclovir.
  ▶ For possible ingestion:
    ○ Naloxone.
    ○ Flumazenil.
    ○ Gastric lavage/activated charcoal.
  ▶ For possible increased intracranial pressure (ICP):
    ○ Mannitol.
  ▶ For possible nonconvulsive status:
    ○ Lorazepam.
    ○ Phenytoin or equivalent.

Conclusion

Patients admitted to the ICU are more sick with multiorgan dysfunction and require round-the-clock monitoring. The ICU can be either open type, closed type, or hybrid type. Management of an unconscious individual requires proper history-taking, examination, diagnostic evaluation, and delivery of appropriate medications.

Section VII
Equipment in Anesthesia

CHAPTER 45

Anesthesia Workstation

Damarla Haritha and Akhil Kant Singh

Introduction

After the public demonstration of ether anesthesia by William Thomas Greene Morton in 1846, the need for an apparatus that will be able to deliver a fixed proportion of anesthetic vapor at an appropriate flow raised. The first anesthesia machine was built by James Taylor Gwathemy, the first president of the American Association of Anesthetists in 1912. But the machine which caught most of the public interest was the one made by Henry Edmund Gaskin Boyle in 1917, as it was publicly demonstrated at the Royal Society of London. Later on, the Boyle's machine was patented by British Oxygen Company (BOC), and several advances from Boyle basic to Boyle E, Boyle F, Boyle G, Boyle H, Boyle M, Boyle Major, and international models were released in the market.

However, the modern anesthesia delivery systems are no longer referred to as anesthesia machines, but rather as "anesthesia workstation" (**Fig. 45.1**). American Society of Testing and Materials (ASTM) describes anesthesia workstation as "*a system for administering anesthesia to the patients consisting of gas supply devices, ventilator, monitoring devices, and various safety features.*" Although the modern anesthesia workstation is well advanced than the traditional Boyle's machine, it retains the basic architecture and the working principle put in a technologically advanced manner. A thorough understanding of the working of the anesthesia machine and various troubleshooting maneuvers is one of the necessary skills of the anesthesiologist.

There are many different companies manufacturing anesthesia workstations like Penlon, Drager, Datex Ohmeda, Space Labs, etc., all of which have a different look. Still, the basic design of all the workstations is similar. All the modern anesthesia workstations can perform essential functions such as providing oxygen, inhalational anesthetic vapors in a precise mixture, providing mechanical ventilation, monitoring of the patients' hemodynamic parameters as well as anesthetic gas concentrations and also effectively preventing theater pollution by foolproof scavenging systems. All these components are mounted on a box-shaped metallic structure and antistatic wheels, which gives it stability and prevents the generation of static electricity. The modern anesthesia workstation gets operated electrically, but it has a battery backup that supplies enough to work up to 60 minutes in case of power failure. While one wonders what other safety features the modern anesthesia workstation offer, it is wise to remember that each and every component of anesthesia workstation has its own significance and puts a foot forward for the safety of patients.

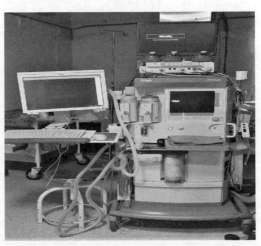

Fig. 45.1 Modern anesthesia workstation (Drager).

All the modern anesthesia workstations consist of a series of pipelines that deliver the oxygen and the various carrier gases like medical air or nitrous oxide (N_2O) from a higher pressure in the hospital's supply to a lower pressure amenable to patient's safety. The components of the modern anesthesia workstation can be broadly classified as follows:

- High-pressure system.
- Intermediate-pressure system.
- Low-pressure system.

The schematic arrangement of the above components is shown in **Fig. 45.2**.

High-Pressure System

The high-pressure system starts from the cylinders attached to the anesthesia workstation and ends at the primary pressure regulator. Each machine has at least two slots for attachment of the cylinders at the back, which is called the yoke. The medical-grade cylinders are made up of an alloy of molybdenum and steel, which is stronger and thinner, making them lighter and easy to carry around. Each cylinder has a body, shoulder, and stem and is generally color-coded. The standard color coding used in India is shown in **Table 45.1**.

Apart from the color coding, the contents of the cylinder, chemical symbol, physical state of the contents, size code, etc., are mentioned in the label on the cylinder. The stem of the cylinder also has a valve and pressure-regulating device to prevent bursting of the contents in case of a disaster. *The cylinders can have either gaseous contents like oxygen, nitrogen, air, and helium or liquids like nitrous oxide and carbon dioxide.* The cylinders are labeled according to their sizes from A to J, *A being the smallest and J being the largest.* The size E cylinders are generally attached to anesthesia workstations. A filled E type oxygen

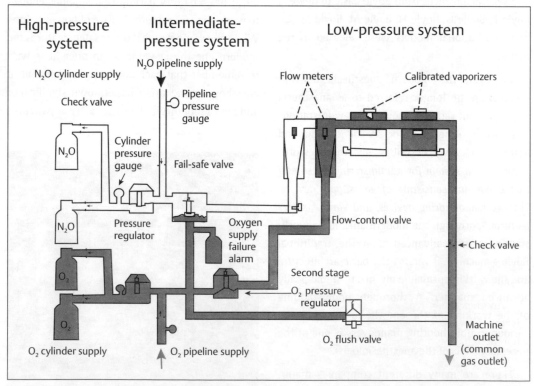

Fig. 45.2 Components of the modern anesthesia workstation.

Table 45.1 Color coding of the common cylinders used

Gas	Color
Oxygen	Black body and white shoulders
Nitrous oxide	Blue
Air	Black body and shoulders with black and white quarters
Carbon dioxide	Grey
Helium	Brown
Entonox	Blue body and shoulders with blue and white quarters
Cyclopropane	Orange

Table 45.2 Pin index of common medical gases

Gas	Pin index
Air	1,5
Oxygen	2,5
Nitrous oxide	3,5
O_2–CO_2 ($CO_2 > 7.5\%$)	1,6
O_2–CO_2 ($CO_2 < 7.5\%$)	2,6
Cyclopropane, carbon dioxide	3,6
Entonox (50% O_2 + 50% N_2O)	7

cylinder has a pressure of 1900 psig (pounds per square inch gauge) and can deliver up to 660 L of oxygen. A full N_2O cylinder has a pressure of 745 psig and can deliver up to 1590 L of N_2O. As oxygen is in the gaseous state in the cylinder, the contents of the oxygen cylinder can be estimated using the pressure. Still, the N_2O cylinder is generally weighed to determine its contents as it is in liquid form. *Checking the cylinder pressure is one of the steps incorporated into the daily anesthesia safety check, and a pressure less than half of the full cylinder is accepted as a cut-off to change the cylinder.*

Another safety feature related to the cylinder is the pin index safety system (PISS). It is a noninterchangeable safety system that prevents attachment of incorrect cylinder to the yoke. The neck of the cylinder has two small holes, which are positioned in a way that they fit into the pins in the hanger yoke of the anesthesia workstation. The position of the pins around the cylinder outlet port of the yoke is in the manner of a circle with an arc of radius 9/16th inch. They are labeled as 1 to 7 and 1 to 3 on the right-hand side, 4 to 6 on the left-hand side, and 7 in the center. The pin index of the commonly used medical gases is described in **Table 45.2**.

The cylinders attached to the hanger yoke of the anesthesia workstation act as a backup in case of emergency when the other pipeline supply fails. So, they should be checked regularly and kept closed after checking in order not to empty the contents after pipeline failure without knowing it. The attachment of the cylinder to the yoke is protected by a gas-tight seal, which allows only unidirectional flow of contents into the workstation but not vice versa. Once the contents of the cylinder open up into the workstation, there is a filter that prevents the delivery of grease and debris from the neck of the cylinder into the machine, and there are pressure gauges which depict the pressure of the cylinder at the front of the workstation. Next to the pressure gauge is the primary pressure regulator, which reduces the pressure of the gas to as low as 45 psig and marks the end of the high-pressure system of the workstation. *This pressure is lower than that of the central pressure system, that is 55 psig, which allows preferential utilization of pipeline supply even when the cylinder is open.*

Intermediate-Pressure System

The intermediate-pressure system of the anesthesia workstation consists of the *pipelines which come from the manifold, oxygen pressure failure devices, oxygen flush, auxiliary oxygen flow meters, and secondary pressure regulators.* The pipelines are generally the main source of supply throughout the hospital and have a pressure of 50 to 55 psig, depending on the country's guidelines.

The pipeline supply is generally accessed by a series of wall mounts attached through quick connectors. *Each quick connector is again color-coded with oxygen being white, N_2O being blue, and vacuum being yellow* to add up to the safety features of the anesthesia workstation. These pipelines get connected to the workstation through a special set of connectors called diameter index safety system (DISS) in the United States or non-interchangeable screw thread (NIST) in the United Kingdom. These connectors prevent the attachment of the incorrect gas into the workstation.

As soon as the gas from the pipeline enters the workstation, there is a filter that prevents the entry of any particulate matter into the workstation. The pipeline pressure gauge follows the filter and displays the pipeline pressure on the front of the machine. One of the main goals of the workstation should be not to deliver a hypoxic mixture to the patient even if one attempts to do so. *The ASTM standards state that any anesthesia workstation should be designed so that when the oxygen supply is reduced to the minimum allowed by the manufacturer, the oxygen concentration at the common gas outlet should not be less than 19%.* So, a sensor is placed in the intermediate-pressure system, which gives an audible and visible alarm to the anesthesiologist once the pressure falls below the manufacturer-set minimum.

The other interesting feature of the intermediate pressure is the oxygen failure protection device, also popularly known as the "fail-safe." Depending on the manufacturer, the device either proportionately decreases the flow of other gases or shut down other gases in case of an oxygen failure. But it is not as foolproof as it sounds, because it depends only on the pressure in the oxygen pipeline and can be overcome if some other gas passes through that line with the same pressure.

Oxygen Flush Valve

One more safety feature added in the intermediate-pressure system would be the oxygen flush valve, which upon activation delivers 100% oxygen at a flow rate of 35 to 70 L/min directly from the pipeline bypassing the low-pressure system and the vaporizers. *Several hazards such as improper activation of the flush valve, leading to dilution of the anesthetic gases, causing awareness, and risk of barotrauma in case of a stuck valve in the open position, have been described.* To prevent these, the oxygen flush valve is always not easily accessible in the modern anesthesia workstations unless someone activates it voluntarily. It also is useful in case of jet ventilation when oxygen at a higher pressure is needed, but most modern anesthesia workstations do not have the fresh gas outlets accessible. *Oxygen flush and auxiliary flow meter are the parts of the workstation which works even when the machine is not electrically powered but connected to a pipeline system.*

Auxiliary Oxygen Flow Meter

It is a separate flow meter mounted on the machine, which provides oxygen directly from the intermediate-pressure system, bypassing the low-pressure system. It is useful in the following:

- Administering oxygen via a Hudson facemask or a venturi mask during regional anesthesia or sedation.

- For apneic oxygen administration in case of a difficult airway.

- During fiberoptic intubation.

- Jet ventilation.

One must be cautious to ensure that the source of oxygen here is the same as the pipeline, and this cannot be used in case of failure of pipeline supply, or suspicion of any crossover of pipelines wherein the backup cylinder will be helpful.

Finally, the intermediate-pressure system ends with secondary pressure regulators, which reduce the pressure to 15 to 30 psig before passing the anesthetic gases into the low-pressure system.

Low-Pressure System

The low-pressure system consists of *flow control valves, flow meters, vaporizers, and fresh gas outlet. It is the most vulnerable of the three systems for leaks and misconnections.*

Flow Meter Assembly

The flow meter assembly consists of flow control knobs that control the precise flow rate of gases and the flow meters, which are calibrated individually for each gas. The flow control knobs on the inner side contain flow control valves, which allow gas to pass at a precise flow to push the bobbin in the flow meters. *As an additional safety, the flow control knob of the flow meter is fluted and broader to give a distinctive tactile feeling than that of the others.* In all the modern anesthesia workstations, a minimum mandatory oxygen flow of 200 or 250 mL/min is set, and the flow of oxygen cannot be reduced beyond this. The flow tubes also referred to as "Thorpe's tubes" are transparent, glass, vertical tubes arranged in series above the flow control valves, with markings of the flow rate on them. All the flow tubes used in the anesthesia workstation are known as "variable orifice flow meters," as these glass tubes are narrowest at the bottom and wider at the top. An indicator float or bobbin gets lifted by the gas coming from the bottom and represents the flow rate. Space through which the gas flows is called the annular space. *At lower flow rates, the viscosity of the gas, and at higher flow rates, the density of the gas plays a role in determining the flow characteristics.* The flow tubes have to be perfectly vertical, and even a slight tilt can alter the gas flows.

The bobbin can be either circular or cylindrical and generally rotates with the gas flow. A dot or mark on the bobbin gives a visual confirmation that the bobbin is turning, and the gas flow

is undisturbed. The main challenges with the traditional flow meter assembly are the leaks and inaccuracy, even with slight dirt or tilting. The oxygen flow meter is always placed downstream toward the patient to prevent delivery of hypoxic mixture even in case of accidental breakage of the other two flow tubes (**Fig. 45.3**). A few modern anesthesia workstations do not have traditional flow meter assembly but rather have electronic flow sensors that are prone to lessen leakage.

Proportioning Systems

They are probably the most important and interesting safety features of the workstation. The *ASTM standards state the workstation has to be provided with a device that does not allow an oxygen concentration below 21% at the fresh gas outlet when any amount of oxygen and N_2O mixture is being delivered.* So, different manufacturers have different sets of devices that either shuts off the N_2O than a particular maximum or increases oxygen proportionately to N_2O. The most widely used safety system is called *"Link-25 Proportion Limiting Control System"* by Datex Ohmeda (**Fig. 45.4**). It is based on the mechanical linking between the flow control valves of oxygen and N_2O through a chain. A 15 tooth sprocket to N_2O flow control valve and a 29 tooth sprocket to an oxygen flow control valve are integrated with a chain that controls the flow knobs in a manner that when the N_2O valve rotates twice, oxygen knob rotates once due to 2:1 gear ratio. Finally, due to the difference in the tapering of the flow control valves of both the gases, a ratio of 3:1 ratio for N_2O and oxygen is maintained at the fresh gas outlet.

The Drager workstations employ a device called sensitive oxygen ratio controller (SORC), which shuts off the flow of N_2O when the flow of the oxygen is reduced to less than 200 mL/min. The proportioning systems are not complete protection against the delivery of hypoxic mixture, because they are purely dependent on

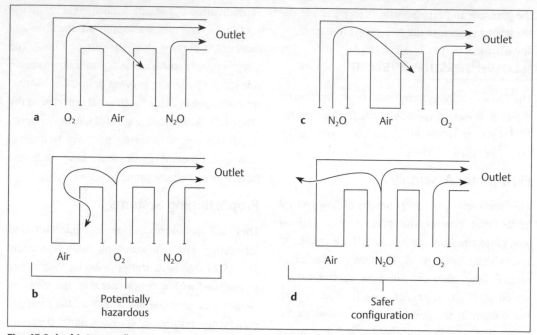

Fig. 45.3 (a, b) Oxygen flow meter at the upstream location; breakage in tubes lead to the delivery of hypoxic mixture. **(c, d)** Oxygen at the downstream position; safer configuration.

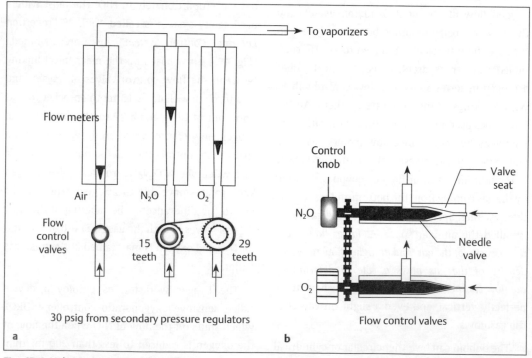

Fig. 45.4 Link-25 proportionating system.

the pressure and can still act the same in case of the wrong supply of gas. Also, there can be leaks downstream to them, which may lead to the delivery of the hypoxic mixture.

Ritchie Whistle was also an age-old oxygen failure warning device in the older anesthesia machine. As the pipeline pressure drops below 30 psig, the flow of anesthetic gases are cut off, and a whistle like the alarm is given, which continues till the pressure falls to 6 psig. Modern anesthesia workstations also employ a visual and audible alarm, which is activated at low-oxygen pressures.

Vaporizer Mount and Vaporizers

As we know, all the inhalational agents are very potent, and a means to accurately regulate their concentration at any temperature and pressure is a necessity. A vaporizer is a device that generates vapor from the liquid inhalational agent, and they are built individually for each agent. *They are color-coded, which adds to the safety features of the workstation.* The colors assigned to each vaporizer are described in **Table 45.3**.

The modern vaporizers are all temperature compensated and are referred to as TEC vaporizers. Desflurane, owing to its boiling point of 22.8°C and saturated vapor pressure of 660 mm Hg, needs a specialized vaporizer (TEC 6), which requires to be electrically heated. Modern anesthesia workstations have a vaporizer mounting bar, which allows easy attachment and detachment of the vaporizers. *Also, an interlock system that prevents the usage of two inhalational agents simultaneously is a safety system.* Most modern vaporizers also have filling systems that prevent

Table 45.3 Color coding of the vaporizers

Agent	Color
Halothane	Red
Isoflurane	Purple
Sevoflurane	Yellow
Desflurane	Blue

administering a different inhalational agent in a vaporizer.

Ahead of the vaporizer is the outlet check valve, which prevents the backflow of anesthetic gases during positive pressure ventilation. It minimizes the fluctuations of anesthetic gases due to changes in pressure ahead. Downstream to the check valve is the fresh gas outlet, which is not visible outside in many of the modern anesthesia workstations to which breathing circuits are attached, which help in ventilation of the patient.

Breathing Systems

Breathing systems can be defined as an arrangement of few components together, which connects the patient's airway to the workstation, creating a conduit through which the patient breathes in and out. The most common elements of the breathing systems include:

- A breathing tube which acts as a conduit.
- Reservoir bag.
- Pressure relief valve.
- Connectors, adaptors.
- CO_2 absorber.
- Humidification system.
- Monitoring devices.

There is no ideal system in existence. The ideal features of a breathing system should be:

- Low resistance to the flow of gases.
- Smooth and uniform cross-section to prevent turbulent flow.
- Resistant to kinking.
- Transparency.
- Minimal dead space.
- Effective for both spontaneous and controlled ventilation.
- Economical usage of gases.
- Reduction of theater pollution.
- Lightweight.

- Conservation of heat.
- Suitable for both adults and children.
- Minimal rebreathing.

Rebreathing is the inspiration of exhaled CO_2 of the previous breath as part of present breath, leading to a reduction in the inspired oxygen concentration. It depends on:

- Fresh gas flows: Higher the fresh gas flow, lower the rebreathing.
- Design of the breathing system: Closed systems have more rebreathing.
- Mode of ventilation: Spontaneous or controlled.
- Respiratory pattern: Tachypnea increases rebreathing.
- Mechanical dead space: Larger dead space leads to more rebreathing.

Classification

The most traditional and oldest method of classification of breathing systems is the Dripp's classification, dividing the breathing systems into the open with minimal rebreathing and closed with maximal rebreathing (**Table 45.4**).

The ambiguity of the above nomenclature can be observed wherein few systems are considered semi-closed and semi-open, depending on the fresh gas flow. So, a more functional classification by Miller et al came into practice and in use now (**Flowchart 45.1**).

Mapleson Circuits

In 1954, Mapleson classified the semi-closed anesthesia circuits into five categories (**Fig. 45.5**), based on the arrangement of the fresh gas flow inlet, expiratory valve, and the reservoir bag.

Table 45.4 Dripp's classification of breathing systems

System	Rebreathing	Examples
Open	No	Open drop
Semi-open	No, but with a reservoir bag	Mapleson circuits at a high fresh gas flow
Semi-closed	Partial	Mapleson circuits at a low fresh gas flow
Closed	Complete	Closed-circuit of the anesthesia workstation

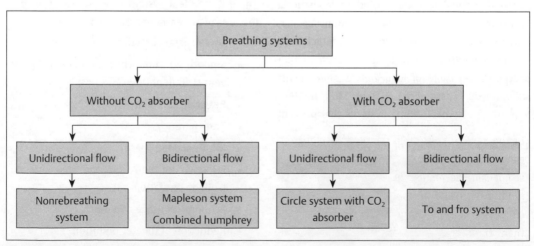

Flowchart 45.1 Miller's functional classification of circuits.

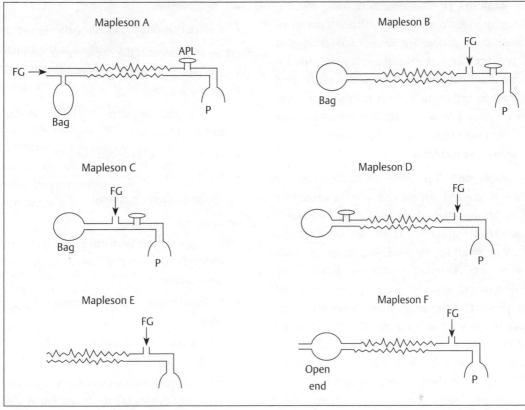

Fig. 41.5 Mapleson circuits. Abbreviations: APL, adjustable pressure limiting valve; FG, fresh gas flow; P, patient end.

The A, B, and C systems are referred to as *afferent systems* in which the expiratory valve is near the patient end, whereas D and E are considered as *efferent systems* in which the expiratory valve is away from the patient end. They are also referred to as T-piece. Mapleson F is originally not included in the classification but is a modification of Mapleson E suggested by Jackson and Rees.

Mapleson A: It is also called as *Magill's system* and *is the best circuit for spontaneous ventilation.* In the case of controlled ventilation, high fresh gas flows are needed to prevent rebreathing. *It is not suitable for use in pediatrics.* The coaxial modification of Mapleson A is known as *Lack's circuit,* which provides no considerable advantage than traditional Mapleson A. Fresh gas flow equivalent to the minute ventilation is required in case of spontaneous ventilation, and 2.5 times the

minute ventilation is required in case of controlled ventilation. Both Magill's and Lack's circuits are not in use at present.

Mapleson B: Mapleson B system is currently obsolete in clinical practice, owing to the advantages of the other circuits being better. Both B and C are functionally similar except that the B system has corrugated tubing, and C does not. Mapleson B is designed to work better for spontaneous ventilation. *The fresh gas flow of 2 to 3 times minute ventilation is required for spontaneous ventilation, and controlled ventilation requires much higher flows.*

Mapleson C: This system is also known as *Water's circuit.* It was previously used with Water's to and fro soda lime canister for delivering field anesthesia. It differs from the B circuit in that it does not have corrugated tubing.

Mapleson D: This system is more efficient when used for controlled ventilation than spontaneous ventilation. The coaxial modification of D type is called *Bain's circuit* and is widely used. *It is often called the universal circuit*, as it can be used for adults and children. *Fresh gas flow equivalent to 1.5 times minute ventilation is required in case of controlled ventilation and 2 to 3 times in case of spontaneous ventilation.*

Mapleson E: It is a T-piece with fresh gas flow inlet at one end, patient end, and the expiratory port at the other. *It is not in use in modern anesthesia practice due to various disadvantages such as small length, more weight, and inability to provide controlled ventilation.* Jackson and Rees's modification of Ayre's T-piece (also called Mapleson F) is commonly used. The reservoir bag attached to the type E provides a visible indication of breathing, acts as a reservoir to some extent, and facilitates controlled ventilation if required. *Flow rate for spontaneous ventilation is 2 to 3 times minute ventilation, and for controlled ventilation, 1.5 times minute ventilation is needed.*

In terms of preventing rebreathing during spontaneous ventilation, the order is A > DFE > CB, and in controlled ventilation, it is DFE > BC > A.

Circle Systems

Circle breathing systems allow the circular, unidirectional flow of gases, which is facilitated with one-way valves. They are essentially closed systems that allow maximal rebreathing with the help of CO_2 absorber incorporated in the system. The components of a circle system are as follows:

- Fresh gas flow source.
- Unidirectional valves in the inspiratory and expiratory limb.
- Corrugated tubes which act as inspiratory and expiratory limbs.
- An adjustable pressure limiting (APL) valve.
- Reservoir or breathing bag.

- CO_2 absorbent.
- Y piece that connects to the patient.

The main advantages of the circle system include:
- Efficient for both spontaneous and controlled ventilation.
- Maintenance of relatively stable inspired gas concentrations.
- Conservation of heat and humidity.
- Elimination of CO_2.
- Minimal theater pollution.

The disadvantages include:
- Complex design with many components, adding to the chance of misconnections and disconnections.
- Malfunctioning of unidirectional valves is fatal.
- Loss of tidal volume due to the compliance of the circuit.
- Interactions of inhalational agents with CO_2 absorbent can lead to the formation of life-threatening compounds.

CO_2 Absorbent

Carbon dioxide in the expired gas of the patient is removed with the help of an absorbent through a series of reactions. The various absorbents in use are soda lime, Dragersorb, barylime, etc. The components of classic soda lime include 80% $Ca(OH)_2$, 16% H_2O, 3% $NaOH$, and 2% KOH. The reaction which removes the carbon dioxide includes:

$$CO_2 + Ca(OH)_2 = CaCO_3 + H_2O + heat$$

However, CO_2 does not react with $Ca(OH)_2$ quickly and hence requires a strong base as a catalyst. The whole series of reactions which occur includes:

$$CO_{2(gas)} + H_2O_{(liquid)} = H_2CO_{3\,(aqueous)}$$

$$H_2CO_3 + 2\,NaOH\,(or\,KOH) = Na_2CO_3\,(or\,K_2CO_3)$$
$$+ 2\,H_2O + Heat$$

$$Na_2CO_3\,(or\,K_2CO_3) + Ca(OH)_2 = CaCO_3 + 2\,NaOH$$
$$(or\,KOH) + Heat$$

The lithium-based absorbents do not require catalysts as LiOH quickly reacts with CO_2. Indicators are added with the absorbents to warn about the exhaustion as they change color. *The most common indicators used are phenolphthalein, which is normally white but changes to pink upon depletion*, ethyl violet, which is white and changes to purple upon exhaustion or ethyl orange, which is normally orange but changes to yellow. The absorptive capacity of soda-lime is 25 L of CO_2 per 100 g.

Interactions with Inhalational Agents

Inhalational agents have been known to react with strong bases such as KOH and NaOH, to form degradation products, especially when the absorbent is dry. One such product of main concern would be compound A (fluromethyl-2,2-difluoro-1-[trifluoromethyl] vinyl ether) formed by sevoflurane, which is nephrotoxic to rats at a normal concentration found in breathing circuits. *However, no such toxicity in humans is demonstrated till now, but the manufacturer recommends limiting patient exposure to less than 2 MAC hours at flow rates between 1 L/min and 2 L/min. A flow of less than 1 L/min is not recommended. Lithium-based absorbents generate a very negligible amount of compound A.*

The other degradation product is carbon monoxide produced by extremely dry, desiccated absorbent reacting with desflurane. A typical event would be seen on Monday when the machine was not turned down over the weekend, and the continuous high flows rendered the absorbent dry. Removal of KOH and NaOH in newer absorbents limits the tendency for carbon monoxide formation. The other life-threatening event would be the extreme exothermic reaction that can lead to fires and explosions, seen mostly due to the interaction of sevoflurane with dry barylime.

Anesthesia Machine Check

The American Society of Anesthesiologists (ASA) recommends a preanesthesia checkout procedure to be followed every day and before every case to ensure the availability of key equipment and to assess the function of the equipment. The various steps to be followed are:

Step 1: Ensuring the presence and functionality of the auxiliary cylinder and self-inflating resuscitation device

The most important and first step to be performed every day before entering the theater is checking for the availability of an extra oxygen cylinder, which is full and functional, and also the presence of a resuscitation bag.

Step 2: Check the suction apparatus

The suction apparatus to be checked every day and also before a new case to ensure that the pressure is enough for the suction of solid contents in the airway. It should be attached to a suction catheter of appropriate length and diameter suitable for the patient.

Step 3: Turn on the workstation and confirm the availability of AC power

The modern anesthesia workstations have a battery backup in case of power failure. Before the start of every day, it has to be ensured that the mains supply is running and the workstation is fully charged.

Step 4: Verify availability of monitors and check alarms

This step ensures that there is no last-minute hassle when a monitor is not functioning, leading to delayed diagnosis of an event. The alarm thresholds for each patient also need to be checked to prevent complications. This step should be performed at the start of each day and also at the beginning of each case.

Step 5: Check the cylinder pressure

At the start of each day, the pressure in the oxygen cylinder connected to the workstation is ensured to be at least half of the maximum.

Step 6: Verify that the pipeline pressure is adequate

This step is followed at the start of each day. The pipeline pressures displayed on the workstation need to be ensured that they are not low.

Step 7: Verify that the vaporizers are filled, and ports are tightly closed

This step is followed before each case and start of the day to ensure an adequate supply of inhalational agents available for the case and avoid theater pollution.

Step 8: Verify leaks between flow meters and common gas outlet

This is to be done every day and also when the vaporizer is changed. *It is done by a universal negative pressure leak test.*

Step 9: Check scavenging system

This step is performed at the start of the day to ensure there is no theater pollution.

Step 10: Calibrate oxygen monitor and check low-oxygen alarm

This step not only ensures that the inspired concentration of oxygen is reflected close to reality but also avoids the delivery of hypoxic mixture in case of supply failure.

Step 11: Verify the exhaustion of CO_2 absorbent

This is done after each use, and the absorbent is recommended to be changed *once one-third of the canister is exhausted or the concentration of inspired carbon dioxide is more than zero.*

Step 12: Breathing system pressure and leak testing

The idea behind this positive pressure leak test is that a leak free-breathing system will be able to hold positive pressure when the APL valve is closed. This ensures that the breathing circuit is intact and should be done at the start of the day and also at the beginning of each case.

Step 13: Verify gas flow in the circuit during inspiration and expiration

This test ensures proper functioning of the inspiratory and expiratory check valves and must be done every time the circuit is used.

Step 14: Document completion of checkout procedures

The anesthesia provider should document the anesthesia checkout procedure at the start of each case as a quality assurance tool.

Step 15: Confirm ventilator settings and evaluate readiness to deliver anesthesia

The ventilator settings for the patient have to be confirmed, and the mask has to be attached to the circuit, according to the size, airway equipment, etc., to be checked.

Conclusion

The modern anesthesia workstation delivers inhaled anesthetic agents, supports patients' respiratory system, and provides an interface for monitoring the patient's vitals. Detailed knowledge of the functioning of anesthesia workstations is required to use them safely and efficiently. A proper checklist of the anesthesia workstation before every case is mandatory and must be practiced to avoid untoward events.

CHAPTER 46

Equipment for Airway Management

Damarla Haritha and Puneet Khanna

Introduction

The airway devices are an integral component of day-to-day anesthesia practice. The airway devices provide oxygen to the patient and may vary from noninvasive devices like nasal prongs to invasive ones like an endotracheal tube. These devices are used in the operating room, postoperative and procedural suites, and intensive care units. This chapter is an overview of the most commonly used airway types of equipment in anesthesia practice.

Face Masks

A face mask acts as an interface for the patient's ventilation without introducing any apparatus into the patient's airway. Mask ventilation is a basic skill for any anesthesiologist. Previously used for administering the whole anesthesia, face masks are now used only for a short time before the placement of a definitive airway or in an emergency. The face mask can be made up of many different substances such as black rubber, plastic, or some elastic material. They are of many sizes which can fit patients of different ages and sizes. Any face mask consists of three main body parts, namely (**Fig. 46.1**):

- **Body:** The body, also called the dome, is the main part of the mask. With a transparent body, the newer masks allow for visualization of the lips of the patient, secretions, blood, and exhaled moisture. It can also be better acceptable to the patient.

- **Seal:** Seal is the rim or edge of the face mask, which comes in direct contact with the patient's face. It can be either a flap type, which is the direct extension of the body, assumes the shape of the face upon pressing, or the cushion type, which is filled with air or material which provides the seal.

- **Connector:** The connector is the opposite end of the seal attached to the circuit. It is made up of a thickened fitting of 22 mm internal diameter, which gets connected to a resuscitation bag or a circuit.

Types of Masks

Rendell–Baker–Soucek (RBS) Mask

This mask has a triangular body, is specifically designed to fit pediatric patients, and has low dead space (**Fig. 46.2**). Some masks are scented, and few have a pacifier. This can also be used for ventilating a patient through the stoma of tracheostomy.

Endoscopy Mask

This mask has a port or diaphragm that allows passage of fiberoptic endoscope and facilitates

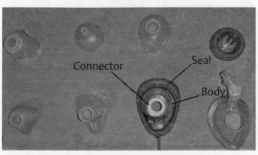

Fig. 46.1 Parts of a facemask.

Fig. 46.2 Rendell–Baker–Soucek (RBS) mask.

ventilating the patient during endoscopy (**Fig. 46.3**).

Techniques of Use

The face mask should form a tight seal around the patient's face to facilitate ventilation. So, appropriate size selection is the first step in mask ventilation. Various techniques of use of face mask are briefly described below.

- **One-handed technique:**

  In this method, the anesthesia provider holds the mask in either of the hand over the patient's face. The thumb and the index finger are pressed over the body of the mask, which forms a "C," and pressure is applied over the patient's face. The remaining three fingers are placed over the mandible, one at the angle of the mandible, one over the body, and the other at the mentum forming an "E." Care should be taken to avoid compression over the eyes or into the soft tissue, which can itself act as an obstruction during ventilation.

- **Two-handed technique:**

  The other method is a two-handed technique with another anesthesiologist

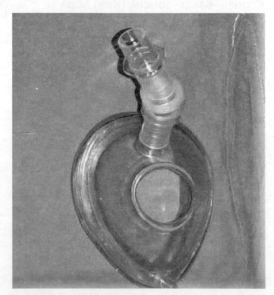

Fig. 46.3 Endoscopy mask.

ventilating the patient. The person who is holding the mask has to place the mask over the patient's face and keep it firm with C and E technique as described earlier with both the hands.

Complications

- Dermatitis due to allergy.
- Nerve compression injuries such as infra-orbital nerve.
- The diaphragm of the endoscopic mask can act as a foreign body and can be aspirated.
- Ventilation with high pressures can lead to gastric insufflation, reduce the functional residual capacity, and increase atelectasis.
- Corneal abrasions.
- Environmental pollution.

Airways

Airways are the devices that help in lifting the tongue and epiglottis away from the posterior pharyngeal wall, thereby preventing the collapse of the airway. It can be achieved via oral or nasal route.

Various other uses of airways include:

- Preventing biting or occlusion of the endotracheal tube.
- Protect from tongue bite during the seizure.
- Facilitate suctioning.
- Help insertion of nasogastric tubes and suction catheters.

Oropharyngeal Airways

It is a curved instrument made up of metal, plastic, or rubber. There is a proximal flange that can be used to fix the airway, thereby preventing from inserting the airway too deep into the airway. Flange continues distally as a bite portion, which is hard and lies in between the lips and teeth. The pharyngeal end is curved and corresponds to the shape of the tongue and palate.

Types of Oral Airways

Guedel Airway

It is a hollow oropharyngeal airway with a large flange and reinforced bite portion. It has a gentle curve that follows the contour of the tongue (**Fig. 46.4**). The hollow part is used for suctioning.

Berman Airway

This airway has the sides cut open, and there is support in the center giving it H-shaped cross-section (**Fig. 46.5**). The open ends allow the tracheal tube to pass and allow suction. It is easier to clean and less likely to be impacted by the foreign body or mucous.

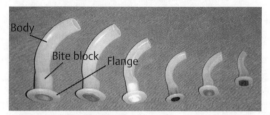

Fig. 46.4 Guedel airway.

Safar Airway

This S-shaped airway consists of two Guedel airways attached to each side with a flange (**Fig. 46.6**). It is designed for mouth-to-mouth ventilation.

Technique for Use

The oral airway is considered to be of appropriate size if it corresponds to the vertical distance between the patient's incisor and the angle of the jaw. If it is too small, it can cause kinking of the tongue, hindering ventilation. It can cause trauma to the larynx or displace epiglottis, causing airway obstruction if it is too big. It is inserted in the mouth with curvature facing the upper lips. Once it is advanced midway, it is rotated to its normal position and advanced further till it attains its position.

Complications

- Airway obstruction.
- Airway edema.

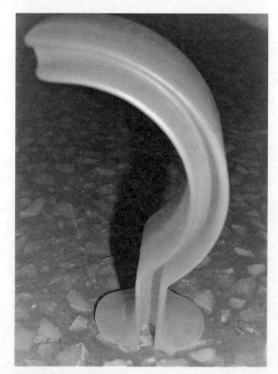

Fig. 46.5 Berman airway.

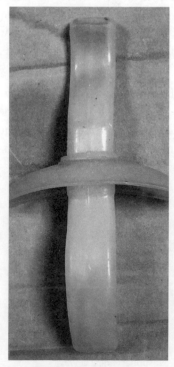

Fig. 46.6 Safar airway.

- Trauma.
- Ulceration and necrosis.
- Dental damage.
- Coughing and laryngospasm.

Nasopharyngeal Airway

Nasopharyngeal airways serve the same purpose as oral airways but are inserted via nostrils. They are soft, pliable, and made up of latex rubber or polyurethane. It has a flange at the proximal end, which is used for fixation of the device, followed by a long, curved body that fits into the nasal cavities (**Fig. 46.7**). The distal end has a bevel that helps in the easy passage and less traumatic insertion. It is available in different sizes and internal diameters.

Technique of Use

The length of the airway can be estimated by measuring the distance between the tragus of the ear to the tip of the nose. The distal end of the airway has to be well lubricated before insertion, and using vasoconstrictor nasal drops prevents bleeding. It is inserted with bevel end first and passed vertically along the floor of the nose with twisting action. The curve of the airway should be directed toward the patient's feet as it is going inside.

Nasal airways are better tolerated in awake patients and are less likely to be accidentally displaced. They are useful in patients with limited mouth opening, fragile dentition, or oral pathology.

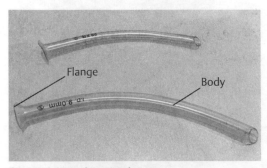

Fig. 46.7 Nasopharyngeal airway.

The complications are almost similar to that of the oral airways, except that nasal bleeding is a possibility. They are absolutely contraindicated in patients with facial fractures (including basal skull fractures) and coagulopathy.

AMBU Bag Resuscitator

Manual resuscitators are portable ventilating devices used for ventilation of the patients during:

- Cardiac arrest.
- Transport of the patients.
- Standby during anesthesia in case of supply failure, leaks, or faults at the workstation.
- Field anesthesia.

There are various types of resuscitators such as artificial manual breathing unit (AMBU) bag resuscitator; Laerdal resuscitator bag of which AMBU bag resuscitator is the most widely used. AMBU is available in three sizes, namely, the following:

- Adult: Used for patients weighing more than 30 kg.
- Child: Used for patients between 7 and 30 kg.
- Neonatal: Used for patients up to 7 kg.

Manual resuscitators have a self-expandable bag that is compressible, a bag refill valve, and a nonbreathing valve at the patient end (**Fig. 46.8**). Neonatal and child sizes also have a pressure relief valve that opens at a pressure greater than 40 cm H_2O and prevents barotrauma. A reservoir bag is also provided with the bag, which increases the FiO_2 delivered.

The concentration of inspiratory oxygen depends on the flow rate, absence or presence of reservoir bag, frequency of compressions, and the ventilation technique. Manual resuscitator is decontaminated by washing ad rinsing, followed by sterilization with either autoclaving or immersing in glutaraldehyde solution for 60 minutes.

Laryngoscopes

Laryngoscopes are devices used for visualization of the larynx during intubation. They also serve other purposes, such as removing a foreign body, biopsy of a lesion in the upper airway, and insertion of a nasogastric tube. They are of different sizes and types but essentially have the same parts which include (**Fig. 46.9**):

- *Handle*: It is the large, vertical portion of the laryngoscope which supplies leverage to the blade. It has a rough surface that provides grip and has a slot for batteries of the light bulb inside it. When the handle and blade come in contact during operation, it completes an electric circuit, and the light bulb glows.
- *Blade*: It is the rigid component that is introduced into the mouth of the patient. It helps to elevate the tongue, soft tissue, and epiglottis to facilitate intubation. The blade further consists of a base, heel, flange, and tip. The tip of the blade also has a light bulb that glows in the operating position.

Types of Laryngoscopes

- **Macintosh laryngoscope:** This is the most common laryngoscope used in adult patients (**Fig. 46.9**). The curved blade offers a distinct advantage in pushing the soft tissues away from the line of sight. It has a flange to the left to push the tongue out of the way and has a cross-section that resembles reverse Z.
- **Miller's laryngoscope:** It has a straight blade instead of a curved blade with only a small curve at the tip. In cross-section, the flange and the heel make a "C." This blade is more likely to be used in pediatrics as the epiglottis is large and floppy in children and needs to be lifted with the blade during intubation.
- **McCoy laryngoscope:** It is based on standard Macintosh laryngoscope design but with an adjustable tip operated by the lever on the handle. The tip can be flexed in patients in whom there is difficulty visualizing the glottis, thereby elevating the epiglottis and the soft tissues.

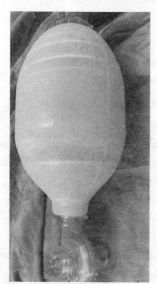

Fig. 46.8 Artificial mandatory breathing unit (AMBU) resuscitator.

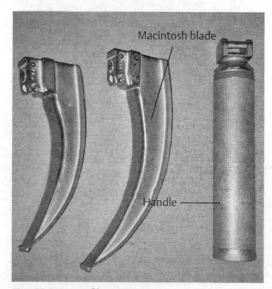

Fig. 46.9 Parts of laryngoscope.

Technique of Use

All the laryngoscopes are universally designed for anesthesiologists with the dominant hand as right. So, the laryngoscope has to be held in the left hand with handle, and the blade is introduced into the mouth of the patient through the right side. As the blade is advanced in the mouth, the tongue is pushed to the left, and the advancement is stopped upon the view of the epiglottis. As the epiglottis comes into view, in the case of a Macintosh laryngoscope, the blade is fixed in the pyriform fossa, and the soft tissues are attempted to elevate with force from the shoulder. In the case of a Miller blade, the blade is fixed under the epiglottis, and the epiglottis, along with soft tissues, is elevated. Always remember during elevation, the shoulder has to be kept straight without any bend at the elbow, which can cause impingement of the flange on the upper teeth and cause dental trauma.

Complications

- Dental injury.
- Cervical spinal cord injury in case of undue extension.
- Trauma to lips and soft tissues in the oral cavity and oropharynx.
- Shock or burn due to the light.
- The bulb can detach from the blade and act as a foreign body.
- Circulatory changes: Laryngoscopy causes very severe hemodynamic response with increase in heart rate, blood pressure, and arrhythmias.
- Transmission of prion diseases.

Supraglottic Airway Devices

Supraglottic airway (SGA) devices are airway conduits that stay above the glottis and provide a leak-free way of ventilation and administering anesthesia. Dr Archie Brain developed the first laryngeal mask airway (LMA) in 1982, which is a prototype of all the SGA devices.

Advantages of SGA over Facemask

- Provide a more reliable and secure means of ventilation.
- Anesthesiologist has more free hands to attend to other problems than the airway.
- Can be easily inserted by nonmedical staff, so it has its place in resuscitation.
- It can be used in patients with difficult bag-mask ventilation due to abnormal face contour.
- Lesser risk of aspiration than a facemask.

Comparison with Endotracheal Tube

- Reduced stress response as there is no laryngoscopy involved.
- Minimal increase in intraocular pressure and intracranial pressure.
- A reduced requirement of anesthetic agents.
- Can be inserted even without neuro-muscular blockade.
- Does not require training.
- Easily inserted in patients with cervical spine instability.
- Does not ensure full protection against aspiration.
- Contraindicated in patients with a history of reflux.
- Higher pressure during ventilation can cause gastric insufflation and leak.

Parts

All the SGA devices have a basic structure which includes (**Fig. 46.10**) the following:

- An inflatable cuff that sits over the larynx or above the level of the larynx.
- An airway tube which acts as a conduit for ventilation.

- A proximal 15-mm connector which fits to the circuit.

Classification

First Generation

These are simple airway tubes that have low seal pressures. There is no specific design to reduce the risk of aspiration; for example, LMA classic, LMA flexible, LMA Fastrach, and LMA AMBU Aura.

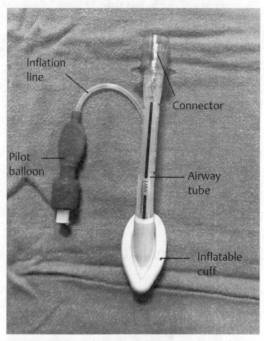

Fig. 46.10 Parts of a supraglottic airway (SGA) device.

Second Generation

These are specifically designed to reduce the risk of aspiration and have high seal pressures, thereby more effective during ventilation. The separate gastric suction port, which runs throughout the airway tube acts, helps suction the contents and separate the esophageal lumen from the glottis; for example, LMA Proseal, I – Gel, and Combitube.

Third Generation

This group serves as an intubation conduit along with features of second-generation SGA devices; for example, Baska Mask.

Types of LMA

- LMA classic (**Fig. 46.10**):
  - ▸ First-generation SGA.
  - ▸ Simple airway tube with a mask at the end.
  - ▸ Comes in various sizes from 1 to 5 (**Table 46.1**).
  - ▸ Maximum seal pressure of 20 cm H_2O.
- LMA flexible:
  - ▸ First-generation SGA.
  - ▸ LMA classic with metallic reinforcement of the airway tube.
  - ▸ Can be fixed away from the surgical field.

Table 46.1 Size selection and maximum cuff inflation volume of LMA

Size	Weight (kg)	Maximum cuff inflation volume (mL)
1	Up to 5	4
1.5	5–10	7
2	10–20	10
2.5	20–30	14
3	30–50	20
4	50–70	30
5	>70	40
6	>100	50

Abbreviation: LMA, laryngeal mask airway.

- ► Can be easily dislodged during movements of the head.
- ► Kinking at the proximal end where there is no metal reinforcement.
- ► Increased airway resistance.
- LMA Proseal (**Fig. 46.11**):
  - ► Second-generation SGA.
  - ► Has an esophageal drain tube for gastric suction.
  - ► Reinforced airway tube with bite block integrated.
  - ► Higher leak pressure of 30 cm H_2O.
- Intubating LMA or LMA Fastrach (**Fig. 46.12**):
  - ► First-generation LMA.
  - ► Rigid stainless steel, anatomically curved body.
  - ► Acts as a conduit for intubation.
- AMBU Aura:
  - ► ′ First-generation LMA.
  - ► Built-in anatomical curve.

- ► Most easy to insert and a device of choice for rescue in the difficult airway.
- Combitube:
  - ► Second-generation device.
  - ► Mostly used by paramedical staff in case of emergency.
  - ► It has two lumens of which one is inserted into glottis and other in the esophagus.
  - ► Not of use in less than 12 years of age.

Complications

- Aspiration of gastric contents.
- Gastric distension.
- Airway obstruction.
- Trauma.
- Dislodgement of the device.
- Bronchospasm.
- Laryngospasm.
- Nerve injury.

Endotracheal Tubes

The endotracheal tube is a device that is inserted into the trachea through the larynx for the purpose of ventilation. It is generally made up of

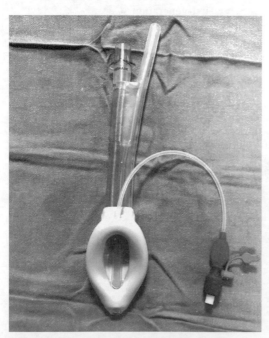

Fig. 46.11 Proseal laryngeal mask airway (LMA).

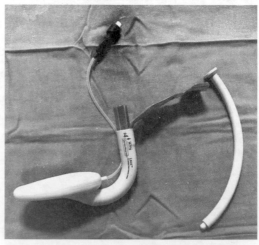

Fig. 46.12 Intubating laryngeal mask airway (LMA).

plastic, polyvinyl chloride or silicone, disposable, transparent for easy visualization of secretions, and with a preformed curve that resembles the airway.

A standard endotracheal tube has two ends, the patient end with a bevel and the machine end which gets attached to the circuit. The bevel faces the left and allows easier visualization of the glottis during insertion. There is a small hole on the opposite side of the bevel called the "Murphy's eye," which helps deliver gases even when the tip is impacted with mucous and secretions (**Fig. 46.13**). There is an inflatable cuff just above the patient's end, which gets inflated with the help of a pilot balloon, preventing displacement and leak of gases. The tube in itself has a curvature, which is shaped like an arc of a circle with a radius of curvature of 140 ± 20 mm. There is a radio-opaque line all along the tube, which helps in visualization upon X-ray and markings at each centimeter, and also helps in knowing the depth of insertion. Also, the inner and outer diameters are mentioned on the surface of the endotracheal tube.

Types of Cuffs

Overinflation of the cuff can lead to excessive pressure on the tracheal mucosa, leading to necrosis. The maximum inflation pressure allowed is approximately 15 to 20 mm Hg. There are two types of cuffs.

- High-volume, low-pressure cuff: This is present on almost all the endotracheal tubes. Upon inflation, the cuff assumes a cylindrical shape, which helps distribute pressure over the walls of the trachea.
- High-pressure, low-volume cuff: This type of cuff assumes a spherical shape upon inflation and puts undue pressure on the tracheal wall. It is present in red rubber tubes and flexometallic tubes.

Important Formulae

- For selecting the size of an endotracheal tube:

  Age less than 6 years

  Size of endotracheal tube (ID) = (age [y]/3) + 3.5

  Age more than 6 years

  Size of endotracheal tube (ID) = (age [y]/4) + 4.5

- For length of fixation = (age/2) + 12 cm.

Methods of Confirmation of Placement

- Proper rise and fall of the chest upon ventilation.
- Visualization of the tube passing through the glottis.
- Auscultation of the chest wall.
- Movement of mist inside the tube.
- Absence of gastric distension.
- X-ray chest.
- Ultrasound.
- Fiberoptic.
- Feel and compliance of the bag.
- End-tidal carbon dioxide tracing—the gold standard.

Types of Endotracheal Tubes

Magill Tipped Endotracheal Tubes

Tracheal tubes without cuffs are called as Magill's tipped endotracheal tubes (**Fig. 46.14**). They were generally used in children because of the sensitive

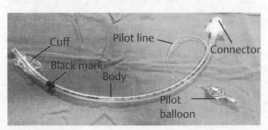

Fig. 46.13 Endotracheal tube and its parts.

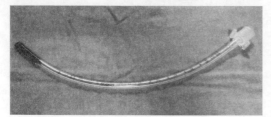

Fig. 46.14 Magill-tipped endotracheal tube.

tracheal mucosa, and the subglottis considered the narrowest portion of the airway.

Ring–Adair–Elwin (RAE) Tubes

These tubes have a preformed curve to facilitate surgery of the head and neck (**Figs. 46.15** and **46.16**). The curve helps in the fixation of the tube away from the surgical field. The oral version, popularly referred to as the south pole, has a bend toward the chin, so that tube can be fixed over the chest. It is used in surgeries of the upper lip, maxilla, and sinus. The nasal version, also called the north pole, is fixed over the forehead. It is used in surgeries of cleft lip, palate, mandible, dental surgeries, etc. The tube's distal end is similar to the normal endotracheal tube with a bevel and Murphy's eye.

Flexometallic/Reinforced/Armored Endotracheal Tubes

These tubes are made up of silicone or PVC but with a steel or nylon wire embedded in the wall of the tube, making them flexible and nonkinkable (**Fig. 46.17**). As they are flexible, they have to be always inserted with the help of a stylet and can be easily dislodged from the glottis due to the elastic recoil force. The patient end does not have a Murphy's eye. It is used in head and neck surgeries where the neck is rotated, such as neurosurgery, thyroid surgeries, airway surgeries, spine surgeries, etc.

Microlaryngeal Tube

This tube has a smaller external diameter and internal diameter compared to that of the normal

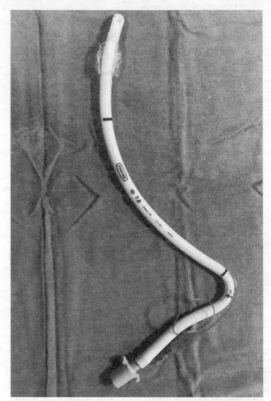

Fig. 46.15 North pole Ring–Adair–Elwin (RAE) tube.

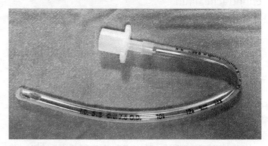

Fig. 46.16 South pole Ring–Adair–Elwin (RAE) tube.

endotracheal tube but with the length of an adult tube. As the tube is narrow, it can be used in patients in whom the glottic aperture is narrow, such as vocal cord nodules, carcinoma larynx, microlaryngeal surgeries, etc.

Complications

- Trauma to the oral mucosa, lips, teeth, and tongue.

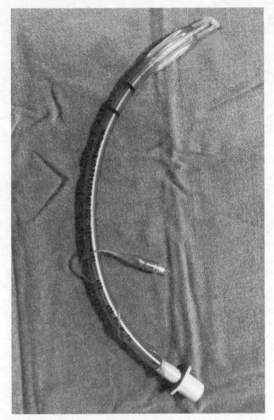

Fig. 46.17 Flexometallic endotracheal tube.

- Hyperextension can cause injury to the cervical spine.
- Intubation response, leading to tachycardia, elevated blood pressure, and arrhythmias.
- Bronchospasm.
- Esophageal intubation.
- Raised intracranial and intraocular pressure.
- Dislodgement of bacterial flora from the upper airway.
- Disconnection and dislodgement.
- Endobronchial intubation.
- Obstruction due to blood, secretions, and kinking.
- Cuff-related problems.
- Sore throat, hoarseness, and vocal cord injury.

Flexible Fiberoptic Bronchoscope

A flexible fiberoptic endoscope is used in anesthesia practice for the following purposes:

- To evaluate the placement of the endotracheal tube.
- Check patency of the endotracheal tube.
- Evaluation of airway.
- Removal of foreign body and mucus.
- As a conduit for endotracheal tube in difficult airway.

Parts

The various parts include:

- Light source: A handle with halogen light bulb and batteries is convenient and inexpensive.
- Handle: This is generally held in hand during use. It also includes the eyepiece, focusing ring, working channel, and the tip-controlling lever.
- Insertion rod: This portion is inserted into the patient and is a long, flexible tube-like structure. It consists of an image-transmitting bundle, light-conducting bundles, and the angulation wires and working channel protected with an outer wire mesh or vinyl coating.
- Tip: Tip consists of the endpoint of all the fiberoptic bundles along with the working channel and is mobile.

Complications

- Discomfort to the patient.
- Inability to view in case of blood or secretions.
- Fogging in case of active breathing by the patient.
- Laryngeal or tracheal trauma.
- Damage to the fiberoptic bundle in case of excessive rotation and kinking.

Conclusion

The practice of anesthesia cannot be imagined without thorough and sound knowledge of airway equipment. The airway equipment is used in preoxygenation, delivery of inhaled anesthetic agents, and securing of an unprotected airway. Choosing an appropriate airway device for a given patient and tailoring it to the clinical scenario is an art that every anesthesia provider should master.

CHAPTER 47

Oxygen Delivery Devices

Damarla Haritha and Puneet Khanna

Introduction

Oxygen therapy forms a major part of an anes-thesiologist's premise and is also a basic skill for all other specialties. The indications for oxygen therapy are as follows:

- Cardiac and respiratory arrest.
- Hypoxemia defined by SpO_2 < 90% or PaO_2 < 60 mm Hg.
- In patients with limited oxygen-carrying capacity—severe anemia, hypotension or shock, very low ejection fraction, and meta-bolic acidosis.
- Respiratory distress due to any other reason.
- After partial recovery from anesthesia.
- Patients with shivering.
- Severe cardiorespiratory disease.

In all these situations, the primary reason for the indication has to be identified and treated appropriately while oxygen is being given.

The oxygen delivery devices can be classified as follows:

- Low-flow devices: Nasal prongs, face mask.
- High-flow devices: Venturi mask, high-flow nasal cannula.

Low-Flow Devices

Low-flow devices deliver oxygen at a flow rate less than the patient's inspiratory flow rate, leading to air entrainment. The FiO_2 depends on the patient's inspiratory flow rate. It is of two types: nasal cannula and face mask.

Nasal Cannula

It consists of two soft prongs that arise from the oxygen supply tubing, which are inserted into the nares of the patient, and tubing is secured to the face by an adjustable strap (**Fig. 47.1**). The nasopharynx acts as an anatomical reservoir, and the FiO_2 depends on the flow rate, patient's minute ventilation, inspiratory flow, and volume of the nasopharynx. Approximate FiO_2 with different flow rates are as follows:

- 1 L/min: 24%.
- 2 L/min: 28%.
- 3 L/min: 32%.
- 4 L/min: 36%.
- 5 L/min: 40%.

Higher flow rates can cause irritation of the nasal mucosa and can result in bleeding and headache. Increased patient compliance and the ability to speak, eat, and drink are the advantages. Inability

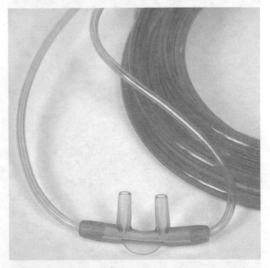

Fig. 47.1 Nasal cannula.

to control the FiO_2 and easier displacement are the disadvantages.

Hudson Face Mask

A plastic reservoir designed to fit over the patient's nose and mouth and secured with a strap around the patient's neck (**Fig. 47.2**). An oxygen delivery tube is present at the base of the mask, and vent holes for the exhaled gases are present on the side of the mask. FiO_2 depending on the flow rate is as follows:

- 5 to 6 L/min: 40%.
- 6 to 7 L/min: 50%.
- 7 to 8 L/min: 60%.

Flow rate less than 4 to 5 L/min increases the rebreathing of exhaled gases and poses more risk to the patient's life, and flow rates more than 8 L/min does not increase oxygen concentration. It is quick and easy to set up, but unpredictable oxygen concentration and an inability to increase oxygen concentration after a certain flow are the disadvantages.

High-Flow Devices

High-flow devices can meet the oxygen requirement of the patient by increasing the flows exceeding the requirement. There is no specific flow rate at which low- and high-flow devices are differentiated, but the most acceptable is more than 10 L/min. It is of two types: Venturi mask and high-flow nasal cannula.

Venturi Mask

They work on the principle of the Venturi effect, which is, in turn, based on the Bernoulli principle. The Venturi effect states that when a fluid flows through the small aperture, the velocity must increase to satisfy the reduction in the pressure. This reduced pressure, in turn, can act as suction and entrain air. A plastic mask that fits over the patient's nose and mouth comes with a strap to fit around the patient's head (**Fig. 47.3**).

The oxygen under pressure is forced to pass through a small jet orifice entering the mask;

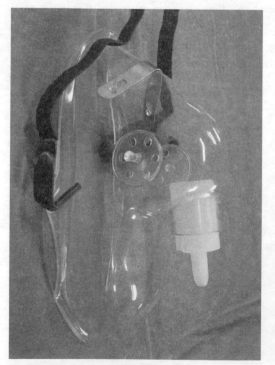

Fig. 47.2 Hudson face mask.

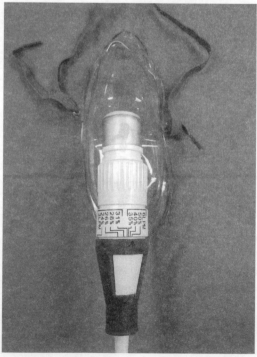

Fig. 47.3 Venturi mask.

negative pressure is created, which causes room air to be entrained via apertures. The Venturi part of the mask is color-coded and labeled with the inspired concentration of oxygen that they deliver and the flow required for it.

High-Flow Nasal Cannula

High-flow nasal cannula consists of an air/oxygen blender with an active humidifier and a nasal cannula. It can deliver an oxygen concentration of approximately 90 to 95% with flows up to 60 L/min. Advantages compared to other oxygen delivery devices are reduced anatomical dead space, positive end-expiratory pressure (PEEP), constant FiO_2, and humidification. It is used in critically ill patients with the following:

- Hypoxemic respiratory failure.
- Chronic obstructive pulmonary disease (COPD).
- Postextubation.
- Preoxygenation.
- Obstructive sleep apnea.

Aerosol generation leading to contamination of the atmosphere is a disadvantage.

Humidification Systems

Humidification of inspired gases is an essential part of oxygen therapy. It is the process of adding water vapor and heat to the inspired gases. Normally, this is the function of nasal mucosa, which adds up the water vapor and heat from the expired gases to the inspired gases. *Administration of dry gases at a flow of more than 4 L/min can cause heat and water loss from the upper airway, leading to the structural damage to the epithelium.* Recommended heat and humidity levels at the trachea are 100% relative humidity and 36 to 40 mg/L of absolute humidity with a temperature of 32 to 35°C.

A humidifier is a device that adds water to the inhaled gas by evaporation of water from a surface. They are of two types: active and passive humidifiers.

Active Humidifiers

They actively add heat and humidity to the inhaled gases. They are of the following two types:

1. *Bubble humidifier:* It breaks the underwater gas stream into small bubbles. Unheated bubble humidifiers are commonly used with oxygen delivery systems to raise water vapor content. They provide an absolute humidity of 15 to 20 mg/L. Their efficiency decreases with higher gas flows due to the limited contact time of gas with water.

2. *Heated humidifier:* They can be either simple reservoir type or wick humidifiers. Both have heating elements that provide heat and moisture to the dry gases using electricity. There can be accidental burns, impaction of mucous, and electromagnetic interference.

Passive Humidifiers

These devices add up the exhaled moisture to the inhaled gases of the next breath. They typically function as an artificial nose. The heat and moist exchangers are the most common passive humidifiers in anesthesia as well as critical care setup.

Heat and moisture exchangers (HME): They are disposable devices with exchanging medium enclosed in a plastic housing. The medium can be either hydrophobic or hygroscopic. Hydrophobic HME are very efficient in even filtering virus particles. Hygroscopic HME can be impregnated with water particles. Both HME lose their efficiency if they become wet. They add up to the dead space of the circuit, leading to higher resistance of breathing.

Conclusion

The oxygen delivery devices are the most commonly used devices by every anesthetist during the perioperative period. The choice of device is based on patient's requirements (FiO2 and inspiratory flows). The oxygen devices should be used wisely to avoid patients, who do not need oxygen, being unnecessarily exposed to a higher concentration of oxygen (risk of oxygen toxicity).

CHAPTER 48

Sterilization of Anesthesia Equipment

Ankur Sharma

Introduction

For an anesthesiologist, cleanliness of equipment is as important as anesthetizing the patients. Precautions and appropriate steps must be practiced by every anesthesiologist to prevent the transmission of infection from one patient to another and also to themselves. Sterilization is the process of making an object or equipment free from all the living microorganisms. Disinfection is the process of destroying most of the microorganisms but not spores.

The foremost crucial step in decontamination is cleaning. If the article is not cleaned properly, the process of sterilization and disinfection can also be affected. Blood and body fluids have to be rinsed thoroughly from the surface of the object by presoaking with detergent and water for at least 3 minutes. The chloride ions from normal saline and sodium hypochlorite solutions can cause corrosion to metals. Therefore, metallic devices should not be rinsed with such solutions. *Each device's manufacturer's instructions with respect to cleaning should be thoroughly followed to prevent damage to the equipment.*

The most common method of sterilization used is autoclaving. It utilizes saturated steam under pressure, which increases the boiling point of water. The minimum time used is 15 minutes at 121°C. After sterilization is done, the items must be dried before being removed from the autoclave. Glutaraldehyde has excellent sterilization capability, even in the presence of organic matter. Soaking for 20 to 30 minutes leads to high-level disinfection. Ethylene oxide, being colorless with a sweet odor, is generally used for sterilization of needles.

Sterilization of Individual Items

1. Anesthesia carts:
   - Cover the top of the cart with a clean sheet at the start of each case.
   - Clean all the vertical surfaces at the end of the day.

2. Remove all the equipment from the drawers once every month, and clean the drawer with a germicide.

3. Cylinders:
   - Before taking into the operation theater, the cylinder has to be washed with water and detergent and wiped with germicide.

4. Anesthesia machines:
   - Same as anesthesia cart.
   - Knobs should be cleaned frequently.
   - Equipment from the drawers should be frequently removed and disinfected.

5. Breathing tubes:
   - Disposable tubes are widely used.
   - Reusable tubes should be cleaned and sterilized with pasteurization or chemical disinfection after proper cleansing.

6. Face masks:
   - Disposable masks have to be used in case of contaminated cases.
   - After use, masks should be cleaned with rinsing and scrubbing.
   - Autoclaving, ethylene oxide, or pasteurization can be used.

7. Airways:
   - They must be kept in a suitable container after use.
   - Airways should be rinsed with cold water immediately after use and be placed in a solution of water and detergent.
   - Pasteurization, ethylene oxide, or liquid chemical sterilization has to be used for airways.
   - Rubber airways are autoclaved.

8. Rigid laryngoscopes:
   - After use, the laryngoscope and the blade have to be placed on a separate surface to prevent contamination.
   - The handle is wiped with water and detergent; the batteries removed and sterilized with autoclave, plasma, or ethylene oxide.
   - The blade should be immersed in water with detergent and washed gently with a soft brush, followed by ethylene oxide, plasma, or autoclaved.

9. Flexible endoscope:
   - They are fragile structures with the potential to transmit infection among the patients.
   - The external surface of the scope has to be wiped with a disinfectant in a gentle manner and then to be immersed in an enzymatic detergent solution and allowed for a time of 2 to 5 minutes.
   - Later on, sterilization with glutaraldehyde and hydrogen peroxide is done.

10. Supraglottic airway devices:
   - Immediately after use, the supraglottic device is washed thoroughly with water and detergent till the visible organic matter is removed.
   - Autoclaving is the only recommended method of sterilization for laryngeal mask airway (LMA).

11. Resuscitation bags:
   - The bag should be disassembled and cleaned if possible after each use.
   - The most common method of sterilization is autoclaving or plasma.

Conclusion

The hygiene of anesthesia equipment must not be ignored. Contaminated equipment will spread infection from one patient to another. Sterilization of anesthesia equipment with the appropriate agent or technique should be done at a regular interval (guided by the manufacturer's brochure).

Index